Orofacial Supportive Care in Cancer

Raj Nair
Editor

Orofacial Supportive Care in Cancer

A Contemporary Oral Oncology Perspective

Springer

Editor
Raj Nair
Oral Medicine and Oral Oncology
Griffith University
QLD
Australia

Haematology and Oncology
Gold Coast University Hospital
Queensland Health
QLD
Australia

ISBN 978-3-030-86509-2 ISBN 978-3-030-86510-8 (eBook)
https://doi.org/10.1007/978-3-030-86510-8

This Springer imprint is published by the registered company Springer Nature Switzerland AG
The registered company address is: Gewerbestrasse 11, 6330 Cham, Switzerland

I dedicate this book to my grandfather,
Dr (Capt.) K N Pillai and my father,
Dr N G Nair for teaching me,
when I was a boy,
the true meaning of empathy in patient care.

Preface

Cancer has become a global term signifying apprehension, a cause of superfluous concern and a significant diagnosis. As a disease, it is distressing us, affecting someone who is close to our hearts, a friend or a stranger. Cancer diagnosis makes an individual a (cancer) survivor due to the nature and course of the disease process. Supportive care becomes a critical facet in their lives whether during active treatment, remission or palliation.

This book, first of its kind as far as I am aware, intended to deliver contemporary updated knowledge and information in orofacial supportive care of cancer patients. This book is a companion for clinicians, nursing fraternity, allied health professionals, trainees in haematology, oncology, radiation oncology, oral medicine and oral oncology.

I have made a conscious effort with the help of my colleagues—contributing authors—in making this book an easy read. When preparing the topics, I have taken into consideration every aspect of cancer care including the hectic nature of dedicated professionals at a cancer centre. The contributing authors are experts in their respective fields and leaders with a wealth of knowledge and experience in cancer care and many of them are international authorities in clinical consensus and guideline development in supportive care in cancer.

I wish to express my sincere gratitude to all of the contributing authors for their excellent contributions and valuable time dedicated towards creating this book. I also extend my thanks to all at Springer, especially Alison Wolf for initially contacting me regarding this book, Beauty Christobel Gunasekaran and the editors for their patience and support.

I hope you will enjoy this book as I did creating it. This unique book will help you understand the full practice of oral oncology in supportive care in cancer thus abetting to provide better cancer care.

Gold Coast, QLD, Australia — Raj Nair

Contents

Editors and Contributors

About the Editor

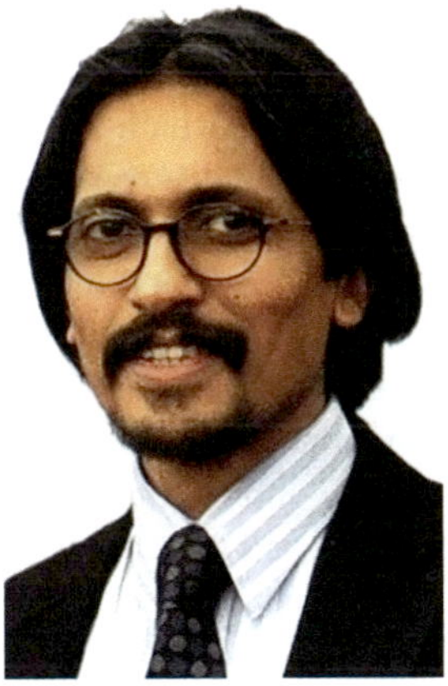

Raj Nair is an internationally known academic and clinician in Oral Medicine and Oral Oncology. He was Deputy Head of School (Research) and Higher Degree Research (HDR) Convenor and is the Discipline Head of Oral Medicine, Oral Pathology and Human Diseases at Griffith University, Australia. He is Senior Oral Oncology Consultant, Haematology and Oncology (Cancer Services), Gold Coast University Hospital (GCUH), Queensland Health, Gold Coast, Australia. He is a member of the Menzies Health Institute Queensland with over 100 publications, books and book chapter contributions. He holds honorary faculty position at the University of Queensland, Brisbane, Australia.

He obtained his PhD in Oral Medicine and Microbiology from the University of Hong Kong in 1996. He received his oral medicine/oncology clinical training as a fellow at Harvard and affiliated hospitals, USA and the University of London, England, UK and recipient of research scholarship from Centre for Blood Disorders, Harvard Medical School. He was awarded membership in the special stream of Oral Medicine by the Royal Australasian College of Dental Surgeons (RACDS) in 2008.

His clinical training and interests are in the field of oral medicine, oral oncology, management of orofacial diseases, orofacial manifestations in patients with medically complex diseases, HIV disease and orofacial supportive care in cancer therapy and haematopoietic stem cell transplantation. Raj has established and maintains out-patient oral medicine practices providing much needed care for complex orofacial diseases, biopsy service and cancer screen for patients from northern New South Wales and southern Queensland. He provides out-patient and in-patient care to cancer patients at the GCUH as senior oral oncology consultant.

His current research projects include but not limited to (1) biomarkers for cancers using precision oncology techniques and microbiome studies; (2) photomedicine in cancer therapy-induced complications; and (3) oral mucositis and other complications amongst cancer patients. He maintains external research collaborations with universities in the USA and Europe. He has presented a number of original research papers at international conferences and has given invited lectures worldwide since 1994.

Raj is the convenor of courses in the discipline of oral medicine, oral pathology and human diseases (internal medicine) which are designed and implemented by Raj. He contributes to education of specialist trainees and nurses at the GCUH and lectures at School of Pharmacy, Griffith University.

Raj holds membership in both professional and research bodies including the International Association for Craniofacial Research (IADR since 1994), the American Academy of Oral Medicine (since 1998), the International Society of Oral Oncology (ISOO), Multinational Association of Supportive Care in Cancer (MASCC since 1999) and Harvard Club of Australia.

He has been an invited consultant and member of international consensus bodies such as World Workshop in Oral Medicine, World Workshop in Oral Health and Diseases in AIDS and Oral Mucositis Group of MASCC/ISOO. He is a Founding Member of the Oral Medicine Academy of Australasia (OMAA).

His senior international leadership positions include (1) Immediete-Past President, Oral Medicine/Pathology Group of international peak research body, IADR; formerly Chair of Membership Recruitment Committee, and Fellowship Committee and currently member of Publication Committee of the IADR, (2) Past Vice President, Editor and Director Board Member of the ISOO (re-elected three terms) and (3) founding Board Member of International Group in Light in Oncology-Barcelona (iGLOB). He was the first Australian-Indian in the fifty years history of RACDS to serve as an elected Director/Councillor (2012–2014).

Contributors

Waseem Abboud, DMD Department of Oral and Maxillofacial Surgery, Sheba Medical Center, Tel-Hashomer, Israel

Institute of Movement Disorders, Department of Neurology, Sheba Medical Center, Tel-Hashomer, Israel

Ragda Abdalla-Aslan, DMD Department of Oral and Maxillofacial Surgery, Rambam Health Care Campus, Haifa, Israel

Department of Oral Medicine, Sedation and Maxillofacial Imaging, Hebrew University-Hadassah School of Dental Medicine, Jerusalem, Israel

Sunday O. Akintoye, DDS, MS Department of Oral Medicine, School of Dental Medicine, University of Pennsylvania, Philadelphia, PA, USA

Amal Bajonaid, DMD Division of Oral Medicine and Dentistry, Brigham and Women's Hospital and Dana Farber Cancer Institute, Boston, MA, USA

Department of Oral Medicine Infection and Immunity, Harvard School of Dental Medicine, Boston, MA, USA

Department of Diagnostic Dental Sciences, College of Dentistry, Jazan University, Jazan, Saudi Arabia

Elena Bardellini, AF, DDS Department of Medical and Surgical Specialities, Radiological Sciences and Public Health, Dental School, University of Brescia, Brescia, Italy

Rene-Jean Bensadoun, MD, MSc, HDR Department of Radiation Oncology, Centre de Haute Energie, Nice, France

Leah M. Bowers, DMD, DABOM Department of Stomatology, Division of Oral Medicine, College of Dental Medicine, Medical University of South Carolina, Charleston, SC, USA

Michael T. Brennan, DDS, MHS, FDS RCSEd Department of Oral Medicine, Atrium Health's Carolinas Medical Center, Charlotte, NC, USA

George Dimitroulis, MDSc, PhD Maxillofacial Surgery Unit, Department of Surgery, St. Vincent's Hospital—University of Melbourne, Melbourne, VIC, Australia

Sharon Elad, DMD, MSc Division of Oral Medicine, Eastman Institute for Oral Health, University of Rochester Medical Center, Rochester, NY, USA

Harry M. Gasper, BSc (Hon.), MBBS Medical Oncology, Gold Coast University Hospital, Gold Coast, QLD, Australia

Michael R. Hamblin, PhD Laser Research Centre, University of Johannesburg, Doornfontein, Johannesburg, South Africa

Radiation Biology Research Center, Iran University of Medical Sciences, Tehran, Iran

Manidhar Reddy Lekkala, MBBS Division of Hematology and Oncology, Wilmot Cancer Institute, University of Rochester Medical Center, Rochester, NY, USA

Jane Liesveld, MD Division of Hematology and Oncology, Wilmot Cancer Institute, University of Rochester Medical Center, Rochester, NY, USA

Alessandra Majorana, FP, MD Department of Medical and Surgical Specialities, Radiological Sciences and Public Health, Dental School, University of Brescia, Brescia, Italy

Kyle Mannion, MD Department of Otolaryngology, Vanderbilt University Medical Center, Nashville, TN, USA

Mel Mupparapu, DMD, MDS, DipABMOR Department of Oral Medicine, School of Dental Medicine, University of Pennsylvania, Philadelphia, PA, USA

Barbara A. Murphy, MD Medical Oncology, Department of Medicine, Vanderbilt University Medical Center, Nashville, TN, USA

Raj Nair, MS, PhD, MRACDS(OralMed) Oral Medicine and Oral Oncology, Griffith University, QLD, Australia

Haematology and Oncology, Gold Coast University Hospital, Queensland Health, QLD, Australia

Ramil Nair, BMedSt, MD Queensland Health, Gold Coast University Hospital, Gold Coast, QLD, Australia

Kenneth Niermann, MD Department of Radiation Oncology, Vanderbilt University Medical Center, Nashville, TN, USA

Ian Olver, AM, MD, PhD Medical Oncology, Faculty of Health and Medical Sciences, University of Adelaide, Adelaide, SA, Australia

Jillian Rigert, DMD, MD Department of Oral Medicine, Atrium Health's Carolinas Medical Center, Charlotte, NC, USA

Jasotha Sanmugarajah, MD Medical Oncology, Gold Coast University Hospital, Gold Coast, QLD, Australia

Stephen T. Sonis, DMD, DMSc Division of Oral Medicine, Brigham and Women's Hospital and Dana Farber Cancer Institute, Boston, MA, USA

Department of Oral Medicine Infection and Immunity, Harvard School of Dental Medicine, Boston, MA, USA

Alessandro Villa, DDS, PhD, MPH Department of Orofacial Sciences, University of California San Francisco, San Francisco, CA, USA

Hannah Wardill, PhD Department of Paediatric Oncology/Haematology, University Medical Centre Groningen The University of Groningen, Groningen, The Netherlands

School of Biomedicine, The Faculty of Health and Medical Sciences, The University of Adelaide, Adelaide, Australia

Precision Medicine (Cancer) The South Australian Health and Medical Research Institute, Adelaide, Australia

Yuanming Xu, DDS Division of Oral Medicine and Dentistry, Brigham and Women's Hospital and Dana Farber Cancer Institute, Boston, MA, USA

Department of Oral Medicine Infection and Immunity, Harvard School of Dental Medicine, Boston, MA, USA

Noam Yarom, DMD Oral Medicine Unit, Sheba Medical Center, Tel-Hashomer, Israel

School of Dental Medicine, Tel-Aviv University, Tel-Aviv, Israel

1 Introduction to Modern Cancer Diagnosis and Survivorship

Raj Nair, Ramil Nair, and Stephen T. Sonis

There is virtually no one who has not been impacted by cancer. We all have relatives or close friends who have had cancer, many who have died from cancer. And the incidence of the disease is increasing from 13.4 million people in 2006 to 18.1 million in 2018 ([1]; Fig. 1.1). That number is projected to be close to 24 million new cases by 2035 [2]. Despite innovative treatments, cancer caused the deaths of 9.6 million people last year (2018) which is equivalent in number to the total populations of Hungary, Austria, or Switzerland and equal to the sum of the populations of Norway and Ireland or Kuwait and Uruguay. Consider that just cancers of the respiratory tract (trachea, bronchus, and lung) were themselves the sixth leading cause of death globally. All cancer diagnoses were the second leading cause of death. But cancer burden is not equally dispersed around the world. While the number of new cases is increasing in less developed countries, it is decreasing in developed countries, and, conversely, cancer deaths are increasing in less developed countries compared to developed countries. The reasons for these disparities are multifold and have been well described and continue to be studied but include risk factor awareness, diet, tobacco and alcohol use and overall lifestyle, access to care, and quality of care.

R. Nair (✉)
Oral Medicine and Oral Oncology, Griffith University, QLD, Australia

Haematology and Oncology, Gold Coast University Hospital, Queensland Health, QLD, Australia
e-mail: r.nair@griffith.edu.au

R. Nair
Queensland Health, Gold Coast University Hospital, Gold Coast, QLD, Australia

S. T. Sonis
Division of Oral Medicine, Brigham and Women's Hospital and Dana Farber Cancer Institute, Boston, MA, USA

Department of Oral Medicine Infection and Immunity, Harvard School of Dental Medicine, Boston, MA, USA
e-mail: ssonis@biomodels.com

R. Nair (ed.), *Orofacial Supportive Care in Cancer*,
https://doi.org/10.1007/978-3-030-86510-8_1

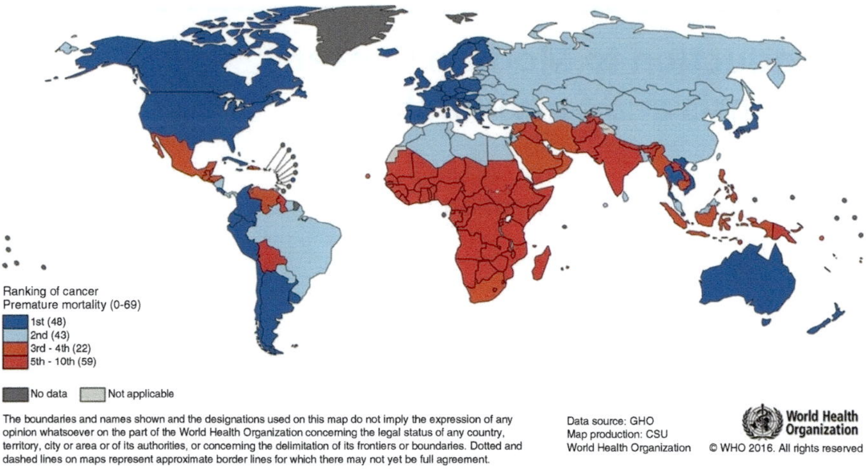

Fig. 1.1 National ranking of cancer as a cause of death at ages below 70 years in 2015 in different countries

The incidence of specific cancers varies geographically, but worldwide lung cancer is both the most common and most deadly accounting for over 2 million new cases in 2018 and more than 1.75 million deaths. Close behind in frequency was breast cancer but with fewer deaths (626,000). Interestingly, new cancers of the head and neck (oral cavity, larynx, nasopharynx, oropharynx, hypopharynx, and salivary glands) impacted almost 1 million patients (907,000) with the same diagnoses associated with more than 450,000 deaths.

Men are more likely (by 20%) than women to develop cancer. Not unexpectedly, given the cancer type distribution by sex, men have a death rate that is 50% higher than women. This is most likely associated with differences in the incidence of lung and liver cancers in men vs. women (Table 1.1).

1.1 Cancer Control

Recognition of many of the environmental and lifestyle cancer risk factors has been known for years. Certainly, tobacco and betel nut use, ultraviolet light exposure, alcohol consumption, excess body weight, air pollution, HPV status, and poor diets have long been associated with increasing the likelihood of an individual developing a malignancy. More recently, the potential importance of the microbiome has been implicated [3], particularly with respect to its contribution to the metabolism of carcinogens. In aggregate, Islami et al. [4] estimated that for patients aged 30 or older in the United States, 42% of diagnosed cancers and 45% of cancer deaths were associated with modifiable risk factors.

Given the breadth of our understanding of identifiable causes of cancer, progress in the development and implementation of programs designed to control risk would

Table 1.1 New cases and deaths for 36 cancers and all cancers combined in 2018

Cancer site	No. of new cases (% of all sites)	No. of deaths (% of all sites)
Lung	2,093,876 (11.6)	1,761,007 (18.4)
Breast	2,088,849 (11.6)	626,679 (6.6)
Prostate	1,276,106 (7.1)	358,989 (3.8)
Colon	1,096,601 (6.1)	551,269 (5.8)
Nonmelanoma of skin	1,042,056 (5.8)	65,155 (0.7)
Stomach	1,033,701 (5.7)	782,685 (8.2)
Liver	841,080 (4.7)	781,631 (8.2)
Rectum	704,376 (3.9)	310,394 (3.2)
Esophagus	572,034 (3.2)	508,585 (5.3)
Cervix uteri	569,847 (3.2)	311,365 (3.3)
Thyroid	567,233 (3.1)	41,071 (0.4)
Bladder	549,393 (3.0)	199,922 (2.1)
Non-Hodgkin lymphoma	509,590 (2.8)	248,724 (2.6)
Pancreas	458,918 (2.5)	432,242 (4.5)
Leukemia	437,033 (2.4)	309,006 (3.2)
Kidney	403,262 (2.2)	175,098 (1.8)
Corpus uteri	382,069 (2.1)	89,929 (0.9)
Lip, oral cavity	354,864 (2.0)	177,384 (1.9)
Brain, nervous system	296,851 (1.6)	241,037 (2.5)
Ovary	295,414 (1.6)	184,799 (1.9)
Melanoma of skin	287,723 (1.6)	60,712 (0.6)
Gallbladder	219,420 (1.2)	165,087 (1.7)
Larynx	177,422 (1.0)	94,771 (1.0)
Multiple myeloma	159,985 (0.9)	106,105 (1.1)
Nasopharynx	129,079 (0.7)	72,987 (0.8)
Oropharynx	92,887 (0.5)	51,005 (0.5)
Hypopharynx	80,608 (0.4)	34,984 (0.4)
Hodgkin lymphoma	79,990 (0.4)	26,167 (0.3)
Testis	71,105 (0.4)	9507 (0.1)
Salivary glands	52,799 (0.3)	22,176 (0.2)
Anus	48,541 (0.3)	19,129 (0.2)
Vulva	44,235 (0.2)	15,222 (0.2)
Kaposi sarcoma	41,799 (0.2)	19,902 (0.2)
Penis	34,475 (0.2)	15,138 (0.2%)
Mesothelioma	30,443 (0.2)	25,576 (0.3)
Vagina	17,600 (0.1)	8062 (0.1)
All sites excluding skin	17,036,901	9,489,872
All sites	18,078,957	9,555,027

Source: GLOBOCAN 2018

be expected to have a marked and favorable impact on cancer statistics. Recognizing the value of cancer control programs, the WHO's developed a Global Action Plan for the Prevention and Control of Noncommunicable Diseases (2013–2020) [5], which has served as a guidance in the United States for programmatic development and implementation.

Cancer control strategies have historically focused on modifying lifestyle behaviors and environmental factors known to impact cancer risk. Probably the most notable have been programs to reduce and eliminate tobacco use. Importantly, the success of these programs is illustrative of the importance of integration of and support between policy makers and lawmakers that effectively influence outcomes. As a measure of effectiveness, smoking prevalence in the United States has declined from 55% of adult men in 1955 to 17.5% in 2016 and 35% of adult women in 1965 to 13.5% in 2016 [6]. Among tactics that have been effective are the levying of high taxes on tobacco products, mandates for smoke-free environments (workplace, restaurants, hotels, etc.), public information programs, restrictions on advertising tobacco products on television, and black box warnings on tobacco product packaging [5]. Other prevention/control programs focused on cessation have also been helpful. Nonetheless, it is important to acknowledge that cancer control programs' effectiveness has varied depending on the demographics of the target population. For example, with respect to smoking, the impact of cancer control programs has been markedly more impressive among patients with higher level education compared to those with less. Thus, like treatment, it is unlikely that a "one-size-fits-all" approach to cancer control programs is realistic. Rather, directed approaches seem likely of having the most utility.

Likewise, initiatives to reduce pollutants associated with cancer risk have had success. One of the most visible programs is associated with radon, the leading cause of lung cancer among US nonsmokers [7]. Increased awareness, home testing, and remediation coupled with policy and legal initiatives have demonstrated efficacy. In addition to radon, the US National Cancer Institute lists 26 other environmental carcinogens as part of their effort to increase awareness and mitigate risk.

An alternative strategy for cancer control has focused on the development of vaccines which target known etiologic agents. Among the most successful of these have been vaccines directed against HPV and hepatitis B (HBV). HPV is a known cause of cervical, vaginal, vulvar, anal, and oropharyngeal cancers, and Gardasil, a 9-valent HPV vaccine, has been approved by the US FDA as a preventive intervention. HBV has been associated with liver cancer risk. Consequently, anti-HBV vaccination mitigates that risk.

1.2 Screening and Early Diagnosis

Screening for cancer and cancer survivors are equally important. Considering the varied types of cancer and their early clinical and biological presentations, it is difficult to come up with a common general screening process for all cancers. In an ideal situation, screening for cancer must be at a primary care setup though that is not the case due to known reasons. When it comes to early diagnosis, those cancers with a known early clinical presentation or a molecular marker have the advantage.

At present, breast and cervical cancer among females and prostate cancer in males and colon cancer screening for those above the age of 50 years in certain parts of the developed world are probably the only cancers with funded screening process. Even though there is a month—April—dedicated to oral cancer screening and awareness internationally, not much has been done to make it mandatory for high-risk individuals.

The gold standard for many cancer screenings still relies upon clinical evaluation by trained individuals, followed by qualitative or quantitative evaluation of additional molecular markers either in the blood or from tissue sampling such as smears or biopsies and imaging techniques. If one were to take oral cancer as an example, dentifying high risks such as (1) high-risk individual based on history or family history of cancer; (2) high-risk activities such as habits, diet, and others; and, finally, (3) high-risk areas, for example, the nonkeratinized oral mucosae in general and floor of the mouth or posterior-lateral borders of the tongue for oral squamous cell carcinomas. The other major hurdle for early cancer screening, indeed, is the financial burden, especially in developing or underdeveloped countries. The best tackle is still prevention and early detection especially when it comes to overall survival.

In recent years, there are several articles on a broader term "liquid biopsy" in the detection of cancer. This method simply refers to detection of tumor cells in body fluids like blood in which free-circulating nucleic acids (cftDNA or cftRNA) originating from tumor cells are to be detected [8]. The basic principle of these noninvasive laboratory-based techniques is with the use of biosensors that can detect cancer biomarkers. It is evident that there are several biomarkers specific to various cancers which are in different phases of refinement and commercialization. For example, inhibitor of apoptosis proteins (IAP) such as surviving has become an important prognostic biomarker for a number of cancers [9].

Broadly, the applications of liquid biopsy are (1) **early detection** of tumor-specific genetic alterations, (2) **forecasting** absence of cftDNA after surgery with a better prognosis and quantification of cftDNA on tumor burden, (3) **prediction** of therapeutically relevant target structures, and (4) **monitoring** of patients using quantification of cftDNA toward tumor burden under therapy, quantification of therapy response, and early identification of resistance mutations [8].

These analyses are expected to provide minimally invasive information about certain properties of the tumor and its metastases, for example, the presence of a therapeutically relevant resistance mutation. However, the term also encompasses other body fluids such as CSF and urine as well as the detection of circulating tumor cells, nucleic acid-containing membrane vesicles (exosomes), or "tumor-educated platelets".

MicroRNAs (miRNAs) have been reported to have a potential to be early markers with both upregulating and downregulating miRNAs in cancer patients compared with normal healthy controls. Another aspect to be mentioned is the role played by the microbiomes, especially in oral cancers [10–15].

1.3 Survivorship

"Survivor" is a word commonly used in the professional field of oncology denoting anyone who has been diagnosed with cancer. This is not the case among cancer survivors as they may not like the idea or the word attached to themselves for varying reasons. In other words, it denotes someone who is living with a known diagnosis of cancer.

The survivors may belong to two groups, those that have no signs of cancer, clinically or through common markers, or those that are living with cancer through therapy. We may be able to define three phases of cancer survivorship such as the following: (1) acute survivorship starts at diagnosis and goes through to the end of initial treatment, (2) extended survivorship starts at the end of initial treatment and goes through the months after, and (3) permanent survivorship is when years have passed since cancer treatment ended.

1.4 Opportunities for Precision Medicine and Oncology

It is abundantly clear that cancer risk, behaviors, and response to treatment vary dramatically across individuals. Likewise, patients' risk of treatment-related toxicities is not uniform. Why is it that one person can smoke a pack of cigarettes for years and live into her 90s, while another develops oral cancer in his 50s? Why is there such variability in response to standard cytotoxic cancer regimens? While one patient with oropharyngeal cancer lives far beyond his concomitant chemoradiation therapy, another with exactly the same demographic, tumor diagnosis, and comorbidities has a recurrence within 2 years of completing initial therapy. How come some patients develop severe oral mucositis following induction chemotherapy, while others sail through treatment with hardly a bump in their quality of life?

Historically, oncology risk and diagnosis were based on averaging overall patient experiences. Tumor characterization and behavior were associated with histological criteria. Hence, all patients with a particular cancer were assumed to have a similar disease. We now know that this is not the case. Advances in technology have permitted scientists to characterize individual tumors [16]. By far, the most significant and clinically meaningful targets have been somatic mutations. Although still relatively new, these discoveries have already had an impact on individualizing tumor diagnosis and, importantly, guiding treatment to specific patients, rather than the "one-size-fits-all" approaches of the past. The results have been profound. Take, for example, the case of checkpoint inhibitors, a form of immunotherapy. At the broadest level, only 20% of patients treated with these drugs respond. Thirty years ago a clinical trial which evaluated an anti-cancer drug based on general histological diagnosis, lung cancer for example, may have concluded that the experimental agent was ineffective. In contrast, further defining patients' cancers genetically might have revealed that patients with cancers having a specific genetic signature did respond to the drug, whereas others did not. However, by recognizing that tumor susceptibility was genomically determined and by being able to screen patients for markers associated with response, the development of the drug for a targeted population where the likelihood of response was high was permitted [17]. Not only was this a huge win for patients and their providers but also for payers who could feel assured that the drug was most likely to be effective in patients treated.

Furthermore, it has become clear that genomic similarities are more important in assessing tumor response than are histomorphological similarities. This provides the basis for novel clinical trial designs in which inclusion criteria are based on common genomic mutations.

Recognition of the genomic diversity of head and neck cancers has provided a platform for both risk prediction and treatment response. Wang et al. noted somatic mutations and HPV in the saliva and blood of patients with head and neck carcinomas [18]. By extension, it is not difficult to imagine a screening application of technologies to detect any of the mutations associated with head and neck cancer [19–21].

Whereas somatic mutations are most associated with tumor diagnosis, behaviors, and treatment response, not much attention has been given to germline mutations—those mutations that are inherited. Tumors have been largely considered to be autonomous. They may be biologically active, but that activity has been considered to be a one-way affair emitting from the tumor and impacting the host. In fact, it seems more realistic that the host affects the tumor in many ways. Consequently, there exists a significant opportunity to assess both somatic and germline mutations and to better understand how they mutually interact. Putting one's eggs into a single basket seems naïve—there is more going on to determine an individual's response than genomics. Future studies will need to assess patients' unique profiles consisting of proteomics, microbiomics, metabolomics, and epigenomic elements and consider how they simultaneously interact to determine an individual's risk and response to treatment.

Germline genomics is especially an important determinant of patients' risk of developing treatment regime-related toxicities and side effects. While, as noted above, other elements contribute to this risk, it is clear that genomics play an important part in determining how well patients tolerate specific drug and radiation regimens. Predicting a patient's risk profile to a variety of treatment options before starting therapy will provide patients and oncologists actionable information to guide individualized treatment [22].

1.5 Challenges in Cancer Supportive Care

Cancer supportive care has emerged as a critical component in tumor management. While still markedly underreported and underappreciated, regimen-related toxicities (RRTs) impart a dramatic burden of illness in overall cancer management. Not only do patients suffer a range of debilitating symptoms including emesis, pulmonary fibrosis, lymphedema, mucositis, arthralgia, neuropathy, and cognitive dysfunction, but their ability to comply with optimal cancer therapy is compromised which threatens their survival. Furthermore, patients with toxicities require additional care resulting in incremental costs that add to the financial burden of their treatment.

Last year, over $11 billion dollars was spent on drugs associated with regimen-related toxicities.

Anyone who has cared for a cancer patient knows that many of the toxicities listed above often happen simultaneously. This observation speaks to the likelihood of common pathobiologic features and provides opportunities for the development of interventions that target multiple toxicities, rather than just one. Better understanding of the biological underpinnings which are associated with toxicity risk and development is critical. But studies that focused on a single toxicity lose the potential value of broader applications. A simple example is the way the epidemiology of RRTs has been studied in so directed ways that characterization of a toxicity constellation—the course, severity, and incidence of multiple toxicities in the same patient over time—has not been achieved. Further compounding RRT assessment has been a lack of standardized reporting criteria. This has extended to frequency of assessment, aggressiveness of RRT evaluation, and inconsistencies in RRT scales.

Oncology remains the number one indication for pharmaceutical development. The activity in field represents the compelling need for effective treatments and the commercial potential for successful interventions. From a supportive care standpoint, this means that the identification, characterization, and interventions for RRTs are a moving target. Mouth sores associated with a cytotoxic agent might be entirely pathobiologically and clinically from mouth sores associated with a targeted therapy as is the case with mucositis caused by melphalan versus stomatitis caused by mTOR inhibitors. Thus, RRTs represent both a continually changing group of challenges and, importantly, opportunities.

RRTs will likely never disappear. Our challenge is to actively engage in finding ways to effectively mitigate or attenuate them so they did not pose a threat to the delivery of optimum cancer care.

Oral oncologists play a significant role in amelioration of cancer complications from diagnosis through hospital stay and survivorship.

Bibliography

1. Bray F, et al. Global cancer statistics 2018: GLOBOCAN estimates of incidence and mortality worldwide for 36 cancers in 185 countries. CA Cancer J Clin. 2018;68(6):394–424.
2. AACR 2018 Annual Report.
3. Ahn J, et al. Oral microbiome and oral and gastrointestinal cancer risk. Cancer Causes Control. 2012;23:399–404.
4. Islami F, et al. Proportion and number of cancer cases and deaths attributable to potentially modifiable risk factors in the United States. CA Cancer J Clin. 2018;68:31–54.
5. Gapstur SM, et al. A blueprint for the primary prevention of cancer: targeting established, modifiable risk factors. CA Cancer J Clin. 2018;68:446–70.
6. Jamal A, et al. Current cigarette smoking among adults—United States 2016. MMWR Morb Mortal Wkly Rep. 2018;67:53–9.
7. Neri A, et al. Radon control activities for lung cancer prevention in National Comprehensive Cancer Control Program Plans, 2005–2011. Prevent Chronic Dis. 2013;10:120337.
8. Lehmann U, Bartels S. Liquid biopsy in tumor diagnostics. Pathologe. 2019; https://doi.org/10.1007/s00292-019-0604-5.
9. Stobiecka M, Ratajczak K, Jakiela S. Toward early cancer detection: focus on biosensing systems and biosensors for an anti-apoptotic protein survivin and survivin mRNA. Biosens

Bioelectron. 2019;137:58–71. https://doi.org/10.1016/j.bios.2019.04.060. [Epub ahead of print].
10. Hung KF, et al. MicroRNA-31 upregulation predicts increased risk of progression of oral potentially malignant disorder. Oral Oncol. 2016;53:42–7.
11. Sharma DC. Salivary bacteria linked to oral cancers. Lancet Oncol. 2005;6:547.
12. Herrero R, et al. Human papillomavirus and oral cancer: the International Agency for Research on Cancer multicenter study. J Natl Cancer Inst. 2003;95:1772–83.
13. Sohrabi M, Nair RG, Samaranayake LP, et al. The yield and quality of cellular and bacterial DNA extracts from human oral rinse samples are variably affected by the cell lysis methodology. J Microbiol Methods. 2016;122:64–72.
14. Fadhil RS, Wei MQ, Nikolarakos D, Good D, Nair RG. Salivary microRNA miR-let-7a-5p and miR-3928 could be used as potential diagnostic biomarkers for head and neck squamous cell carcinoma. PLoS One. 2020;15(3):e0221779. https://doi.org/10.1371/journal.pone.0221779. eCollection 2020.
15. Fadhil R, Nair RG, Nikolarakos D, Wei M. Next Generation Sequencing Identifies Novel Diagnostic Biomarkers for Head and Neck Squamous Cell Carcinoma. Oral Cancer. 2019; https://doi.org/10.1007/s41548-019-00019-5.
16. Tsimberidou AM, et al. Review of precision cancer medicine: evolution of the treatment paradigm. Cancer Treat Rev. 2020;86:102019.
17. Al-Samadi A, et al. In vitro humanized 3D microfluidic chip for testing personalized immunotherapeutics for head and neck cancer patients. Exp Cell Res. 2019;383:111508.
18. Wang Y, et al. Detection of somatic mutations and HPV in the saliva and plasma of patients with head and neck carcinomas. Sci Transl Med. 2015;7:293ra104.
19. Nor JE, Gutkind JS. Head and Neck Cancer in the new era of precision medicine. J Dent Res. 2018;97:601–2.
20. Agrawal N, et al. Exome sequencing of head and neck squamous cell carcinoma reveals inactivating mutations in NOTCH1. Science. 2011;333:1154–7.
21. Polverini PJ, et al. Precision therapy of head and neck squamous cell carcinoma. J Dent Res. 2018;97:614–21.
22. Bachour P, Sonis ST. Predicting the risk of mucositis associated with cytotoxic cancer treatment regimens: rationale, complexity and challenges. Curr Opin Support Palliat Care. 2018;12:1998–210.

Hematologic Malignancies, Classification, and Update on Modern Interventions

2

Manidhar Reddy Lekkala and Jane Liesveld

2.1 Introduction

Hematologic malignancies as a combined group are the fourth largest group of cancers in terms of the incidence rates in both men (after prostate, lung, and colorectal) and women (after breast, lung, and colorectal).

Malignancies of the hematopoietic and lymphoid tissues include the lymphomas, leukemias, myeloproliferative neoplasms (MPNs), plasma cell dyscrasias, histiocytic tumors, and dendritic cell neoplasms.

2.2 Classification

There have been different classification schemes that were used through the years. WHO 2016 classification system is the most commonly used, which encompasses features of morphology, immune phenotype, genetics, and clinical features to classify these diagnoses. The full classification of these tumors is beyond the scope of this chapter. Whenever possible, different tumors are grouped by lineage.

Myeloid Neoplasms: These are the neoplasms which are derived from progenitor cells in the bone marrow which develop into erythrocytes, megakaryocytes, granulocytes (neutrophils, basophils, and eosinophils), or monocytes. These include acute myeloid leukemia (AML), MPNs, and myelodysplastic syndromes (MDS).

Lymphoid Neoplasms: These are the neoplasms which are derived from the progenitors of the B cell (bone marrow derived) or T cell (thymus derived) lineages or from mature B or T lymphocytes. The WHO classification generally classifies

M. R. Lekkala · J. Liesveld (✉)
Division of Hematology and Oncology, Wilmot Cancer Institute, University of Rochester Medical Center, Rochester, NY, USA
e-mail: manidhar_lekkala@urmc.rochester.edu; jane_liesveld@urmc.rochester.edu

R. Nair (ed.), *Orofacial Supportive Care in Cancer*,
https://doi.org/10.1007/978-3-030-86510-8_2

Table 2.1 Some examples of mature B cell neoplasms

Chronic lymphocytic leukemia/small lymphocytic leukemia (CLL/SLL)
Lymphoplasmacytic lymphoma (LPL)
Mantle cell lymphoma
Follicular lymphoma
Diffuse large B cell lymphoma (DLBCL)
Marginal zone lymphoma

these neoplasms depending on whether they are derived from progenitor lymphoid cells or from mature T or B cells.

(a) Precursor lymphoid neoplasms: Includes precursor B lymphoblastic leukemia/lymphomas (B-ALL) and precursor T lymphoblastic leukemia/lymphomas (T-ALL).
(b) Mature lymphoid neoplasms: Includes mature B cell (Table 2.1) and mature T cell neoplasms. These are generally called the non-Hodgkin lymphomas.
(c) Hodgkin lymphoma: These lymphomas are pathologically and clinically distinct B cell lymphomas and thus are classified separately.

Neoplasms with Myeloid and Lymphoid Lineage: These are the tumors which presumably are derived from multipotent stem cells and show evidence of both myeloid and lymphoid differentiation. They are grouped in a separate category.

Histiocytic/Dendritic Neoplasms: These neoplasms are derived from cells that develop into dendritic cells or histiocytes which are the antigen-presenting cells and connective tissue macrophages, respectively.

NK Cell Neoplasms: These neoplasms are derived from the natural killer cells which are part of the innate immune system which recognizes virus and other pathogens.

2.2.1 Leukemias

There are four major types of leukemia classified by their rapidity of growth (acute vs. chronic) and by the cell of origin (myeloid vs. lymphoid). They are AML, acute lymphoid leukemia (ALL), chronic myeloid leukemia (CML), and chronic lymphoid leukemia (CLL). There are also other leukemias which are very low in incidence.

Acute leukemia	Chronic leukemia
AML	CML
ALL	CLL

2.2.1.1 Clinical Features

Most of the signs and symptoms of acute leukemia occur due to the infiltration of organs with leukemic blasts which are proliferating in an uncontrolled fashion.

Fatigue, dyspnea, bleeding, and life-threatening infections are some of the common features. In some patients, especially with a myelomonocytic or monocytic leukemia, involvement of the spleen, liver, lymph nodes, skin, or gums where these cells accumulate and cause enlargement can be observed. CNS involvement is noted especially in patients with ALL. Laboratory workup can show anemia and thrombocytopenia with normal, low, or elevated white cell counts. Most leukemia patients present with blasts in the blood, but some will present with low blood counts due to replacement of the marrow with the abnormal blast cells.

Chronic leukemias, on the other hand, present with indolent features. Chronic myelogenous leukemia can manifest symptoms of fatigue, night sweats, weight loss, and abdominal discomfort over many weeks to months. Sometimes these are found on a routine blood work performed for other reasons. In CML, the elevated white count can include a spectrum of myeloid progenitors. CML may transform into accelerated or blastic phase. Chronic lymphocytic leukemia can present with enlarged lymph nodes, splenomegaly, and an increased number of mature lymphocytes on a blood smear.

2.2.1.2 Diagnosis

The diagnosis of leukemia is usually facilitated by examination of the peripheral smear for blasts or other precursor cells, but for the most part in order to make a definitive diagnosis, a bone marrow biopsy and aspirate is required. Morphology, immunohistochemistry, and flow cytometry for immunophenotyping help to further distinguish these leukemias. All patients suspected of leukemia should undergo cytogenetic analysis which aids in diagnosis, treatment, and posttreatment monitoring. Molecular studies for abnormalities in certain genes are important which confer prognostic significance. For example, TP53, ASXL1, and MECOM gene mutations are associated with adverse risk in AML, and NPM1 without FLT3-ITD mutation is associated with favorable risk AML. Karyotype analysis also helps in predicting outcomes, for example, t(8;21), inv(16), and t(15;17) predict good outcome, and monosomy 5 or 7 or a 17p abnormality predicts adverse outcome.

2.2.1.3 Management

Acute Leukemia

Acute leukemias, if untreated, are usually fatal, leading to death in weeks to months. Initial treatment is directed at decreasing the number of leukemic cells. For many years, this was achieved using chemotherapy. In AML, the first or induction therapy is often with continuous infusion cytarabine for 7 days and an anthracycline drug given for 3 days, the so-called "7 + 3" regimen, which has been in use for many decades. Depending on specific mutations, other medications, for example, midostaurin for the fms-like tyrosine kinase 3 (FLT3 mutation), are used. Acute promyelocytic leukemia (APL), a subtype of AML, has a unique feature where it shows high sensitivity to all-trans retinoic acid (ATRA) and arsenic trioxide, which can sometimes be used without chemotherapy. CPX-351, a liposomal formulation of cytarabine and daunorubicin co-encapsulated to maximize the synergy between these agents, has recently been shown to improve the overall survival in certain subtypes of AML. Post-remission, these patients are usually offered high-dose cytarabine to consolidate the remission, or they undergo allogeneic hematopoietic stem cell transplant (allo-HCT). If medically unfit, low-intensity chemotherapy approaches such as the combination of 5-azacitidine, a hypomethylating agent and venetoclax, an inhibitor of Bcl-2 are used.

In ALL, a standard induction chemotherapy regimen with vincristine, anthracycline, prednisone, and asparaginase is often utilized. About 90% of the patients achieve complete remission with this regimen, but if no further therapy is administered, the duration of remission is very short-lived. Post-remission therapies for consolidation and prevention of central nervous system involvement are used, and allogeneic HCT can be considered for those who are fit and who have high-risk features. TKI inhibitors like imatinib or dasatinib are added to the regimen in patients with Philadelphia chromosome-positive ALL which is present in about one third of adults with ALL, and anti-CD20 antibodies like rituximab can improve responses in CD20-positive ALL.

Chronic Leukemia

The treatments in chronic leukemia have evolved over the last few years. In CML, since the development of oral tyrosine kinase inhibitors (TKIs), they are the treatment of choice for initial treatment, where the overall survival was found to be greater than 85% after 4–6 years. Some of the commonly used BCR/ABL TKIs are imatinib as well as second- and third-generation TKIs such as nilotinib and dasatinib. Failure to respond to multiple TKIs with disease progression is an indication for allogeneic HCT.

In CLL, the standard treatment is moving away from chemoimmunotherapy as a first-line treatment to Bruton's tyrosine kinase (BTK) inhibitors like ibrutinib. In patients with relapsed or refractory disease, monotherapy with ibrutinib, idelalisib with rituximab, and venetoclax with or without rituximab are some of the treatment options. Also, more selective second-generation BTK inhibitors like acalabrutinib are currently being studied. Venetoclax is a BCL-2 inhibitor which showed high response rates especially in patients with 17p deletion with previous failure of ibrutinib. Also, CD19-directed chimeric antigen receptors (CAR)-modified T cell therapies also showed encouraging early results. Rarely, these patients undergo HCT with advanced and high-risk CLL which has not responded to other drugs.

2.2.2 Lymphomas

There are multiple types of lymphomas classified into the broad groups as discussed above and shown in Table 2.1. Clinically, we tend to classify these tumors into indolent lymphomas and aggressive lymphomas.

- Indolent: These lymphomas are characterized by slow growth which sometimes occurs over years. The most common are the follicular lymphoma, small lymphocytic lymphoma, marginal zone lymphoma, lymphoplasmacytic lymphoma (LPL), and some cases of mantle cell lymphoma. In these lymphomas, there is a lifetime risk of about 30% chance of transformation into an aggressive form of lymphoma. They are associated with prolonged survival, though relapses are common.

- Aggressive: These lymphomas are characterized by rapid growth associated with related symptoms. The most common subtypes are the diffuse large B cell lymphoma (DLBCL), mantle cell lymphoma, and other rare T and B cell lymphomas which represent a small fraction of all lymphomas.

2.2.2.1 Clinical Manifestations

Clinical presentation of lymphoma varies from asymptomatic patients with associated lymphadenopathy, organomegaly, or lymphocytosis detected during a routine examination which is usually seen in indolent lymphomas to constitutional symptoms like weight loss, low-grade fever, and drenching night sweats associated with rapid growth of aggressive lymphomas. Some of the symptoms can be related to compression of different organs leading to neurologic, urinary, or lung problems. LPL produces paraprotein, an abnormal protein detected on blood chemistries, usually a monoclonal IgM. In this subtype of lymphoma, symptoms related to hyperviscosity are common especially when the levels are high. Cytopenias are seen commonly in these patients especially when bone marrow is involved. Marginal zone lymphoma causes symptoms depending on the organ involved. Gastric marginal zone lymphoma, the most common MZL, typically presents with abdominal discomfort, nausea, vomiting, or bleeding. Splenic MZL presents with symptomatic splenomegaly, sometimes associated with associated lymphocytosis and marrow infiltration.

2.2.2.2 Diagnosis

Diagnosis of lymphoma requires adequate tissue for hematopathology review, architectural assessment, immunohistochemistry, and flow cytometry. An excisional biopsy is the gold standard as fine needle biopsies often do not adequately define nodal architecture for accurate diagnosis. Cytogenetic analysis and chromosome rearrangements may be diagnostic and also help support the diagnosis of particular subtype of lymphoma. In about 50% of patients, bone marrow is involved by the lymphoma, which requires a bone marrow biopsy and aspiration to document.

2.2.2.3 Staging

Staging is important as it aids in treatment decisions. Lugano staging is currently used for staging NHL.

Stage	Involvement	Extranodal
I	One node or group of adjacent nodes	Single extranodal lesions without nodal involvement
II	Two or more nodal groups on the same side of the diaphragm	Stage I/II by nodal extent with limited contiguous extranodal involvement
III	Nodes on both sides of the diaphragm; nodes above the diaphragm with spleen involvement	Not applicable
IV	Additional noncontiguous extralymphatic involvement	Not applicable

2.2.2.4 Treatment

Indolent Lymphomas

Follicular Lymphoma: Most of the indolent lymphomas especially in their early stages with no associated symptoms do not require treatment. Patients who are symptomatic, have high tumor burden, or are in advanced stages can be treated with immunotherapy, chemoimmunotherapy, or radiation. Rituximab and obinutuzumab are anti-CD20 monoclonal antibodies which are used alone or in combination with chemotherapy. R-CHOP (cyclophosphamide, doxorubicin, vincristine, and prednisone plus rituximab) and BR (bendamustine and rituximab) are the common chemoimmunotherapy regimens in use. There is a role of radiation especially in the early stages. In the advanced stages, radiation is used for palliation purposes. In relapsed follicular lymphoma, alternative chemoimmunotherapy modalities are used, sometimes with the addition of stem cell transplantation. Anti-CD19-directed CAR-T therapies are also being explored in follicular lymphomas.

LPL: As with other indolent lymphomas, treatment is usually indicated only in symptomatic and advanced disease. First-line treatment options include rituximab, a BTK inhibitor ibrutinib, chemoimmunotherapy, or bortezomib-based therapy.

Marginal Zone Lymphoma: In the early stages of gastric marginal zone lymphoma, the treatment is focused on *H. pylori* eradication, with triple therapy (proton pump inhibitor (PPI) plus two antimicrobials) or quadruple therapy (PPI, bismuth, tetracycline, metronidazole). Patients who are resistant to this therapy or have negative *H. pylori* should receive second-line options like rituximab monotherapy, rituximab plus chlorambucil, or ibrutinib which are especially used in advanced/relapsed disease. Historically, splenectomy was considered in splenic marginal zone lymphoma, but rituximab or fludarabine can be used in patients to avoid surgery.

SLL: This is the tissue counterpart to CLL, and treatment is similar to CLL as discussed above.

Aggressive Lymphomas

DLBCL: About 20% of patients present with limited stage disease (stage 1 or non-bulky stage II). Chemoimmunotherapy with involved field radiotherapy is commonly used in limited stage disease. Chemoimmunotherapy alone is an acceptable alternative especially when radiation therapy is thought to cause long-term toxicities depending on the disease sites. R-CHOP is the preferred chemoimmunotherapy regimen in DLBCL. Advanced stage disease (bulky stage II, stages III and IV) cannot be contained within one radiation field. These patients account for about 70–80% of DLBCL. R-CHOP has been the standard of care in advanced DLBCL, with an OS of approximately 60% at 5 years. The overall survival was found to be inferior especially in patients with double-hit DLBCL (translocations of the MYC gene together with rearrangement of BCL2 and/or BCL6), in whom a more aggressive regimen called dose-adjusted etoposide, doxorubicin, and cyclophosphamide with vincristine, prednisone, and rituximab (DA-EPOCH-R) is used. Currently, there are multiple clinical trials evaluating adding lenalidomide, ibrutinib, and bortezomib to the R-CHOP base, especially in the advanced and activated B cell (ABC) type of

DLBCL. Even though there is an improved cure rate in DLBCL, slightly less than half of these patients relapse or have primary refractory disease. These patients are treated with salvage chemotherapy with plan for hematopoietic stem cell transplant, in patients who show response. Recently, CAR-T cell therapy is being considered in patients who do not show significant response to chemotherapy or have a relapse after a previous stem cell transplant.

Mantle Cell Lymphoma: Initial treatment in mantle cell lymphoma depends on whether the patient is eligible for HSCT. Conventional chemoimmunotherapy with autologous HCT and maintenance rituximab showed improved progression-free survival. Patients who are not eligible for HSCT showed complete remission with chemoimmunotherapy and maintenance rituximab. Intensive chemoimmunotherapy with hyper-fractionated cyclophosphamide, vincristine, doxorubicin, and dexamethasone (hyper-CVAD) alone is another option in younger patients who do not want to undergo HSCT. Relapse is common and seen in almost all patients who enter remission. These therapies are not curative, but an occasional patient may be cured after allogeneic stem cell transplantation. Some of the potential salvage regimens include ibrutinib and acalabrutinib, which are BTK inhibitors, lenalidomide, an immunomodulatory thalidomide derivative, and bortezomib, a proteasome inhibitor. CAR-T therapy has also been approved for use in mantle cell lymphoma.

Burkitt Lymphoma: This is one of the most aggressive lymphomas, and these patients require an intensive, multiagent, short-duration chemotherapy with CNS prophylaxis. Common regimens used are CODOX-M with IVAC (cyclophosphamide, vincristine, doxorubicin, high-dose methotrexate with ifosfamide, cytarabine, etoposide) with intrathecal methotrexate and dose-adjusted EPOCH (infusional etoposide, vincristine, and doxorubicin with oral prednisone and bolus dose-escalated cyclophosphamide chemotherapy) can also be used. Prognosis in cases not associated with the human immunodeficiency virus (HIV) is favorable.

Hodgkin Lymphoma (HL)

Hodgkin lymphoma has been separated from other B cell lymphomas due to its special clinicopathologic features. It has a unique cellular composition, wherein there are minimal neoplastic cells in an inflammatory background. The selection of treatment for HL is usually based on presenting stage. Doxorubicin, bleomycin, vinblastine, and dacarbazine (ABVD) for three to four cycles followed by involved field irradiation are the preferred treatment in early stage (I–II) HL. In advanced stages (III–IV), combination chemotherapy with ABVD for a maximum of six cycles is the main treatment. About 15% of patients have refractory HL, and about 15% relapse after complete remission. These patients are generally treated with salvage chemotherapy (e.g., ifosfamide, carboplatin, etoposide (ICE), dexamethasone, high-dose cytarabine, cisplatin (DHAP), or gemcitabine, cis-platinum, and dexamethasone (GDP)), and patients who show a complete response on restaging proceed to autologous HCT, if eligible. Targeted therapy (e.g., brentuximab, an anti-CD30 conjugated monoclonal antibody) and immunotherapy (e.g., nivolumab or pembrolizumab) are also used especially in patients who relapse after autologous HCT or after two prior multiagent chemotherapy regimens. HL survivors are at risk of developing late complications related to the therapy like second malignancies, cardiac disease, radiation side effects, and others.

There are many other lymphoma subtypes which are rare in incidence and beyond the scope of this chapter.

2.2.3 Myeloma

Multiple Myeloma: MM is a neoplastic process where there is uncontrolled proliferation of plasma cells producing monoclonal immunoglobulin.

Clinical Features: The clinical signs and symptoms are related to the infiltration of the plasma cells into different organs and deposition of the monoclonal proteins in various organ systems. The most common clinical features noted are anemia, bone pain, kidney dysfunction, fatigue, weight loss, and symptoms of hypercalcemia with a minority of patients having symptoms of paresthesias and organomegaly. It is very important to distinguish multiple myeloma from other plasma cell disorders such as light chain amyloidosis for prognostic purposes and treatment.

2.2.3.1 Diagnosis

When multiple myeloma is suspected, patients should be tested for the presence of monoclonal protein. Serum protein electrophoresis (SPEP), serum immunofixation (SIFE), urine protein electrophoresis (UPEP), urine immunofixation (UIFE), and serum free light chain assay will aid in detecting the monoclonal proteins. A bone marrow biopsy and aspirate with immunohistochemistry and flow cytometry are needed for diagnosis. Examination of all bones using plain radiography or preferably whole-body low-dose CT scan is required to diagnose lytic lesions. MRI is the most sensitive modality of bone involvement, while PET/CT may be more sensitive for extramedullary involvement.

2.2.3.2 Management

The initial treatment in MM depends on whether a patient is eligible for autologous stem cell transplant (ASCT). In patients who are not eligible for ASCT, VRd (bortezomib/lenalidomide/dexamethasone) is the standard of treatment for initial therapy followed by Rd (lenalidomide and dexamethasone) as maintenance. VCd (bortezomib/cyclophosphamide/dexamethasone) and VTd (bortezomib/thalidomide/dexamethasone) are other options to use especially if lenalidomide is not available. The anti-CD38 antibody, daratumumab is also being added to upfront treatment regimens. The same regimens are used in induction in patients eligible for ASCT, but they are given for only a few cycles before transplant commences.

Almost all patients with MM will eventually relapse. There is no clear standard regimen to use in relapsed patients. Generally, an alternative regimen than the regimen used in induction is used. Many newer drugs are currently being evaluated regarding their optimal role in myeloma treatment. Some of the newer drugs include proteasome inhibitors like carfilzomib and ixazomib, monoclonal antibodies like daratumumab and elotuzumab, and histone deacetylase inhibitors like panobinostat.

Venetoclax is also being examined as are CAR-T cells directed to the BCMA (B cell maturaton) antigen. Present studies do not provide us with a clear indication of which of these medications and combinations are optimal for treatment of relapsed myeloma. They are often used in succession. Also, patients with MM may receive bisphosphonates like pamidronate or zoledronic acid once per month to prevent bone disease.

2.2.4 Myeloproliferative Neoplasms

Myeloproliferative Neoplasms (MPNs): MPNs exhibit proliferation of the terminal myeloid cells resulting in erythrocytosis, leukocytosis, thrombocytosis, bone marrow fibrosis, and, in some cases, splenomegaly. The common MPNs seen in practice are polycythemia vera (PV), CML, essential thrombocythemia (ET), and primary myelofibrosis (PMF). Most of these patients have mutations in the JAK2, CALR (calreticulin), or MPL (thrombopoietin receptor) genes. CML has a characteristic reciprocal translocation between chromosomes 9 and 22 called the Philadelphia chromosome which results in a bcr/abl fusion gene. These disorders tend to progress and can transform into an acute leukemia over the years. PV and ET can transform into a secondary myelofibrosis.

2.2.4.1 Clinical Features

Patients are usually symptomatic in the advanced stages with associated fatigue, fever, weight loss, night sweats, and organomegaly. RBC counts are elevated in PV, and thrombocytosis is seen in ET. It is important to rule out secondary causes of elevation of these blood cell types. Symptoms related to elevated RBC counts like headache, fatigue, visual changes, and pruritus can occur. In ET, erythromelalgia, a painful burning in the pads of fingers and toes, can occur. If platelet counts are extremely high (>1,000,000/μL), abnormal bleeding rather than thrombosis can occur. Early satiety due to splenomegaly is also often seen in patients with myelofibrosis. Patients especially with myelofibrosis can develop bone pain due to skeletal changes associated with marrow fibrosis.

2.2.4.2 Treatment

The goal of treatment in MPNs is to alleviate symptoms and prevent complications like thrombosis or bleeding and to decrease the progression to myelofibrosis and transformation into an acute leukemia. For low-risk PV patients, usually antiplatelet therapy like aspirin is recommended as well as phlebotomies to decrease the hematocrit to <45%. In high-risk PV patients, cytoreductive therapy is recommended in addition to the above. Hydroxyurea is usually the first choice of cytoreductive agent. Other second-line agents like interferon-alpha and anagrelide are used in patients resistant or intolerant to hydroxyurea. Ruxolitinib, a JAK-2 inhibitor, has been approved in PV which is superior to standard treatment in those who progress or are intolerant of hydroxyurea. In patients with low-risk ET, low-dose aspirin to decrease the thromboembolic complications is recommended, whereas in high-risk ET, hydroxyurea is used for cytoreduction. For low-risk PMF, close observation or hydroxyurea may be appropriate, but for high-risk PMF, allogeneic HCT should be considered in patients of appropriate age who have available donors. Ruxolitinib has shown substantial benefit in both primary and secondary myelofibrosis, by decreasing spleen size and systemic symptoms. CML has been discussed above in Sect. 2.1.

2.2.5 Myelodysplastic Syndrome (MDS)

MDS are a group of hematopoietic disorders characterized by ineffective hematopoiesis. This is most commonly seen in older adults >65 years and rarely seen in those <50 years of age.

2.2.5.1 Clinical Features

Most of the patients present with nonspecific symptoms related to low counts like fatigue, bleeding, or infections. Peripheral smear and bone marrow examination shows dysplastic cells with hypercellular marrow.

2.2.5.2 Treatment

Treatment strategies primarily depend on the risk group. Erythropoietin is shown to improve anemia in 20–30% of patients with MDS. Lenalidomide has been used in transfusion-dependent MDS with 5q-deletion, and it showed transfusion independence and cytogenetic response in many patients. Azacytidine and decitabine, both hypomethylating agents, are approved in MDS, and these have shown overall survival benefit and decrease in transformation to AML. Allogeneic HCT is the only curative therapy in MDS. Patients who are old and frail and who cannot undergo the above therapies are given supportive care with RBC and platelet transfusions as needed. Infections are also common, often requiring antibiotic therapy.

Recent Advances in the Field of Hematologic Malignancies

In the last few years, the field of hematologic malignancies has seen significant discoveries and advances. Advances in drug development helped in discovery of multiple drugs, especially immunotherapy and molecular targeting agents. Immunotherapies are being incorporated into multiple disease treatment regimens. These include TKIs, antibody therapies, immune checkpoint inhibitors, and CAR-T cell therapy, among others.

CAR-T Cell Therapy

Genetically modifying the T cells to target the cancer is a new disruptive cancer treatment option that is approved currently in some B cell malignancies. CAR-T cells that target CD-19 were recently approved by the FDA for treatment of the advanced ALL in children and large cell non-Hodgkin lymphoma in adults. Since then, CAR-T cells are being developed to target different receptors in other cancer cells. Most of this work remains investigational, but clinical trials in several hematologic malignancies are under way.

With new treatments come unique side effects. Cytokine release syndrome (CRS) and neurotoxicity are the common side effects noted with CAR-T cell therapy. CRS occurs in the first few days after the T cell infusion and in its severe form causes very high fever, tachycardia, hypotension, coagulopathy, and respiratory compromise. Neurotoxicity is seen with symptoms of headaches, seizures, focal neurological deficits, and in some cases loss of consciousness, which is often treated with steroids.

Side Effects of Therapies Used in Hematologic Malignancies

Chemotherapy is long known to have significant side effects related to damage of the normal cells along with malignant cells. Some of the common side effects seen with chemotherapeutic agents are cumulative fatigue, nausea, vomiting, decreased blood counts, increased infections, effects on organs like liver and kidney causing elevated liver function tests (LFTs) and elevated creatinine, respectively, neuropathies, and skin rash. Some of the side effects are specific to a particular chemotherapy regimen or agent used.

We now have multiple new drugs being developed and used in these cancers. Immunotherapy and targeted therapy are being used more and more frequently, and thus it is important to know the side effect profile of these medications. Treatment with the immunotherapy is associated with immune-related adverse effects. Some of the common side effects noted are mild fatigue; infusion-related reactions; dermatologic toxicities; inflammation of the organ systems causing colitis, hepatitis, and pneumonitis; and endocrinopathies.

Hematopoietic stem cell transplant patients are subject to toxicity affecting multiple organ systems sometimes even warranting intensive care admission. Anemia, neutropenia, and thrombocytopenia are common. Nausea, vomiting, and diarrhea are the common gastrointestinal system-related side effects. Infections are a major risk in transplant patients. Bacterial infections with gram-positive and gram-negative organisms and fungal infections with candida and viral infections with herpes simplex virus and cytomegalovirus are commonly seen in transplant patients.

Acute graft versus host disease (acute GVHD) is usually restricted to allogeneic transplant patients, seen in the first 3 months after transplant. The typical presentation will be skin involvement with erythematous or maculopapular rash and GI tract involvement with nausea, vomiting, diarrhea, and abnormal liver function tests. Less commonly eyes, kidneys, hematopoietic system, and lungs are involved. Sometimes symptoms of acute GVHD are seen beyond the 3-month period post-transplantation, called late-onset GVHD. Skin involvement manifests as lesions resembling scleroderma, and liver involvement is suggested by elevated alkaline phosphatase and bilirubin levels. GI tract involvement manifests as dry oral mucosa with ulcerations, dysphagia, chronic diarrhea, and malabsorption. This is dealt with in detail in a separate chapter.

Oral Side Effects

Oral side effects are common with these agents, and these include acute and long-term side effects. Mucositis is the most common acute side effect causing dysphagia, odynophagia, and impaired nutrition. Late side effects include mucosal atrophy and xerostomia. Gingival bleeding is seen especially in patients with low platelets. Bacterial, fungal, and viral infections are commonly seen. Osteonecrosis is seen in patients who are treated with bisphosphonates, often in multiple myeloma patients. A referral to a dentist is important before initiation of some of these medications. These are dealt in more detail in the later sections of this textbook.

Bibliography

1. Swerdlow SH, et al. The 2016 revision of the World Health Organization classification of lymphoid neoplasms. Blood. 2016;127(20):2375–90. Web 24 Nov 2018.
2. Döhner H, et al. Diagnosis and management of AML in adults: 2017 ELN recommendations from an international expert panel. Blood. 2017;129(4):424–47. Web 25 Nov 2018.
3. Cortes J, Kantarjian H. How I treat newly diagnosed chronic phase CML. Blood. 2012;120(7):1390–7. Web 25 Nov 2018.
4. Hallek M, et al. iwCLL guidelines for diagnosis, indications for treatment, response assessment, and supportive management of CLL. Blood. 2018;131(25):2745–60. Web 25 Nov 2018.
5. Cheson BD, et al. Recommendations for initial evaluation, staging, and response assessment of Hodgkin and non-Hodgkin lymphoma: the Lugano classification. J Clin Oncol. 2014;32(27):3059–68.
6. Rumi E, Cazzola M. Diagnosis, risk stratification, and response evaluation in classical myeloproliferative neoplasms. Blood. 2017;129(6):680–92. Web 25 Nov 2018.

Solid Tumours and Update on Modern Medical Oncology Interventions

3

Ian Olver

3.1 Introduction

Systemic therapy in oral squamous cell cancers which most often present as locoregional disease can be used alone or in combination with radiation therapy. Single agent induction chemotherapy prior to definitive treatment has been tested. Systemic therapy has been used in combination with radiation therapy as the definitive treatment. If surgery is the definitive treatment, combined chemoradiotherapy has been trialled as adjuvant therapy post-surgery [1]. Systemic therapy can also be used for recurrent disease or metastatic disease [2].

There has been a paradigm shift in the options for systemic therapy. In the setting of head and neck cancer, the conventional systemic therapy has been cytotoxic chemotherapy with single agents or combinations. However, targeted therapies, such as the monoclonal antibody cetuximab, target protein receptors responsible for the cancer cell's growth and can be used alone or combined with radiotherapy or chemotherapy [3]. Then there is immunotherapy with checkpoint inhibitors such as pembrolizumab which allow the body's own immune system to attack the cancer [4]. These agents are being combined into the multimodality therapy for head and neck cancer.

The response to therapy in head and neck cancers can be predicted by prognostic factors such as the volume of the tumour and the stage of the disease at presentation [5]. More recently, when the cancer arises as a result of human papilloma virus (HPV—often assessed by the HPV-associated p-16 expression) rather than environmental carcinogens such as tobacco and alcohol, it is more likely to have a better prognosis [6]. This may lead to refining the dosing of systemic therapy in these patients. However, p-16 does not appear to predict therapy response to agents like cetuximab [7].

I. Olver (✉)
Medical Oncology, Faculty of Health and Medical Sciences, University of Adelaide, Adelaide, SA, Australia

R. Nair (ed.), *Orofacial Supportive Care in Cancer*,
https://doi.org/10.1007/978-3-030-86510-8_3

Before reporting how systemic therapies are used in head and neck cancers, we will explore the new targeted and immunotherapies and how they differ from conventional cytotoxics.

3.2 The Evolution of Targeted and Immunotherapies

Systemic cancer therapies are moving from conventional chemotherapy to targeted therapies, including immunotherapy, which allows "personalised" medicine.

Conventional chemotherapy kills cells that are dividing when it is administered, by disrupting the cell's DNA and therefore the mechanisms of cell division. It is not specifically targeted to cancer cells but kills normal cells that are dividing as well. The cancer usually has a higher percentage of cells dividing than normal tissues, and the normal tissues can recover between chemotherapy doses far better than the cancer, thereby gaining a differential effect. This also explains why the side effects of chemotherapy appear in tissues with higher growth fractions, including the bone marrow, the mouth and gastrointestinal mucosa and the hair follicles.

The aim was to develop therapies that would target cancer specifically. Early targeted therapies were developed more than 50 years ago, in 1967, after the discovery of the oestrogen receptor on breast cancers. Of women with breast cancer, 70% have these receptors, which are targeted by oestrogen that signals the growth of the cancer. Blocking the receptor with tamoxifen stopped the cancer growth.

Cancers are caused by mutations in the DNA. Some are inherited, and some are acquired when we are exposed to agents in the environment such as tobacco smoke. In each case, the mutation interferes with the body's normal controls over cell growth. If the mutations can be identified, and the proteins that are associated with them and the signalling pathways involved, then therapies can be designed which will block the pathways and stop the cancer growing [8].

The development of genomics has made this possible. Genetics considers single-gene mutations, while genomics looks at the whole genome and how the genes interact with each other and affect the growth of tissues. In 2001, the human genome was sequenced [9]. This revealed individuals' variations in the DNA sequences. This information could be used to reveal susceptibility to developing cancers. Pharmacogenomics explained different responses to drugs as gene expression dictated differences in the ability to metabolise drugs between individuals.

Next-generation DNA sequencing has allowed rapid sequencing of the genome of a cancer [10]. The pattern of mutations of each cancer can be identified. The process creates large datasets (a whole genome sequence would create about 1 terabyte of data), but new bioinformatic techniques and increased computational capacity have been developed to handle this demand. Furthermore, high-throughput screening techniques can test thousands of compounds at once for their activity on a target [11]. Potential treatments can be identified as those that are likely to block the growth of a cancer while not affecting surrounding normal tissues.

3.3 Targeted Therapies

One the first targeted therapies was a tyrosine kinase inhibitor, imatinib. It was featured on the cover of *Time* magazine as proof of principle of this therapeutic strategy. This worked in a couple of tumour types. The tyrosine kinase product of a mutated C kit when blocked by imatinib resulted in the shrinkage of a rare cancer, the gastrointestinal stromal tumour. This was remarkable because this tumour was quite resistant to conventional chemotherapy and radiotherapy. Similarly, imatinib blocked the tyrosine kinase product of the BCR-ABL (Philadelphia chromosome) which resulted in a major advance in the treatment of chronic myeloid leukaemia [12]. In both cases, the mutation was the driving mutation involved in the growth of the tumours.

Another example of a targeted therapy having significant impact was in metastatic melanoma. Conventional chemotherapy with dacarbazine achieved a response in up to 15% of patients, but it was uncommon for this to improve survival [13]. In the early 2000s, a mutation in a cancer-promoting gene BRAF, which was found in half of all melanomas, caused activation of the BRAF kinase protein which was part of the signalling path which regulated cell growth. The drug vemurafenib inhibited this protein and did result in a survival advantage when compared to conventional therapy with dacarbazine [14]. This reinforced the therapeutic potential of small molecules that target the protein products of mutated genes, which were part of the growth signalling pathway.

3.4 Immunotherapies

An increased understanding of the role of the body's own immune system and how it interacts with cancers has led to a series of immunotherapies. For example, antibodies target proteins on foreign invaders such as bacteria and viruses. Monoclonal antibodies which are antibodies all of the same type can be produced which target proteins on a cancer cell and result in its death. An early example focusses on the HER 2 gene which is overexpressed in 20% of breast cancers and therefore can be used as a biomarker that indicates the presence of this aggressive form of breast cancer. The antibody trastuzumab was produced to target HER 2 [15]. When added to adjuvant chemotherapy for HER 2-positive breast cancer, the 3-year survival increased from 75% to 84%, a result which received a standing ovation at the American Society of Clinical Oncology meeting in 2005 when it was first presented [16].

A further example of an early monoclonal antibody is rituximab which targets the CD20 protein on lymphomas and has improved the outcomes of low- and intermediate-grade lymphomas by about 13% [17].

There are other uses for monoclonal antibodies in cancer therapy, given that they target the cancer cell and not the surrounding normal tissue. They can be used to deliver cytotoxic drugs or even radioisotopes to the cancer cell. The therapy TDM-1 links the cytotoxic emtansine to trastuzumab to target breast cancer [18]. Likewise, the antibody ibritumomab tiuxetan which targets CD20 can carry the isotope yttrium-90 to lymphomas [19].

The cancer cell does not have to be the sole target for monoclonal antibodies. Growing cancers stimulate neovascularisation so that nutrients can get to the cells and the new vessels can be a pathway for cells to metastasise to distant sites. The vascular endothelial growth factor (VEGF) is a target for the monoclonal antibody bevacizumab [20]. This has improved survival outcomes when added to therapy for lung cancer and bowel cancer.

The answer to the question of why the immune system is not more successful in fighting cancer has led to a very important therapeutic advance. In addition to antibodies, the T cells have an important role in attacking invading organisms. However, it has been found that T cells and also cancer cells exhibit proteins that block the T cells from attacking the cancer. Antibodies have been produced to block these proteins and allow the T cells to attach the cancer cell.

To give examples, one of the blocking proteins on T cells is PD-1 (programmed cell death protein 1); its function in the normal body is to stop the T cells causing autoimmune reactions by attacking normal tissues, but in doing so it blocks the T cells from attacking the cancer [21]. Two newer antibodies pembrolizumab and nivolumab target the PDF-1 protein and stop it blocking the T cell from attaching to the cancer cell [4]. These immunotherapies have been found to improve survival in metastatic melanoma, where chemotherapy was ineffective, and they are also being utilised in lung cancer and likely to be useful in a range of cancers [22]. However, this comes at the cost of several toxicities including autoimmune reactions in multiple tissues, particularly in endocrine organs.

A further example of this class of antibodies, known as checkpoint inhibitors, is ipilimumab. This targets the CTLA-4 (cytotoxic T-lymphocyte-associated protein 4) found on T cells which similarly blocks the T cells from attacking cancer cells. Ipilimumab allows the T cell to function as it should against the invading cancer. One fifth of the patients with metastatic melanoma who have received this drug have survived for 3 years or more [23].

Much research is being directed at producing cancer vaccines which could ultimately be used to prevent cancer but can also be developed to treat it. For treatment, proteins from the cancer are used to stimulate an immune response to kill the cancer [24].

Chimeric antigen receptor (CAR) T cell immunotherapy is an adoptive immunotherapy which has been associated with small series of patients achieving dramatic results in patients with haematological malignancies, particularly childhood acute lymphoblastic leukaemia and adults with lymphoma which has become unresponsive to chemotherapy [25, 26]. In CAR T cell therapy, the T cells are extracted from the patient where they are genetically altered to express CAR. They are grown in large numbers and then reinfused back into the patients. When the CAR T cells come in contact with the protein targets on the cancer cells, the CAR T cells are activated, and the cancer cell is killed. There are significant toxicities associated with this therapy, and more clinical trials are required.

The targeted therapies, either small molecules or immunotherapies, have ushered in the era of personalised medicine. We will now explore their application to head and neck cancers.

3.5 Systemic Treatments to Manage Head and Neck Cancer

Chemotherapy as a single modality cannot cure cancers of the head and neck, and so it is combined with local treatments, either surgery or radiotherapy. These are the definitive treatments, since head and neck cancer stays local for much of its natural history. When given with radiotherapy, chemotherapy not only contributes to cell kill locally and for distant disease but can act as a radiosensitiser. Chemotherapy is not usually given for early-stage (T1, T2) head and neck cancer.

3.5.1 Neoadjuvant Chemotherapy

The concept behind giving chemotherapy prior to radiotherapy or surgery in head and neck cancer was to shrink the cancer to make radiotherapy more effective by reducing the volume and reducing the radioresistant hypoxic areas. If surgery was contemplated, a good response to chemotherapy may allow radiotherapy to be used instead and preserve an organ like the larynx. Giving therapy in this way is called neoadjuvant or induction therapy. This was trialled in the Veterans trial where patients received two courses of cisplatin and 5-fluorouracil treatment and if they responded were given chemoradiotherapy rather than a laryngectomy [27]. It was also hoped that the response to chemotherapy would provide prognostic information and predict the response to subsequent therapy.

However, a meta-analysis of 93 studies which included in excess of 17,000 patients showed no overall survival advantage for patients who had received induction chemotherapy [28]. A study just considering nasopharyngeal cancer included 19 trials and 4806 patients who had received neoadjuvant therapy prior to chemotherapy and radiotherapy and showed a survival advantage [29]. In oral cancer in highly selected patients, a reduction in distant metastases can be found, and there can be a higher incidence of preserving the mandible [30]. So, there may be subgroups of patients who benefit from neoadjuvant therapy, but, overall, chemotherapy alone is not recommended for neoadjuvant (or induction) therapy.

The question remains as to whether more effective therapy in general would improve its use in the neoadjuvant setting. For example, the initial randomised studies of adding a docetaxel to cisplatin and 5-fluorouracil did improve survival but also increased the toxicity [31, 32]. A newer taxane cabazitaxel has entered a phase I trial in combination with cisplatin and 5-fluorouracil [33]. However, randomised studies have not confirmed that these neoadjuvant therapies offer a survival benefit [34–36].

It remains to be seen whether the efficacy of induction therapy will change if newer targeted and immunotherapies form part of the induction regimen. For example, the monoclonal antibody cetuximab is active when added to chemotherapy in recurrent and metastatic disease [37]. It has been trialled as part of induction therapy. One study added cetuximab to docetaxel/cisplatin/fluorouracil (TPF) for induction therapy and then followed with cisplatin and cetuximab given concomitantly with radiotherapy. The response rate to the induction therapy was 88.4% with 32 of 36 completing the course, which was judged as tolerable [38]. However, there followed a randomised phase II trial where induction therapy was again TPF plus cetuximab, and then the patients were randomised to either radiotherapy with cetuximab and carboplatin or cetuximab and cisplatin. The outcome was that cetuximab added to full-dose TPF led to unacceptable complications and only 34 of 46 patients completed four cycles [39].

The checkpoint inhibitor pembrolizumab is showing activity in head and neck cancer resistant to cisplatin and cetuximab [40]. In the future, this could be trialled in the neoadjuvant setting.

3.5.2 Primary Chemoradiotherapy

Patients with localised stage I and II disease can be treated with surgery or radiotherapy which results in similar disease control. Locally advanced disease which invades surrounding tissue and neck nodes but does not spread to distant sites is treated with chemoradiotherapy [41]. The chemotherapy is both cytotoxic and acting as a radiosensitiser. Definitive chemoradiotherapy is also employed for organ preservation. Long-term follow-up of the approach in hypopharyngeal squamous cell cancers showed a 62% 5-year survival and 43% 10-year survival [42].

In the MACH-NC trial, chemoradiotherapy was compared to radiotherapy alone and resulted in a survival advantage with mortality improved by 6.5% at 5 years [28]. The most common drug to use with radiotherapy is cisplatin. As a single agent cisplatin and radiotherapy showed a survival advantage over radiation alone post-surgery (overall survival 40 vs. 53%) and reduced the rate of the disease recurring. The scheduling of the cisplatin does not seem to have a major impact on the outcomes, with a retrospective review comparing standard-dose 3-weekly with low-dose weekly showing similar outcomes [43]. 5-Fluorouracil can be added to cisplatin, but adding both drugs to radiation increases the toxicity [44]. Although a study of higher dose cisplatin versus cisplatin/5-fluorouracil with radiation showed similar efficacy and toxicity, patients on the higher dose cisplatin had to have their renal function monitored closely [45]. Sometimes patients with renal impairment receive carboplatin instead of cisplatin [46]. Taxanes have also been used as part of the chemoradiotherapy with cisplatin for unresectable locally advanced head and neck cancer [47]. Intra-arterial delivery of the chemotherapy to be given with radiotherapy represents a further attempt to achieve better local control by increasing the concentration of chemotherapy delivered to the tumour and ultimately allowing greater preservation of organ function [48].

The monoclonal antibody cetuximab has also been added to chemotherapy concurrently with radiation [38, 39]. In patients who are not fit to receive cisplatin concurrently with radiotherapy, cetuximab and carboplatin were used as the concurrent chemotherapy. It was found to be feasible and safe.

A randomised study set out to determine whether cetuximab could be administered as a single agent with radiation after a standard induction regimen TPF was used, by comparing this with just standard carboplatin/5-fluorouracil and radiation for head and neck carcinomas. The induction therapy with cetuximab/radiation did not improve the outcome over standard chemoradiotherapy alone [49].

Cetuximab chemoradiotherapy has been substituted for cisplatin chemoradiotherapy in the off-trial use of cetuximab in this setting for good prognosis p16-positive oropharyngeal cancers where this p16-positive subset, unlike p16-negative, may need less treatment and where the p16 status may also predict response to cetuximab. This showed that the more conventional cisplatin arm had significantly better survival outcomes [50]. However, more formal randomised studies are yet to be reported.

Another strategy to be used with radiation to improve the response is to administer hypoxic cell radiosensitising drugs such as tirapazamine to reduce radioresistance. A randomised study of adding tirapazamine to chemoradiotherapy in head and neck patients, who had not been selected because hypoxia was present, showed no benefit to this approach, but other studies are ongoing [51].

There are many regimens that have been reported as treatment of locally advanced head and neck cancer. Iocca and colleagues performed a systematic review and Bayesian meta-analysis of the treatment options [52]. They included 57 trials that reported on 26 treatments. They concluded that concurrent cisplatin with radiation was the gold standard but suggested that taxanes may also have an impact. Certainly, the strategy of using chemoradiotherapy was found to be superior to just altering the fractionation schedule of the radiotherapy.

3.5.3 Adjuvant Therapy

Systemic therapy has been given after surgery to try to improve survival. There is no established role for adjuvant chemotherapy alone after surgery. A meta-analysis that included 2567 patients, including oral cancers, from six studies showed no benefit for adjuvant chemotherapy alone [28]. However, chemotherapy given concurrently with radiation therapy has been reported as more successful in patients at higher risk of recurrence after surgery, although results have been equivocal.

The EORTC 22931 trial randomised 334 patients to either radiation alone or with high-dose cisplatin (100 mg/sq. m) once every 3 weeks [53]. Their criteria for high risk were extracapsular extension, positive margins, perineural invasion or vascular tumour embolism. They found that chemoradiotherapy improved both progression-free survival and overall survival.

Identical treatments were compared in RTOG 9501 in 459 patients. They used different criteria for high risk [54, 55]. This included having positive margins, extracapsular extension or two or more nodes involved. They demonstrated improved disease-free survival but only in the patients with positive margins or extracapsular extension in nodes. Both studies included over 25% of patients with oral cancer.

These studies suggest benefit for adjuvant chemoradiotherapy after surgery for selected patients based on specific risk factors. Outside of these criteria, there may be no benefit. For example, a review of the National Cancer Database showed no benefit for adjuvant chemoradiotherapy over radiotherapy for patients with stage IV T4N0 disease [56].

High-dose cisplatin is associated with a number of side effects which can persist, including renal dysfunction and peripheral neuropathy. Lower dose concomitant cisplatin has been reported as effective in the adjuvant setting when combined with radiation, but the absence of randomised studies comparing it to the higher dose makes it difficult to recommend for routine use in the adjuvant setting [57].

Just as in the preoperative setting it is possible to include other cytotoxic agents such as docetaxel in adjuvant chemoradiotherapy regimens, cetuximab could also be studied in this setting based on its role in primary treatment, as could other immunotherapies. RTOG-0234 was a randomised phase II trial in patients with positive margins or extracapsular extension in the lymph nodes, where patients received cetuximab plus radiation with either weekly cisplatin or docetaxel. The regimens were found to be feasible, and because of better outcomes than historical controls, the docetaxel arm will be taken into a phase III trial [58]. However, a retrospective single institution experience with cetuximab and postoperative radiation in high-risk patients showed poor outcomes [59].

Another epidermal growth factor inhibitor lapatinib has been trialled in the adjuvant setting in high-risk patients in a randomised study [60]. It was added to high-dose cisplatin and radiotherapy postoperatively and then given as maintenance. The study accrued 688 patients. Lapatinib did not improve the outcome and simply added toxicity.

An important issue with adjuvant chemoradiotherapy is that there is an increased risk of death if the adjuvant therapy is delayed. A delay of more than 14 weeks in overall treatment time from surgery to the completion of the radiotherapy was found to compromise survival when the outcomes of 16,733 patients were reviewed [61].

3.6 Recurrent or Metastatic Head and Neck Cancer

The management of recurrent disease will depend on whether it is a local recurrence only or there is distant metastatic disease. For local recurrence after surgery and adjuvant therapy, salvage surgery may be appropriate, but a systematic review shows that the prognosis is poor [62]. Photodynamic therapy can also be considered as adjuvant treatment to surgery for superficial recurrences in the oral cavity and larynx [63, 64]. It is also possible to consider re-irradiation or combined chemoradiotherapy as salvage therapy, and small volumes of metastatic disease may not preclude these local therapies. The factors associated with patients having a good outcome with salvage therapy are the sites, like laryngeal cancer, low-volume recurrences after long disease-free intervals, and lack of comorbid illnesses which may impact on fitness and performance status [65].

Given the poor prognosis for patients who develop metastatic disease often several months to 1 year after initial therapy, the use of systemic therapy will depend on whether symptoms need controlling, whether there are comorbid illnesses and whether the patients are likely to tolerate the chemotherapy or whether it could decrease their overall quality of life, particularly as it does not have a significant effect on overall survival [2].

The major chemotherapy drug used for recurrent metastatic head and neck cancer is cisplatin, ever since a randomised study with cisplatin and bleomycin showed that cisplatin extended survival by 10 weeks [66]. Carboplatin with its different toxicity spectrum was also found to extend overall survival [67]. Methotrexate was another agent which is still being explored for palliation because in low doses it is well tolerated [68].

Doublet therapy with cisplatin and 5-fluorouracil was then commonly used, but in a randomised trial, although response rates were improved, this did not translate into survival advantage over monotherapy [69]. The taxanes paclitaxel and docetaxel were added, but this increased the toxicity and a randomised trial of cisplatin paclitaxel showed no additional benefit compared to cisplatin/5-fluorouracil [70, 71].

3.7 Monoclonal Antibodies

The monoclonal antibody cetuximab was the next major advance in the treatment of metastatic head and neck cancer. The EXREME study compares cisplatin/5-fluorouracil to this doublet with the addition of cetuximab. The overall survival was 7.4 months vs. 10.1 months ($p = 0.04$) [37], and it has become the gold standard against which newer regimens are compared. This is still a modest survival, and so the newer targeted therapies and immunotherapies are being investigated in the next wave of studies. A previous ECOG trial (SPECTRUM) randomised patients to cisplatin plus or minus cetuximab, but cetuximab did not improve the overall survival [72].

Other anti-EGFR antibodies have been trialled including panitumumab added to cisplatin/5-fluorouracil in a randomised study. No survival advantage was seen, but the p16-positive patients tended to survive longer [73]. Zalutumumab has also been tested in a phase 3 trial in patients with head and neck cancer after cisplatin failure. It was combined with best supportive care and compared to best supportive care only. It extended progression-free survival but not overall survival [74]. A dual-action antibody against EGFR and HER 3 has recently been added to cisplatin/5-fluorouracil or carboplatin/paclitaxel in a phase Ib study and showed encouraging responses but with added toxicity [75].

3.7.1 Tyrosine Kinase Inhibitors

The tyrosine kinase inhibitors erlotinib and gefitinib have been trialled in head and neck cancer as single agents and in combinations where they may have had a synergistic effect in combination with cisplatin. However, there are no improved clinical outcomes to encourage further large trials [76].

3.7.2 Angiogenesis Inhibitors

Bevacizumab is a monoclonal antibody that inhibits VEGF. It has been trialled in locally advanced disease, and a phase III trial in recurrent/metastatic disease is ongoing. A phase II trial in combination with pemetrexed, an antifolate, had some encouraging responses, but bleeding was a frequently reported toxicity [77].

3.7.3 mTOR Inhibitors

The P13K/Akt/mTor pathway is activated in squamous cell cancers of the head and neck. Because the mTor inhibitor everolimus has been effective when paired with cisplatin in other cancers, trials showed that the combination was tolerated by patients with head and neck cancer [78]. Temsirolimus has been added to low-dose weekly carboplatin and paclitaxel for patients with recurrent or metastatic head and neck squamous cell carcinoma and achieved an encouraging 41.7% response rate [79].

3.7.4 Checkpoint Inhibitors and Other Immunotherapies

The initial trials of the checkpoint inhibitors were in patients with recurrent or metastatic head and neck cancer whose cancer had progressed within 6 months of receiving platinum-based chemotherapy. The CheckMate 141 study randomised patients to receiving nivolumab or single agent weekly cetuximab or the cytotoxics methotrexate or docetaxel [80]. There was an improved survival for those receiving nivolumab with the 18 months survival being 21.5% versus 8.3% for the control arm [81]. Greater benefit was seen in patients who had not received prior cetuximab.

Similarly, the KEYNOTE 55 and KEYNOTE 12 studies showed the efficacy of pembrolizumab as first-line therapy after disease progression on cisplatin [40, 82]. In KEYNOTE 055 which treated patients with progression within 6 months of receiving cisplatin and cetuximab, pembrolizumab was associated with a median response duration of 8 months. There was some correlation with the expression of the target biomarker, PD-L1 expression, in that when this was measured at ≥1.0, the response was 18% compared to 12% when <1.0. In KEYNOTE 040, pembrolizumab was randomised against the standard of care, either methotrexate or cetuximab when patients had relapsed within 3–6 months of receiving a platinum containing regimen or presenting with metastatic head and neck cancer. This study did not show a statistically significant advantage for pembrolizumab but was significant for those cancers where 50% or over of the cells expressed the target PD-1 [83].

Another approach to immunotherapy involves activating Toll-like receptor 8. These receptors on monocytes and dendritic cells release inflammatory mediators, and the expression of co-stimulatory molecules on antigen-presenting cells results in better presentation of tumour expressing antigens to the body's T cells [84]. Taking the EXTREME regimen of cisplatin (or carboplatin) plus 5-fluorouracil plus cetuximab, 195 patients with recurrent or metastatic squamous cell head and neck cancer were randomised to the Toll-like receptor 8 agonist motolimod or placebo. Motolimod did not improve progression-free or overall survival across the whole population, but the subset of HPV-positive patients and those with injection site reactions showed a significant benefit [85].

Ongoing phase III trials are moving immunotherapy into first-line therapy [86].

3.8 Conclusions

Systemic therapy for head and neck cancers is not given with curative intent as a single modality. It has had little success as induction therapy prior to definitive local treatments of radiotherapy or surgery but is successful when combined with radiotherapy for the primary treatment of locally advanced disease or as adjuvant chemoradiotherapy after definitive surgery. It is useful for recurrent or metastatic disease either with radiotherapy for local disease or in combinations for metastatic disease.

The major advance in these settings has been the advent of immunotherapies such as monoclonal antibodies or checkpoint inhibitors which can be added to convention chemotherapy in an attempt to improve outcomes.

Bibliography

1. Gold KA, Neskey M, William WN. The role of systemic treatment before, during, and after definitive treatment. Otolaryngol Clin N Am. 2013;46:645–56.
2. Kelly CG. Chemotherapy: United Kingdom National multidisciplinary guidelines. J Laryngol Otol. 2016;130(Suppl 2):S71–4.
3. Bonner JA, Harari PM, Giralt J, Cohen RB, Jones CU, Sur RK, et al. Radiotherapy plus cetuximab for locoregionally advanced head and neck cancer: 5-year survival data form a phase III randomized trial, and relation between cetuximab-induced rash and survival. Lancet Oncol. 2010;11:21–8.
4. Mehra R, Seiwer TY, Gupta S, Weiss J, Gluck I, Eder JP, et al. Efficacy and safety of pembrolizumab in recurrent/metastatic head and neck squamous cell carcinoma: pooled analyses after long-term follow-up in KEYNOTE-012. Br J Cancer. 2018;119:153–9.
5. Yue Q, Zhang M, Chen Y, Zheng D, Chen Y, Feng M. Establishment of prognostic factors in recurrent nasopharyngeal carcinoma patients who received salvage intensity-modulated radiotherapy: a meta-analysis. Oral Oncol. 2018;81:81–8.
6. Solomon B, Young RJ, Rischin D. Head and neck squamous cell carcinoma: genomics and emerging biomarkers for immunomodulatory cancer treatments. Semin Cancer Biol. 2018; https://doi.org/10.1016/j.semcancer.2018.01.008. [Epub ahead of print].

7. Bonner JA, Mesia R, Giralt J, Psyrri A, Keilholz U, Rosenthal DI, et al. p19, HPV, and cetuximab: what is the evidence? Oncologist. 2017;22:811–22.
8. Smith IE, Harris AL, Morgan M, Ford HT, Gazet JC, Harmer CL, et al. Tamoxifen versus aminoglutethimide in advanced breast carcinoma: a randomized cross-over trial. Br Med J (Clin Res Ed). 1981;283:1432–4.
9. International Human Genome Sequencing Consortium. Initial sequencing and analysis of the human genome. Nature. 2001;409:860–921.
10. Shendure J, Hanlee J. Next-generation DNA sequencing. Nat Biotechnol. 2008;26:1135–45.
11. Broach JR, Thorner J. High-throughput screening for drug discovery. Nature. 1996;384(Suppl):14–6.
12. Drucker BJ, Guilhot F, O'Brien SG, Gatmann I, Kantarjian H, Gattermann N, et al. Five-year follow-up of patients receiving imatinib for chronic myeloid leukemia. N Engl J Med. 2006;355:2408–17.
13. Eggermont AMM, Kirkwood JM. Re-evaluating the role of dacarbazine in metastatic melanoma: what have we learned in 30 years? Eur J Cancer. 2004;40:1825–36.
14. McArthur GA, Chapman PB, Robert C, Larkin J, Haanen JB, Dummer R, et al. Safety and efficacy of vemurafenib in BRAF(V600E) and BRAF(V600K) mutation-positive melanoma (BRIM-3): extended follow-up of a phase 3, randomised, open-label study. Lancet Oncol. 2014;15:323–32.
15. Shak S. Overview of the trastuzumab (Herceptin) anti-HER2 monoclonal antibody clinical program in HER2-overexpressing metastatic breast cancer. Herceptin Multinational Investigator Study Group. Semin Oncol. 1999;26(Suppl 12):71–7.
16. Romond EH, Perez EA, Bryant J, Suman VJ, Geyer CE, Davidson NE, et al. Trastuzumab plus adjuvant chemotherapy for operable HER2-positive breast cancer. N Engl J Med. 2005;353:1673–84.
17. Cheung MC, Haynes AE, Meyer RM, Stevens A, Imrie KR, Members of the Hematology, Disease Site Group of the Cancer Care Ontario Program in Evidence-Based Care. Rituximab in lymphoma: a systematic review and consensus practice guidelines for cancer care Ontario. Cancer Treat Rev. 2007;33:161–76.
18. Fabi A, De Laurentiis M, Caruso M, Valle E, Moscetti L, Santini D, et al. Efficacy and safety of T-DM1 in the 'common-practice' of HER2+ advanced breast cancer setting: a multicenter study. Oncotarget. 2017;8:6481–9.
19. Mondello P, Cuzzocrea S, Navarra M, Mian M. 90 Y-ibritumomab tiuxetan: a nearly forgotten opportunity. Oncotarget. 2016;7:7597–609.
20. Keating GM. Bevacizumab: a review of its use in advanced cancer. Drugs. 2014;74:1891–925.
21. Acúrcio RC, Scomparin A, Conniot J, Salvador JAR, Satchi-Fainaro R, Florindo HF, Cardos Guedes R. Structure-function analysis of immune checkpoint receptors to guide emerging anti-cancer immunotherapy. J Med Chem. 2018; https://doi.org/10.1021/acs.jmedchem.8b00541. [Epub ahead of print].
22. Mahoney KM, Freeman GJ, McDermott DF. The next immune-checkpoint inhibitors: PD-1/PD-L1 blockade in melanoma. Clin Ther. 2015;37:764–82.
23. Hodi FS, O'Day SJ, McDermott DF, Weber RW, Sosman JA, Haanen JB, et al. Improved survival with ipilimumab in patients with metastatic melanoma. N Engl J Med. 2010;363:711–23.
24. Menaria J, Kitawat S, Verma V. Cancer vaccine: an overview. SJAMS. 2013;1:161–71.
25. Grupp SA, Kalos M, Barrett D, Aplenc R, Porter DL, Rheingold SR, et al. Chimeric antigen receptor-modified T cell for acute lymphoid leukaemia. N Engl J Med. 2013;368:1509–18.
26. Ramos CA, Heslop HE, Brenner MK. CAR-T cell therapy for lymphoma. Annu Rev Med. 2016;67:165–83.
27. The Department of Veterans Affairs Laryngeal Cancer Study Group. Induction chemotherapy plus radiation compared with surgery plus radiation in patients with advanced laryngeal cancer. N Engl J Med. 1991;324:1685–90.
28. Pignon JP, le Maitre A, Maillard E, Bourhis J, Group M-NC. Meta-analysis of chemotherapy in head and neck cancer (MACH-NC): an update on 93 randomised trials and 17,346 patients. Radiother Oncol. 2009;92:4–14.

29. Ribassin-Majed L, Marguet S, Lee AWM, Ng WT, Ma J, Chan ATC, et al. What is the best treatment in nasopharyngeal carcinoma? An individual patient data network meta-analysis. J Clin Oncol. 2016;35:498–505.
30. Vishak S, Rangarajan B, Kekatpure VD. Neoadjuvant chemotherapy in oral cancers: selecting the right patients. Indian J Med Paediatr Oncol. 2015;36:148–53.
31. Posner MR, Hershock DM, Blajman CR, Mickiewicz E, Winquist E, Gorbounova, et al. Cisplatin and fluorouracil alone or with docetaxel in head and neck cancer. N Engl J Med. 2007;357:1705–15.
32. Vermorken JB, Remenar E, van Herpen C, Gorlia T, Mesia R, Degardin M, et al. Cisplatin, fluorouracil and docetaxel in unresectable head and neck cancer. N Engl J Med. 2007;357:1695–704.
33. Camille N, Rozehnal J, Roy E, Uczkowski D, Olson A, Genden E, et al. A phase I study of cabazitaxel in combination with platinum and 5-fluorouracil (PF) in locally advanced squamous cell carcinoma of head and neck (LA-SCCHN). Oral Oncol. 2017;71:99–104.
34. Cohen EE, Karrison TG, Kocherginsky M, Mueller J, Egan R, Huang CH, et al. Phase III randomized trial of induction chemotherapy in patients with N2 or N3 locally advanced head and neck cancer. J Clin Oncol. 2014;32:2735–43.
35. Haddad R, O'Neill A, Rabinowits G, Tishler R, Khuri F, Adkins D, et al. Induction chemotherapy followed by concurrent chemoradiotherapy (sequential chemoradiotherapy) versus concurrent chemoradiotherapy alone in locally advanced head and neck cancer (PARADIGM): a randomised phase 3 trial. Lancet Oncol. 2013;14:257–64.
36. Lefebvre JL, Pointreau Y, Rolland F, Alfonsi M, Baudoux A, Sire E, et al. Induction chemotherapy followed by either chemoradiotherapy or bioradiotherapy for larynx preservation: the TREMPLIN randomised phase II study. J Clin Oncol. 2013;31:853–9.
37. Vermorken JB, Mesia R, Rivera F, Remenar E, Kaewecki A, Rottey S, et al. Platinum-based chemotherapy plus cetuximab in head and neck cancer. N Engl J Med. 2008;359:1116–27.
38. Chang PM, Lu HJ, Wang LW, Tai SK, Chen MH, Chu PY, et al. Effectiveness of incorporating cetuximab into docetaxel/cisplatin/fluorouracil induction chemotherapy and chemoradiotherapy for inoperable squamous cell carcinoma of the oral cavity: a phase II study. Head Neck. 2017;39:1333–42.
39. Specenier PM, Remenar E, Buter J, Schriivers DL, Bergamini C, Licitra LF, et al. TPF plus cetuximab induction chemotherapy followed by biochemoradiation with weekly cetuximab plus weekly cisplatin or carboplatin: a randomized phase II EORTC trial. Ann Oncol. 2017;28:2219–24.
40. Bauml J, Selwert TY, Pfister F, Worden F, Liu J, Gilbert J, et al. Pembrolizumab for platinum—and cetuximab-refractory head and neck cancer: results from a single-arm phase II study. J Clin Oncol. 2017;35:1542–9.
41. Šeparovic R, Pavlovic M, Silovski T, Tecic Vuger M, Juric A. Systemic therapy of head and neck carcinoma. Lib Oncol. 2016;44:45–9.
42. Juloori A, Koyfman SA, Geiger JL, Joshi NP, Woody NM, Burkey BB, et al. Definitive chemoradiation in locally advanced squamous cell carcinoma of the hypopharynx: long-term outcomes and toxicity. Anticancer Res. 2018;38:3543–9.
43. Lee SY, Choi YS, Song I-C, Park SJ, Keam B, Yang YJ, et al. Comparison of standard-dose 3-weekly cisplatin for concurrent chemoradiation of patients with locally advanced head and neck squamous cell cancer: a multicentre retrospective analysis. Medicine. 2018;97:810778. https://doi.org/10.1097/MD.0000000000010778.
44. Rades D, Seidl D, Janssen S, Bajrovic A, Hakim SG, Wollenberg B, Schild SE. Do we need 5-FU in addition to cisplatin for chemoradiation of locally advanced head- and-neck cancer? Oral Oncol. 2016a;57:40–5.
45. Rades S, Strojan P, Sedl D, Janssen S, Bajorvic A, Kazic N, et al. Radiochemotherapy for locally advanced squamous cell carcinoma of the head and neck: higher-dose cisplatin every 3 weeks versus cisplatin/5-fluorouracil every 4 weeks. J Craniomaxillofac Surg. 2016b;44:1436–40.
46. Nagasaka M, Zak M, Issa M, Kim H, Abrams J, Sukari A. Definitive chemoradiotherapy with carboplatin for squamous cell carcinoma of the head and neck. Laryngoscope. 2017;127:2260–4.

47. Nakahara S, Hanamoto A, Seo Y, Miyaguchi S, Yamaoto Y, Tomiyama Y, et al. Chemoradiotherapy with weekly low-dose docetaxel and cisplatin concurrent with radiation for patients with locally advanced nasopharyngeal carcinoma, followed by adjuvant chemotherapy for selected patients. Jpn J Clin Oncol. 2016;46:903–10.
48. Mitsudo K, Toshiyuki K, Iida M, Iwai T, Nakashima H, Oguri S, et al. Retrograde superselective intra-arterial chemotherapy and daily concurrent radiotherapy for stage III and IV oral cancer: analysis of therapeutic results in 112 cases. Radiother Oncol. 2014;111:306–10.
49. Geoffrois L, Martin L, De Raucourt D, Sun XS, Tao Y, Maingon P, et al. Induction chemotherapy followed by cetuximab radiotherapy is not superior to concurrent chemoradiotherapy for head and neck carcinomas: results of the GORTEC 2007-02 Phase III randomized trial. J Clin Oncol. 2018; https://doi.org/10.1200/JCO.2017.76.2591. [Epub before print].
50. Barney CL, Walson S, Zamora P, Healy EH, Nolan N, Diavolitsis VM, et al. Clinical outcomes and prognostic factors in cisplatin versus cetuximab chemoradiation for locally advanced p16 positive oropharyngeal carcinoma. Oral Oncol. 2018;79:9–14.
51. Rischin D, Peters LJ, O'Sullivan B, Giralt J, Fisher R, Yuen K, et al. Tirapazamine, cisplatin, and radiation versus cisplatin and radiation for advanced squamous cell carcinoma of the head and neck (TROG 02.02, HeadSTART0): a phase III trial of the Trans-Tasman Radiation Oncology Group. J Clin Oncol. 2010;28:2989–95.
52. Iocca O, Farcomeni A, Di Rocco A, Di Maio P, Golusinski P, Pardinas Lopez S, et al. Locally advanced squamous cell carcinoma of the head and neck: a systematic review and Bayesian network meta-analysis of the currently available treatment options. Oral Oncol. 2018;80:40–51.
53. Bernier J, Domenge C, Ozsahin M, Matuszewska K, Lefevbre JL, Greiner RH, et al. Postoperative irradiation with or without concomitant chemotherapy for locally advanced head and neck cancer. N Engl J Med. 2004;350:1945–52.
54. Cooper JS, Pajak TF, Forastierre AA, Jacobs J, Campbell BH, Saxsman SB, et al. Postoperative concurrent radiotherapy and chemotherapy for high-risk squamous-cell carcinoma of the head and neck. N Engl J Med. 2004;350:1937–44.
55. Cooper JS, Zhang Q, Pajak TF, Forastierre AA, Jacobs J, Saxman SB, et al. Long-term follow-up of the RTOG 9501/Intergroup phase II trial: postoperative concurrent radiation therapy and chemotherapy in high-risk squamous cell carcinoma of the head and neck. Int J Radiat Oncol Biol Phys. 2012;84:1198–205.
56. Kirke DN, Qureshi MM, Kamran SC, Ezzat W, Jalisi S, Salama A, et al. Role of adjuvant chemoradiotherapy in T4N0 stage IV head and neck cancer: a national Cancer Database analysis. Head Neck. 2018;40:1174–84.
57. Franchin G, Minatel E, Politi D, Gobitti C, Talamini R, Vaccher E, et al. Postoperative reduced dose of cisplatin concomitant with radiation therapy in high-risk head and neck squamous cell carcinoma. Cancer. 2009;115:2464–71.
58. Harari PM, Harris J, Kies MS, Myers JN, Jordan RC, Gillison ML, et al. Postoperative chemoradiotherapy and cetuximab for high-risk squamous cell carcinoma of the head and neck: Radiation Therapy Oncology Group RTOG-0234. J Clin Oncol. 2014;32:2486–95.
59. Araki D, Redman MW, Martins R, Eaton K, Baik C, Chow L, et al. Concurrent cetuximab and postoperative radiation in resected high-risk squamous cell carcinomas of the head and neck: a single-institution experience. Head Neck. 2016;38:1318–23.
60. Harrington K, Temam S, Mehanna H, D'Cruz A, Jain M, D'onofrio I, et al. Postoperative adjuvant lapatinib and concurrent chemoradiotherapy followed by maintenance lapatinib monotherapy in high-risk patients with resected squamous cell carcinoma of the head and neck: a phase III, randomized, double-blind, placebo-controlled study. J Clin Oncol. 2015;33:4202–9.
61. Tam M, Wu SP, Gerber NK, Lee A, Schreiber D, Givi B, Hu K. The impact of adjuvant chemoradiotherapy timing on survival of head and neck cancers. Laryngoscope. 2018; https://doi.org/10.1002/lary.27.152. [Epub before print].
62. Zenga J, Gross J, Fowler S, Chen J, Vila P, Richmon JD, et al. Salvage of recurrence after surgery and adjuvant therapy: a systematic review. Am J Otolaryngol. 2018;39:223–7.
63. Civantos FJ, Karakullukcu B, Biel M, Silver CE, Rinaldo A, Saba NF, et al. A review of photodynamic therapy for neoplasms of the head and neck. Adv Ther. 2018;35:324–40.

64. Vander Poorten V, Meulemans J, Nuyts S, Clement P, Hermans R, Hauben E, Delaere P. Postoperative photodynamic therapy as a new adjuvant treatment after robot-assisted salvage surgery of recurrent squamous cell carcinoma of the base of tongue. World J Surg Oncol. 2015;13:214–8.
65. Spencer SA, Harris J, Wheeler RH, Machtay M, Schultz C, Spanos W, et al. Final report of RTOG 9610, a multi-institutional trial of reirradiation and chemotherapy for unresectable recurrent squamous cell carcinoma of the head and neck. Head Neck. 2008;30:21–8.
66. Morton RP, Rugman F, Dorman EB, Stoney PJ, Wilson JA, McCormick M, et al. Cisplatinum and bleomycin for advanced or recurrent squamous cell carcinoma of the head and neck: a randomised factorial phase III controlled trial. Cancer Chemother Pharmacol. 1985;15:283–9.
67. Eisenberger M, Hornedo J, Silva H, Donehower R, Spaulding M, Van Echo D. Carboplatin (NSC-241-240): an active platinum analog for the treatment of squamous-cell carcinoma of the head and neck. J Clin Oncol. 1986;4:1506–9.
68. Sharma M, Gupta M, Fotedar V, Sharma A. Methotrexate, an attractive agent for palliation in head and neck cancers. South Asian J Cancer. 2014;3:299.
69. Jacobs C, Lyman G, Velez-Garcai E, Sridhar KS, Knight W, Hochster H, et al. A phase II randomised study comparing cisplatin and fluorouracil as single agents and in combination for advanced squamous cell carcinoma of the head and neck. J Clin Oncol. 1992;10:257–63.
70. Dreyfus AI, Clark JR, Norris CM, Rossi RM, Lucarini JW, Busse PM, et al. Docetaxel: an active drug for squamous cell carcinoma of the head and neck. J Clin Oncol. 1996;14:1672–8.
71. Gibson MK, Li Y, Murphy B, Hussain MH, DeConti RC, Ensley J, et al. Randomised phase II evaluation of cisplatin plus fluorouracil versus cisplatin in advanced head and neck cancer (E1359): an intergroup trial of the Eastern Cooperative Oncology Group. J Clin Oncol. 2005;20:3562–7.
72. Burtness B, Goldwasser MA, Flood W, Mattar B, Forastiere AA, Eastern Cooperative Oncology Group. Phase III randomised trial of cisplatin plus placebo compared with cisplatin plus cetuximab in metastatic/recurrent head and neck cancer: an Eastern Cooperative Oncology Group study. J Clin Oncol. 2005;23:8646–54.
73. Vermorken JB, Stöhlmacher-Williams J, Davidenko I, Licitra L, Winquist E, Villanueva C, et al. Cisplatin and fluorouracil with or without panitumumab in patients with recurrent or metastatic squamous-cell carcinoma of the head and neck (SPECRUM): an open-label phase 3 randomised trial. Lancet Oncol. 2013;14:697–710.
74. Machiels JP, Subramanian S, Ruzsa A, Repassy G, Lifirenko I, Flyglare A, et al. Zalutumumab plus best supportive care versus best supportive care alone in patients with recurrent or metastatic squamous-cell carcinoma of the head and neck after failure of platinum-based chemotherapy: an open-label, randomised phase 3 trial. Lancet Oncol. 2011;12:333–43.
75. Jimenca A, Machiels JP, Wirth L, Specenier P, Seiwert TY, Mardiuadi F, et al. Phase Ib study of duligotuzumab (MEHD7945A) plus cisplatin/5-fluoruracil or carboplatin/paclitaxel for first-line treatment of recurrent/metastatic squamous cell carcinoma of the head and neck. Cancer. 2016;122:3803–11.
76. Siu LL, Soulieres D, Chen EX, Pond GR, Chin SF, Francis P, et al. Phase I/II trial of erlotinib and cisplatin in patients with recurrent or metastatic squamous cell carcinoma of the head and neck. A Princess Margaret Hospital phase II consortium and National Cancer Institute of Canada Trials Group Study. J Clin Oncol. 2007;25:2178–83.
77. Argiris A, Karamouzis MV, Gooding WE, Bransletter BF, Zhong S, Raez LE, et al. Phase II trial of pemetrexed and bevacizumab in patients with recurrent or metastatic head and neck cancer. J Clin Oncol. 2011;29:1140–5.
78. Fury MG, Lee NY, Sherman E, Ho AL, Rao S, Heguy A, et al. A phase I study of everolimus + weekly cisplatin + intensity modulated radiation therapy in head-and-neck cancer. Int J Radiat Oncol Biol Phys. 2013;87:479–86.
79. Dunn LA, Fury MG, Xiao H, Baxi SS, Sherman EJ, Korte S, et al. A phase II study of temsirolimus added to low-dose weekly carboplatin and paclitaxel for patients with recurrent and/or metastatic (R/M) head and neck squamous cell carcinoma (HNSCC). Ann Oncol. 2017;28:2533–8.

80. Ferris RL, Blumenschein G Jr, Fayette J, Guigay J, Colevas AD, Licitra L, Harrington K, et al. Nivolumab for recurrent squamous-cell carcinoma of the head and neck. N Engl J Med. 2016;375:1856–67.
81. Gillison ML, Blumenschein GR, Fayette J, Guijay J, Coeva AD, Licitra L, et al. CheckMate 141: 1-year update and subgroup analysis of nivolumab as first-line therapy in patients with recurrent/metastatic head and neck cancer. Oncologist. 2018; https://doi.org/10.1634/theoncologist.2017-0674.
82. Chow LQ, Haddad R, Gupta S, Mahipal A, Mehra R, Tahara M, et al. Antitumour activity of pembrolizumab in biomarker-unselected patients with recurrent and/or metastatic head and neck squamous cell carcinoma: results from the phase Ib KEYNOTE-012 expansion cohort. J Clin Oncol. 2016;34:3838–45.
83. Cohen EE, Harrington KJ, Le Tourneau C, Dinis J, Licitra L, Ahn M-J, et al. Pembrolizumab (pembo) vs standard of care (SOC) for recurrent or metastatic head and neck squamous cell carcinoma (R/M HNSCC): phase III KEYNOTE-040 trial. Ann Oncol. 2017;28(Suppl 5) https://doi.org/10.1093/annonc/mdx440.040.
84. Dietsch GN. Motolimod effectively drives immune function activation in advanced cancer patients. Oncoimmunology. 2016; https://doi.org/10.1080/2162402X.2015.1126037.
85. Ferris RL, Saba NF, Gitilitz BJ, Haddad R, Sukari A, Neupane P, et al. Effect of adding motolimod to standard combination chemotherapy and cetuximab treatment of patients with squamous cell carcinoma of the head and neck: The active8 randomised clinical trial. JAMA Oncol. 2018; https://doi.org/10.1001/jamaoncol.2018.1888. [Epub before print].
86. Specenier P, Vermorken JB. Optimizing treatments for recurrent or metastatic head and neck squamous cell carcinoma. Expert Rev Anticancer Ther. 2018; https://doi.org/10.1080/14737140.2018.1493925.
87. Stewat JS, Cohen EE, Licitra L, Van Herpen CM, Khorprasert C, Soulieres D, et al. Phase III study of gefitinib compared with intravenous methotrexate for recurrent squamous cell carcinoma of the head and neck [corrected]. J Clin Oncol. 2009;27:1864–71.

Principles and Practice of Radiation Oncology and Modern Radiation Therapy Techniques

4

Rene-Jean Bensadoun and Raj Nair

4.1 Introduction

Radiation oncology uses ionizing radiation to treat cancer (and occasionally a few benign conditions). Radiotherapy or radiation therapy (RT) was initially developed in conjunction with diagnostic radiology but has evolved into a separate specialty. Currently, more than 50% of cancer patients undergo RT at some point during the course of their cancer. Most receive treatment with curative intent (definitive therapy). Patients with incurable disease receive shorter courses of therapy to relieve cancer-induced symptoms designed to minimize acute side effects. The acute side effects of RT are often milder than either chemotherapy or radical surgery; most patients find it the easiest portion of their therapy. While ionizing radiation damages both normal and cancerous cells, normal cells have greater capacity to repair this damage, and carefully administered treatment can eradicate cancer cells while relatively sparing the organ that harbors them. For example, a laryngeal tumor and its draining nodes can be cured while sparing the voice and neck muscles. Although RT can be used alone, it is often combined with surgery and/or chemotherapy in a multimodality regimen that benefits from the unique advantages of each modality. Combined modality therapy does run the risk of increased toxicity because of each treatment's side effects, so these regimens should be carefully designed and tested in clinical studies.

RT consists of two modalities: teletherapy and brachytherapy. Teletherapy utilizes X-ray or subatomic particle beams, delivered by a machine positioned a

R.-J. Bensadoun (✉)
Department of Radiation Oncology, Centre de Haute Energie, Nice, France

R. Nair
Oral Medicine and Oral Oncology, Griffith University, QLD, Australia

Haematology and Oncology, Gold Coast University Hospital, Queensland Health, QLD, Australia
e-mail: r.nair@griffith.edu.au

R. Nair (ed.), *Orofacial Supportive Care in Cancer*,
https://doi.org/10.1007/978-3-030-86510-8_4

distance (typically, a meter) from the patient. Brachytherapy utilizes radiation emanating from radioactive sources implanted inside the patient's body, either temporarily or permanently. Both modalities have been in use for over a century.

In order to deliver safe and effective RT, the radiation oncologist must master five foundation disciplines: clinical oncology, radiobiology, oncologic imaging, computer science, and medical physics.

Effective practice of radiation oncology depends on a sound understanding of clinical oncology and basic sciences.

This knowledge must include:

- Principles of cancer pathology, medical oncology, and surgical oncology.
- Gross anatomy and radiographic anatomy.
- Natural history of each cancer.
- General clinical care of the cancer patient including supportive care, management of cancer symptoms, and treatment effects.

Anatomy, the precise location of tumor in the patient, and the natural history of a cancer are the basis of treatment planning for each patient. For example, careful recording of precise lymph node metastasis locations and risk of involvement of those locations in a study population dictate shape of fields to cover areas at greatest risk of microscopic tumor spread.

4.2 Radiobiology

Radiobiology studies the impact of ionizing radiation on biological molecules, living cells, and tissues. Whether an ionizing ray hits a molecule upon striking a cell is a random event. Statistically, a ray is most likely to strike the most common molecule in the cell, water. The ionizing ray causes water molecules to break apart into ion pairs, producing the highly reactive hydroxyl radical. Free radicals bounce around in the cell and may strike other molecules, usually water, causing a cascade that increases the number and density of free radicals. Ultimately, one or more of these radicals may randomly strike a molecule of DNA, resulting in single- or double-strand DNA breaks. Without functioning DNA, the cancer cells cannot reproduce properly or repair themselves, and the cells transition to apoptosis. Apoptosis (programmed cell death) is the capacity of a cell to destroy itself if its DNA is irrevocably damaged. A cell has several endogenous agents that are protective against radiation damage. The continued existence of free radicals depends on the concentration of the primary cellular defense, glutathione, which destroys free radicals. Enzymes that metabolize reactive oxidative species, including catalase, superoxide dismutase, and glutathione peroxidase, also may protect cells from radiation. Oxygen is a radiosensitizer because it extends the existence of free radicals by a factor of 3. Cells in a hypoxic environment are relatively radioresistant (by the same factor of 3; this is not a coincidence). The body can usually repair single-strand breaks and sometimes can repair double-strand breaks. Lethal damage results in mitotic cell death; damage that can be repaired is called "potentially lethal damage." Death of a cell line after lethal damage may take several mitotic cycles and, therefore, depending on cell cycle time, as long as several months. A cell is most sensitive to radiation when it is undergoing mitosis; conversely, cells in G0 and the late S phase are relatively radioresistant. After cell death, the body must resorb the cell remains, and scars may form. So tumors usually shrink slowly, and sometimes a mass will remain that is simply a scar. RT traditionally has been fractionated, which means delivered in multiple small daily doses, to maximize the effect on tumor cells and minimize the late effects on normal tissues. Acute side effects are largely due to the effect of radiation on the rapidly dividing normal cells of the body, such as skin and mucous membranes. Tumor cells are actively dividing, so tumors tend to respond in the same way as normal cells that actively divide. Due to very different pathophysiology, occurrence of acute effects do *not* predict for occurrence of late effects. Late effects are largely due to microvascular damage that resembles that caused by diabetes mellitus, loss of parenchymal cell function, and scarring. It is important to remember that late effects may occur many years after treatment. The 4 R's of radiobiology, reoxygenation, repair, redistribution, and repopulation, are the reasons radiation oncologists fractionate radiation. Reoxygenation: When a tumor is irradiated, the better-oxygenated cells in the periphery of the tumor deposit are more likely to die. As these cells die during the course of therapy, O_2 penetrates more deeply into the tumor and reach cells that had previously been poorly oxygenated. Hence, fractionated radiotherapy results in the induction of radiosensitivity in cells that had originally been radioresistant by the phenomenon of "reoxygenation." Repair: Potentially lethal damage is damage which may be repaired, both in tumor cells and most importantly in normal, healthy, noncancerous tissue within the radiation field. This process is felt to be largely complete in about 6 h. Repair decreases risk of late effects. Redistribution: Redistribution refers to the movement of cells into different phases of the cell cycle. Since cells in the late S phase and G0 are relatively resistant to radiation, multiple treatments enhance the chance that any given cell will receive treatment during a sensitive phase in the cell cycle. Redistribution makes RT more effective. Repopulation: Hopefully, all tumor cells are encompassed by the treatment, and much normal tissue is not. In that case, normal cells can migrate from unirradiated tissue into the target volume to replace damaged cells. For example, skin cells will migrate into a denuded patch of skin, creating islands of normal skin which will enlarge to cover the open area. Surviving normal cells in the field can repopulate by cell division. Repopulation heals acute effects and also decreases risk of late effects. Unfortunately, surviving tumor cells can also repopulate by cell division; so interruptions or extended treatment duration may decrease the probability of tumor control. Organs that are organized in parallel (lung, kidney, liver) can tolerate the loss of large portions of their volume, while linear organs (spinal cord) cannot. Respecting radiation tolerance of these latter organs is very important. Exceeding tolerance of (sacrificing) portions of lung, liver, or kidney is acceptable, providing enough functional parenchyma is left to sustain the vital function of that organ and the patient's quality of life. For example, the volume of lung that can be safely sacrificed depends on the pretreatment lung function.

A radiation oncologist aims to deliver an effective dose to the tumor while delivering as low a dose as possible to the surrounding normal tissue. Radiation dose is a very complicated concept, as it depends not only on the total dose but also fraction size and treatment duration. For example, 30 Gy delivered in 5 fractions would be more potent than the same dose delivered in 10 fractions, and daily treatments are different than biweekly treatments. Although smaller fraction size tends to decrease late effects, if smaller daily doses are used, a higher total dose is required to achieve the same level of tumor control. However, the longer regimen is likely to decrease both acute and late effects. The volume of irradiated normal tissue has a major impact on treatment tolerance, even though it is not recorded in the prescription or reported in studies. Large fields will tolerate less dose. Fortunately, control of microscopic disease requires less dose than control of gross tumor deposits. Often, smaller fields will be used at the end of treatment to provide adequate dose to the tumor; this is referred to as the "shrinking field technique," and the smaller field is called "the boost." Since radiation cell kill depends on the random distribution of energy deposition in the cell, there is no way to guarantee the effectiveness of a course of radiotherapy, nor can we accurately predict toxicity expected from a certain dose.

Dose response curves are asymptotic to both the 100% and the 0% probability of a given outcome.

Surgery or pre-radiation chemotherapy may improve the risk/benefit calculation by reducing tumor burden, because a lower dose of radiation is needed to eradicate residual microscopic disease than would have been needed to sterilize a bulky tumor.

4.2.1 Radioprotection and Radiosensitization

When the therapeutic ratio is unfavorable, attempts to control the cancer involve protection of normal tissues, radiosensitization of tumor cells, or both. Both radioprotection and radiosensitization are attempts to improve the therapeutic ration, by shifting the late effect curve to the right or the tumor control curve to the left.

Radioprotection: Decreasing the effective dose to normal cells, either by decreasing the fraction size or improving the normal tissue dose distribution (physical radioprotection), will improve the therapeutic ratio. Attempts to develop drugs to chemically protect cells have been largely unsuccessful (with the exception of amifostine, developed by the army for protection against nuclear attack, during the Cold War, and pilocarpine, a cholinergic agonist that protects salivary function to some extent during RT affecting salivary glands).

Radiosensitization: Since oxygen is required for effective radiotherapy, and since tumors almost always contain hypoxic areas, improving delivery of oxygen to tumor cells may improve clinical outcomes. Although pressurized oxygen has not been demonstrated to improve the therapeutic ratio, randomized data suggests that raising depressed hemoglobin levels enhances tumor control, presumably by increasing tissue oxygen levels. Hyperthermia, either before or after irradiation, has been shown to radiosensitize tumor cells. This effect is not related to the presence of oxygen; in fact, cells in a hypoxic environment are more sensitive to hyperthermia.

Delivering and maintaining heat homogenously has been challenging. Very commonly, chemotherapy is administered concomitantly with radiation to sensitize the malignant cells to radiation. The treatment of many cancers, including anal, head and neck, lung, and cervix cancer, has been transformed by the use of concomitant chemoradiotherapy. The effective and safe dose of both drugs and radiation, however, must be determined for each drug or combination regimen, since radiosensitizing agents make normal cells more radiosensitive too.

4.3 Medical Imaging

The effective delivery of RT has always required an anatomic target. Originally, the target was defined by means of physical examination, plain radiographs, surgical findings (metallic clips placed during surgery), and analysis of patterns of disease spread demonstrated in surgical and through autopsy series.

Daily target localization on the treatment machine (image-guided RT—IGRT), either by localizing implanted radio-opaque markers (fiducials) or by imaging with an onboard CT scanner, called cone beam CT, has greatly improved the accuracy of treatment delivery, because the prostate actually moves a bit in a living patient, largely as bowel and bladder variably fill and empty from day to day.

Cone beam CT has also enhanced the accuracy of treatment of lung tumors, permitting greater sparing of normal lung tissue, which is important as most lung cancer patients also have chronic obstructive pulmonary disease to one extent or another.

4.3.1 Computer Science

The great recent advances in radiotherapy (3D conformal RT, intensity-modulated RT—IMRT, IGRT) would not have been possible without the explosion in computer technology. Today, treatment planning is done almost entirely by computer. Computers also control the actual treatment delivery, including the positioning and motion of the leaves that shape and texture the treatment beams. Multi-leaf collimators have replaced lead blocks for beam shaping and can move during the actual treatment (IMRT). IMRT delivers precise dose into the body, permitting tight control of dose distribution within the body by shaping dose around critical structures and the tumor. This technology enables even greater dose conformity and treatment of tiny volumes. This precision allows for safe delivery of much higher doses than possible with traditional treatment planning and delivery techniques.

4.3.2 Medical Physics

The physics of ionizing radiation is paramount in RT. X-rays, heavy particles (such as protons), and electrons are beams produced by machines; gamma rays are the product of radioactive decay.

Remember, from physics, that the density of any radiation (visible light, ultraviolet light, ionizing radiation, etc.) falls off with the square of the distance. This fundamental property is referred to as the inverse square law. Diagnostic radiography typically uses low-energy (kilovoltage) X-rays. Diagnostic energy X-rays (kilovoltage) can treat superficial tumors, but the deposition pattern delivers full dose to the skin and increases acute skin reaction, and preferential absorption of these low-energy beams in bone increases the risk of late bone damage. In addition, the dose delivered by these beams decreases (falls off) rapidly as depth in tissue increases. Today, electrons are more commonly used, because the dose delivered decreases rapidly with increasing depth in tissue, to the point of almost no dose deep in the body. Treatment of deep-seated tumors requires high-energy beams (megavoltage) that have greater penetrating power, so dose delivered at depth falls off more slowly than with kilovoltage radiation. Both the amount of skin sparing and the depth of penetration depend on the energy of the megavoltage beam. Megavoltage X-rays have this greater penetration, are not preferentially absorbed in the bone, and do not deliver full dose to the skin. This skin-sparing effect is due to buildup of the free radicals generated as the beam penetrates into tissues.

The use of multiple megavoltage fields permits protection of overlying tissue. Before IMRT, this was commonly used for the treatment of prostate cancer. These techniques may still be seen in old patient records or in emerging countries, where contemporary technology is not yet available. When patients who have received radiation treatment in the past are seen, it is important to be aware of how they were treated. The ultimate use of many fields is arc therapy, using, in essence, up to 360 fields, where the treatment head rotates around the patient; before IMRT, this was the best tissue-sparing plan available.

Various heavy atomic particles have been used for RT as well; the only one in much use today is the proton. At great cost, proton beams provide great precision of conformal dose delivery, which is felt to be important in treating tumors close to critical structures such as the brainstem and perhaps in children. Brachytherapy (the temporary or permanent implantation of tumors or body cavities with radioactive sources) is a method of focusing high doses of radiation into tumor while reducing dose to surrounding tissues. Dose distribution depends on precise positioning of the radioactive sources and the physical characteristics of the individual isotope disintegration products. Dose rate depends on the initial radioactivity strength of the source and the half-life of the particular isotope.

Precise target definition and patient immobilization are critical. Individually designed restraints are used to assure patient positioning.

Stereotactic treatments (SRS, SRT, SBRT) rely on several technologies:

- Three-dimensional imaging that determines the exact coordinates of the target within the body.
- Systems to immobilize and carefully position the patient.
- Highly focused gamma ray or X-ray beams that converge on a tumor or abnormality.

- Image guidance on the treatment table SRS is usually used for treating small lesions. Both SRS and SRT were originally used to treat brain lesions because the skull is easily immobilized. These treatments have been useful for the treatment of some noncancerous conditions, including intracranial arteriovenous malformations (AVMs) and trigeminal neuralgia.

More recently, stereotactic technology has been applied to treat extracranial lesions, such as the liver and lung; this is called stereotactic body radiotherapy (SBRT). Extracranial lesions are harder to immobilize, as organs move with respiration; 4D planning is necessary where respiratory motion is expected, as in the lung and liver. SRS and SBRT have become much more common in the last few years. SRS replaces whole brain radiotherapy for many cases with limited (one to four lesions) brain metastases. SBRT for small lung lesions without apparent nodal metastases (T1N0M0) appears to have comparable survival to surgical removal of these tumors, with local control in the range of 90%. It is now being used routinely in medically inoperable patients or those who refuse thoracotomy. It has been studied against lobectomy, with comparable results in small studies. Additional studies are ongoing. SBRT is also proving to be useful for treatment of liver tumors, whether primary or metastatic.

The biology of SRS and SBRT is not well understood yet. It is clear that these treatments are ablative—they are designed to entirely kill the volume treated, so treatment of adjacent normal tissue must be minimized, and the new technologies that making these treatments possible. In addition to direct cell kill, vascular damage and immune effects are believed to contribute to the efficacy of SRS and SRT. The biology of ablative therapies is an active area of research in radiobiology.

4.4 Goals of Radical Treatments

Radical RT seeks to permanently control primary tumors (often, with the draining lymph nodes) while limiting toxicity to acceptable levels. If the tumor has not already spread, eradication of the primary (and regional nodes) will cure the patient. RT has the capacity to achieve control while preserving the affected organ, thereby enhancing long-term quality of life.

For example, for mediastinal tumors, reported radiation doses have ranged from 30 to 60 Gy given in 1.8 or 2.0 Gy per fraction daily. The recommended postoperative radiation dose after gross total resection for malignant thymoma is 45–50 Gy in 1.8–2.0 Gy daily fractions. For microscopically positive resection margins and grossly positive margins, higher radiation doses of 54 Gy and 60 Gy, respectively, administered in 1.8–2.0 Gy of daily dose fractions are appropriate. Although one retrospective study did not find any relationship between radiation dose and local control, others have noted that radiation dose was a significant prognostic factor for local control. It is difficult to prove a consistent improvement in local tumor control with higher doses in part due to the rarity of this tumor and prospective clinical trials. However, excellent local tumor control has been reported with doses higher than

40 Gy, and increased local recurrences have been reported with doses lower than 40 Gy. When resection is impossible, doses of 60 Gy or more to gross disease may be required for adequate tumor control but not without higher associated risks of complications such as pericarditis or radiation myelitis. Dose to the spinal cord should be limited to 45 Gy using oblique mediastinal fields. Treatment fields and dose fractionation should be carefully planned and arranged to minimize complications such as pulmonary fibrosis, pericarditis, and myelitis. The typical volume treated should include the entire thymus or tumor bed, mediastinum, and part of the involved adjacent lung if there is parenchymal involvement or as delineated by CT scan or surgical clips, plus a margin of at least 2 cm to account for daily variability during treatment and allow coverage of areas of possible microscopic disease. In general, inclusion of the noninvolved supraclavicular fossa is unnecessary and has not shown consistent therapeutic benefits. Treatment portals may include single anterior field, opposed anterior-posterior fields with differential weighting (1:1, 2:1, or 3:1), wedge pair, and multi-field arrangements. Modern CT simulation with customized treatment planning can yield optimized isodose distribution and avoid geographic misses. Conformal therapy with three-dimensional treatment (3D-CRT) planning may further minimize dose heterogeneity and radiation toxicity to adjacent noninvolved structures while allowing higher doses to be delivered to the tumor.

4.5 Goals of Palliative Treatments

Palliative RT seeks to relieve specific symptoms (such as pain or bleeding) while minimizing patient inconvenience and side effects. It is an effective modality for reducing or eliminating many tumor-associated symptoms requiring relief and is often the most effective, least invasive, and least expensive option. Unfortunately, it has been estimated that half of patients in the United States who might benefit from palliative RT have not been referred to a radiation oncologist. Treatment should relieve the targeted symptom for a significant length of time, often for the remainder of a patient's life, while causing few, if any, side effects. The treatment should be planned to minimize patient imposition and cost (the latter is usually born by society through health insurance). Radiation oncologists must balance efficacy against cost, through the judicious use of fractionation and choice of technique. The use of prolonged therapy is typically unwarranted, as symptom relief requires a lower radiation dose than is necessary for tumor eradication. However, acute normal tissue tolerances must be accounted for; a high daily dose to bowel may cause significant gastrointestinal symptoms, impacting quality of life. The mechanism of palliative radiation is incompletely understood; it is more likely secondary to alteration of humoral factors (perhaps an anti-inflammatory effect) rather than tumor shrinkage, as a patient may enjoy dramatic pain relief without any change in tumor volume. In most cases, the likelihood of response is not dependent on tumor histology (although there are exceptions). On the other hand, maximal pain relief may take 6–8 weeks for some bone metastases. This seems to be due to bone healing after tumor cell death. Partial or complete pain relief can be expected in at least 60% of patients;

reduction or elimination of tumor bleeding occurs in 90%. Certain tumors (e.g., lymphoma) are so radiosensitive that lower doses of radiation can be utilized. Most commonly, radiotherapy is used for palliation of pain; the second most common palliative use is to relieve the symptoms of brain metastases and other neurologic signs and symptoms. It is also useful for relief of tumor bleeding, obstruction (except the biliary tree), and respiratory compromise due to airway obstruction or post-obstructive pneumonia. Disfiguring lesions of Kaposi's sarcoma reliably respond to palliative RT. The efficacy of RT in palliating painful, draining chest wall recurrences of breast cancer was recognized more than a century ago. It is a myth that radiotherapy cannot be repeated. Many patients will require treatment of multiple sites over the terminal portion of their illness, which sometimes can last for several years, particularly for bone metastases, and retreatment of the same site is often possible. The brain will only perceive pain from one to three sites at a time. So it is not uncommon for patients to achieve good pain palliation from a course of radiotherapy and shortly thereafter requiring treatment to another site or sites, sometimes many times over the course of illness.

To summarize this section, radiotherapy is a powerful tool for palliation and can improve the quality of even a short life. Retreatment is often possible, especially in patients for whom late effects are less of a concern.

4.6 Conclusion

Radiation oncology is the medical specialty concerned with the prescription and delivery of RT, one of the three main modalities for treating cancer. Computer technology has revolutionized the field over the past decade, and the physicians who manage cancer patients must keep abreast with the changes so that their patients are not deprived of these advances. Although acute or long-term adverse effects may be a consequence, it is important to balance these risks against the risks of surgery or chemotherapy especially when the goal of the treatment is the best outcome for the patient.

Bibliography

1. Pieters RS, Ding L, Bushe H, Aronowitz J. Principles of radiation oncology. In: Pieters RS, Liebmann J, editors. Cancer concepts: a guidebook for the non-oncologist. 2nd ed. Worcester, MA: University of Massachusetts Medical School; 2017. https://doi.org/10.7191/cancer_concepts.1008.

the demand for labor [illegible]
ambitions for development.

5 Oral Mucositis

Ragda Abdalla-Aslan, Hannah Wardill, and Sharon Elad

5.1 Introduction

Oral mucositis (OM) is defined on MeSH as an inflammation of the mucosa with burning or tingling sensation, characterized by atrophy of the squamous epithelium, vascular damage, inflammatory infiltration, and ulceration. Mucositis generally occurs at the mucous lining of the mouth, the gastrointestinal tract, or the airways due to chemical irritations, chemotherapy (CT), or radiation therapy (RT). Actually, this is relevant to any anticancer therapy including combination of chemoradiotherapy (C-RT) and hematopoietic stem cell transplantation (HSCT) [1].

In accordance with the above definition, the profile of OM extended when the targeted therapies were introduced and soon after the associated oral adverse effects were reported. Targeted therapies include antitumor monoclonal antibodies, small molecules, signal transduction receptor inhibitors, and cancer vaccines [2–7].

R. Abdalla-Aslan
Department of Oral and Maxillofacial Surgery, Rambam Health Care Campus, Haifa, Israel

Department of Oral Medicine, Sedation and Maxillofacial Imaging, Hebrew University-Hadassah School of Dental Medicine, Jerusalem, Israel

H. Wardill
Department of Paediatric Oncology/Haematology, University Medical Centre Groningen The University of Groningen, Groningen, The Netherlands

School of Biomedicine, The Faculty of Health and Medical Sciences , The University of Adelaide, Adelaide, Australia

Precision Medicine (Cancer) The South Australian Health and Medical Research Institute, Adelaide, Australia
e-mail: hannah.wardill@adelaide.edu.au

S. Elad (✉)
Division of Oral Medicine, Eastman Institute for Oral Health, University of Rochester Medical Center, Rochester, NY, USA
e-mail: selad@urmc.rochester.edu

R. Nair (ed.), *Orofacial Supportive Care in Cancer*,
https://doi.org/10.1007/978-3-030-86510-8_5

Targeted therapies may be continuously administered for their long-term ability to inhibit tumor growth, progression, cell proliferation, and angiogenesis, and, as such, even mild adverse toxicity is considered burdensome [8]. If targeted therapies are combined with conventional cancer therapies, previously identified toxicities may be increased in severity or duration [9, 10].

The utmost importance of OM stems from the severity of its associated symptoms. In regard to the significance of OM to the patient, 42% of patients undergoing HSCT identified OM as the most significant transplant-related toxicity [11]. In this study, the second most stressful toxicity was nausea and vomiting, described by 13% of the patients [11]. The difference between the proportion of patients affected by OM and the proportion of patients affected by the nausea and vomiting demonstrated the devastating effect of OM on the patients. In another study, OM was described as the most debilitating toxicity by 65% of patients receiving TBI-based regimens, and 84% of the patients reported OM as more severe than expected [12]. This reflects not only the impact of OM on the ability to perform daily tasks but also the risk of systemic consequences such as infection. This is further complicated by its impact on the delivery of anticancer therapy with OM being a significant driver of dose reductions and complete treatment cessation. As such, OM is translated to significant health-care costs due to the overreliance on supportive care measures and hospitalization. Therefore, there is a surge of research in attempt to identify prevention or treatment for OM [13].

This chapter will present a review about the epidemiology, clinical presentation, consequences, pathogenesis, and management approach of OM.

5.2 Epidemiology

The prevalence of OM varies greatly between cancer subpopulations. Generally, the more toxic the anticancer protocol, the higher the risk for OM. The factors that influence the prevalence of OM include both treatment-related variables and patient-related risk factors.

Treatment variables that may affect the prevalence and the severity of OM include the type, dose, and schedule of systemic cytotoxic medications, radiation dose and field, and concomitant use of CT and radiation [14–17].

5.2.1 Radiotherapy for Head and Neck Cancers (HNCs)

The vast majority of patients treated with RT for HNCs develop severe OM [18, 19]. In HNC patients treated with RT or C-RT to the head and neck (H&N), the incidence of OM ranged from 59.4% [20] to 100% [21–26]. In patients receiving altered fractionation RT or high-dose RT, the incidence of grade 3 or 4 OM is 65–85%, and in patients receiving conventional RT, the incidence of grade 3 or 4 OM is 34% [27, 28]. Special radiation techniques may reduce the severity of OM. Several studies reported that grade 4 OM did not develop following volume-modulated arc therapy

(VMAT) [22], proton beam radiation therapy (PBRT) [20], and intensity-modulated radiotherapy (IMRT) [24].

5.2.2 Chemotherapy

OM affects on average 20–40% of patients receiving conventional-dose cytotoxic CT [14, 29–32]. Overall OM frequency for all grades is reported to be between 14.4% and 81.3% depending on the type of tumor and treatment, with most of them being mild OM (grades 1–2), while severe OM (grades 3–4) is generally less than 5% of cases [33–36]. In a study of patients with advanced cancer, the overall prevalence of OM was 22.3% [37]. Data on OM incidence by type of malignancy are limited. One study evaluating OM secondary to conventional chemotherapy as a single modality reported breast cancer to be most associated with OM (76.5% of cases), followed by HNC (67.7%), colorectal cancer (CRC) (63%), and esophageal cancer (57.8%) [33]. Although less frequently described, the risk of severe OM (≥grade 3) has been reported in prostate cancer (14%) and breast cancer patients (0.98–8%) [31, 33].

The incidence of OM depends also on the specific regimen. When using TAC protocol (docetaxel, adriamycin, and cyclophosphamide) for breast cancer, incidence of low-grade OM was 60% with 5% severe OM [38]. When using dose-dense therapy, in which the interval between successive CT cycles is reduced to minimize the likelihood of tumor regrowth and neoangiogenesis between cycles, incidence of grade 1–2 OM reported to be ranged from 15% in patients who received weekly paclitaxel to as high as 59% dose-dense AC → T (adriamycin-cyclophosphamide with sequential taxane). Severe OM reached 14% among those who were treated with weekly AC [38].

For commonly used platinum/gemcitabine in lung cancer, incidence of grade 1–2 OM was 14%, with 1% grade 3 or higher [38].

In various protocols for CRC, the risk of grade 1–2 OM averages 14% with various regimens including FOLFOX (leucovorin, fluorouracil [5-FU], and oxaliplatin), FOLFIRI (leucovorin, 5FU, and irinotecan), and IROX (irinotecan and oxaliplatin). The risk is higher with FOLFIRI (35%). Grade 3–4 OM is low with incidence of 1.35–4.43% [38].

The toxicity of each drug depends on its dosage and the exposure duration, as well as its intrinsic properties [30, 31] and mode of administration (bolus versus continuous infusion) [39]. Many cytotoxic agents have been reported to produce OM [40]; however, few studies have specifically analyzed incidence and severity of the toxicity in relation to these regimens. It is generally accepted that antimetabolites and alkylating agents are associated with a high OM incidence and worse OM severity, although these views have been largely based on anecdotal reports [40–43]. Furthermore, published data on toxicity of various regimens are sometimes inconsistent [43–46].

Chemotherapeutic agents that are DNA cycle-specific (e.g., bleomycin, 5-FU, and methotrexate) are apparently more stomatotoxic than agents that are cell phase

Table 5.1 Cytotoxic agents which incur mucotoxic effect [15, 32]

Category	Cytotoxic agents
Antimetabolites	Methotrexate, 5-fluorouracil, hydroxyurea, cytosine arabinoside
Topoisomerase II inhibitors	Etoposide, irinotecan
Pyrimidine analogs	Cytarabine
Purine analogs	6-Mercaptopurine, 6-thioguanine
Alkylating agents at high doses	Busulfan, melphalan, cyclophosphamide
Intercalating drugs	Idarubicin, doxorubicin, daunorubicin
Antibiotics	Bleomycin, mitomycin
Taxanes	Docetaxel, paclitaxel
Vinca alkaloids	Vinblastine, vincristine

nonspecific [47]. Certain drugs (e.g., etoposide) may be secreted into the saliva, further increasing the potential for stomatotoxicity [48, 49].

The most recognized mucotoxic agents are listed in Table 5.1 [15, 32]. The literature indicates that treatment regimens containing 5-FU and adriamycin-cyclophosphamide pose high risk for OM [33]. Specifically, 5-FU has been reported to cause grade 3–4 OM with incidence of more than 15% [31].

In selected regimens for solid tumors, the prevalence of OM is reported to be less than 10% [50]. This low prevalence of OM in patients treated for solid tumors is attributed in part to underreporting for various reasons: monitoring protocols in outpatients that is less intensive, low- and moderate-level OM that may not require palliative treatment, and patient's and clinician's preference to avoid cancer treatment interruption [1].

Of note, when CT is administered in multiple cycles, the risk of OM increases at each course owing to residual changes in the biological structure of the oral mucosa (e.g., angiogenesis) [31, 33, 51].

OM was found in 90% of all patients diagnosed with acute leukemia who were treated with induction CT, with grades 3–4 in 20%, and in 12.5% for consolidation CT with 0% grades 3–4 [52]. Patients with acute myeloid leukemia (AML) treated with standard anthracycline-based regimens develop profound myelosuppression and OM (10–15% of cases) [53]. In this setting, liposomal daunorubicin seems to reduce the incidence of mucositis [54], while more aggressive protocols were associated with a higher incidence. The FLAG (fludarabine, cytarabine, G-CSF) protocol induces mucosal damage in 50% of patients [55], a rate that rose to 70% in patients treated with idarubicin-containing FLAG [56]. In patients with acute promyelocytic leukemia treated with trans-retinoic acid (ATRA) and idarubicin, the incidence of OM is about 10% [57, 58].

In non-Hodgkin's lymphoma (NHL), OM was reported in 2–11% for various CT protocols [15, 59, 60]. Other studies in NHL patients reported a higher incidence of 22.2% [52] and up to 42.9% [33]. Grade 3–4 OM in NHL patients is reported to range from 0 [33, 52] up to 6.6% [38].

As for various protocols in NHL patients, grade 3–4 OM has been reported in 4–5% of CHOP-treated patients (cyclophosphamide, doxorubicin, vincristine, and prednisone) [38, 61]. The addition of rituximab (R-CHOP) does not appear to modify the risk for OM [31]. Dose intensification of the CHOP regimen, achieved by increasing the cyclophosphamide dose, results in a slight increase in the risk (7.9%) [38]. The addition of etoposide to CHOP, however, more than doubles the risk for grade 3–4 OM in a similar patient population (10.4%). Other protocols CEOP/IMVP-Dexa (cyclophosphamide, epirubicin, vincristine, prednisone, ifosfamide, methotrexate, etoposide, dexamethasone) produce similar rates of grade 3–4 OM to those reported with CHOP (4.17%) [38].

The differences in incidence of OM between acute leukemia and NHL patients may be related to the underlying degree of immunosuppression. The first induction of CT is aggressive, aiming to eradicate malignant clones. Furthermore, in most studies, NHL patients were admitted for a short stay at the hospital with limited follow-up during the ambulatory period [33, 52].

In regard to Hodgkin's lymphoma, OM incidence was reported to be 3% in patients who received the ABVD protocol (doxorubicin, bleomycin, vinblastine, and dacarbazine) and 8% in patients treated with hybrid multidrug regimens [62].

5.2.3 Hematopoietic Stem Cell Transplantation (HSCT)

OM is undoubtedly one of the most debilitating toxicities of hematopoietic stem cell transplantation and reported in up to 99% of patients undergoing HSCT, 67.4% of which are grade 3 or 4 [11, 46, 63–65]. This was consistently reported in other studies in HSCT patients with all OM grades being 70–86.8% [66–68]. OM grade 3 was reported to be 12.9% and 30.5% [67, 68], and OM grade 4 is reported to be 8.2% and 13.7% [67, 68].

Factors associated with the development of OM during HSCT are summarized in Table 5.2 [12, 31, 46, 69–77]. Multivariate analysis showed that the conditioning regimen is the most significant determinant of OM [15, 71]. Regimens containing

Table 5.2 Factors associated with the development of OM during HSCT [12, 31, 46, 69–77, 299]

Class	Factor
Conditioning regimen administered	CT type and dose and use of TBI
Hematopoietic progenitor source	PBPC leads to higher OM incidence compared to allo-BMT, which leads to higher OM incidence compared with auto-BMT
Previous exposure to drugs	Methotrexate for prophylaxis of GVHD, as well as other drugs such as anthracyclines, vinca alkaloids, cyclophosphamide, fludarabine, platinum analogs, and etoposide in the mobilizing regimen
Gender	Female
Type of disease	Leukemia (compared to various indications for allo-BMT and auto-BMT) NHL (compared to MM and HD undergoing auto-BMT)

CT chemotherapy, *TBI* total body irradiation, *PBPC* peripheral blood progenitor cells, *allo-BMT* allogeneic bone marrow transplant, *auto-BMT* autologous bone marrow transplant, *GVHD* graft versus host disease, *MM* multiple myeloma, *HD* Hodgkin's disease, *NHL* non-Hodgkin's lymphoma busulfan or melphalan or total body irradiation (TBI) were associated with the worst OM [15, 71].

The type of HSCT may also be related to severity of OM. While some studies reported an increased severity of OM in allo-BMT compared to auto-BMT patients, others found no differences in OM severity and duration [43, 45, 46]. Incidence of OM in auto-BMT was reported to be 40–86.8%, with 9.6–44.2% grade 3 or 4 OM [67, 78–80]. In contrary, in allo-BMT, OM incidence was 70.4–95.7% for all-grade OM and 20–51.3% for grade 3 or 4 OM [81–84].

In reduced intensity conditioning (RIC) protocols, the treatment rationale is largely based on triggering an immunity-mediated graft-versus-malignancy effect rather than by the cytotoxic treatment itself [85]. Accordingly, OM incidence in myeloablative conditioning is higher than in RIC. Specifically, the OM incidence in myeloablative conditioning is reported to be 83.4%–88.2% with 33.4–78.4% grade 3–4 OM [81, 82, 86, 87]. In contrast, the OM incidence in RIC is 56.3–75.7% for all OM grades and 4–32.9% for grade 3–4 OM [81, 82, 86–88].

Interestingly, a systematic review found that RIC regimens led to a high incidence of OM similar to that of myeloablative regimens [66]—86.5% vs. 73.2% for all grades of OM and 57.4% vs. 63.2% for grade 3 or 4, respectively. Moreover, it was found that there is an increased risk of developing grade 3 and 4 OM over grade 1 and 2 OM in the RIC group. Of note, none of the included studies reported whether radiation therapy was included in the conditioning regimen, and only some studies included information regarding previous cycles of CT or HSCT. Therefore, these results should be interpreted with caution due to possible residual confounding factors [66].

5.2.4 Targeted Therapy

The epidemiology of mucositis or stomatitis due to targeted therapy is summarized in Table 5.3. The oral complications associated with these new classes of anticancer agents are distinctly different compared to those induced by traditional cytotoxic agents. Despite this, they are largely referred to as OM.

Epidermal growth factor receptor inhibitors (EGFRI) have been investigated in the treatment of epithelial cancers including breast, colorectal, oropharyngeal, non-small cell lung cancer, and renal cell carcinoma (RCC) [89–94], with oral complications remaining poorly characterized.

Cetuximab is a recombinant human/murine mAbs directed toward EGFR and is FDA approved for treatment of head and neck squamous cell carcinoma (HNSCC) and CRC [95, 96].

In a trial of metastatic CRC (mCRC) comparing irinotecan plus cetuximab to cetuximab alone, fewer patients experienced grade 3 or 4 stomatitis in the cetuximab alone group (0.9%) versus cetuximab plus irinotecan (2.4%, nonsignificant difference, $p = 0.67$) [97].

In recurrent or metastatic HNSCC, cetuximab may be used alone or in combination with RT [98]. Concurrent administration of cetuximab and RT makes the

Table 5.3 Targeted therapy-induced oral mucositis/stomatitis

Mode of action	Agent	Brand name	FDA-approved indications	OM/stomatitis-related clinical signs and symptoms	
EGFRI	Cetuximab	Erbitux	HNSCC and CRC	Stomatitis	0.9% grades 3–4 [97]
				Mucositis, HNCSCC	93% (Cetuximab with RT) 56% grades 3–5 94% (RT alone) 52% grades 3–5 [8]
				Mucositis, various indications	52.7% all-grade RT plus EGFR [99]
				Mucositis, concurrent RT HNC	23% <grade 2 77% grade 3 [100]
	Panitumumab	Vectibix	Wild-type RAS mCRC	Stomatitis	7–23% [113–115]
	Erlotinib	Tarceva	mNSCLC Metastatic pancreatic cancer Malignant gliomas	Stomatitis	19% vs. 3% placebo 1% >grade 3 [119]
	Afatinib	Gilotrif	mNSCLC	Stomatitis	72% all-grade, 9% ≥grade 3 [122]
mTORI	Everolimus	Afinitor, Zortress	Advanced RCC after failure with sunitinib or sorafenib Hormone receptor-positive, HER2-negative breast cancer Progressive NET in pancreas and nonfunctional NET of GI or lung TSC: renal angiomyolipomas and subependymal giant cell astrocytoma Kidney and liver transplant rejection	Stomatitis	40–44% vs. 8% in placebo 3–5% grade 3 [103, 125–127]
				Mucosal inflammation	14% grade 2 vs. 2% in placebo 1% grade 3 [103]
	Sirolimus	Rapamune	Kidney transplant rejection Lymphangioleiomyomatosis	Stomatitis	71% ≥grade 2 4% grade 3 [130]
	Temsirolimus	Torisel	Advanced RCC	Various	19–41% stomatitis/mucositis 1–3% grades 3–4 4% aphthous stomatitis, 3% ulcers [132, 133]
	Deforolimus	None	Has not been approved to date	Ulcerations • Include oral pain, mucosal inflammation, and stomatitis	63% grades 1–2 16% grades 3–4 [134]

(continued)

Table 5.3 (continued)

Mode of action	Agent	Brand name	FDA-approved indications	OM/stomatitis-related clinical signs and symptoms	
TKI, MKI and others	Imatinib mesylate TKI of abl-bcr fusion gene, PDGF-R, and c-kit kinases	Gleevec/ Glivec	Philadelphia chromosome positive ALL and CML Myelodysplastic/myeloproliferative diseases with specific PDGF-R gene rearrangements Hypereosinophilic syndrome and/or chronic eosinophilic leukemia Metastatic dermatofibrosarcoma protuberans Aggressive systemic mastocytosis Advanced malignant GIST	Various	10.6% stomatitis [138] 2.8% mouth ulcers 0.7% mucosal sensitivity [135]
	Sorafenib tosylate MKI of VEGF, PDGF, and TK	Nexavar	Advanced RCC Hepatocellular carcinoma Advanced thyroid cancer refractory to radioactive iodine treatment	Stomatitis/ mucositis	11–38% 2–9% ≥grade 2 [96, 142–147]
				Mucosal sensitivity	14.5% [135]
	Sunitinib malate TKI of VEGF and PDGF	Sutent	Advanced RCC GIST after failure with imatinib Advanced pancreatic NET	Stomatitis	17–38% grades 1–2 1–4% grade 3 [156–159]
				Mucosal sensitivity	23% [135]
				Ulcers	8.7% [135]
				Aphthous-like ulcers	33–43% [150]
	Bevacizumab Anti-VEGF mAbs	Avastin, Mvasi	mRCC (in combination with interferon alfa-2a) mCLC (in combination with 5-fluorouracil) Advanced mNSCLC Metastatic cervical cancer (with combination CT) Ovarian, fallopian tube, or peritoneal cancer (with combination CT) Recurrent glioblastoma	Various	5.7% ulcers 6.3% mucosal sensitivity [135]
	Pazopanib TKI of VEGF and PDGF	Votrient	Advanced RCC Advanced soft tissue sarcoma	Various	4.6% ulcers 10.6% mucosal sensitivity [135]
	Cabozantinib MKI of RET, MET, VEGFR-1, VEGFR-2, and VEGFR-3, KIT, TrkB, FLT-3, AXL, and TIE-2	Cometriq, Cabometyx	Advanced RCC Metastatic medullary thyroid cancer	Various	26.1% ulcers 34.8% mucosal sensitivity [135]
	Lapatinib TKI of EGFR and HER2	Tykerb	HER2-overexpressing metastatic breast cancer (in combination with capecitabine) Hormone-positive and HER2-positive advanced breast cancer (in combination therapy with letrozole)	Stomatitis	13% grade 1 [162, 163] 21% grade 2 [164]

EGFRI epidermal growth factor receptor inhibitor, *HNSCC* head and neck squamous cell carcinoma, *CRC* colorectal cancer, *RT* radiation therapy, *mNSCLC* metastatic non-small cell lung cancer, *mTORI* mammalian target of rapamycin inhibitor, *RCC* renal cell carcinoma, *NET* neuroendocrine tumor, *GI* gastrointestinal, *TSC* tuberous sclerosis complex, *PDGF-R* platelet-derived growth factor receptor, *GIST* gastrointestinal stromal tumor, *TKI* tyrosine kinase inhibitor, *MKI* multikinase inhibitor, *VEGF* vascular endothelial growth factor, *mAbs* monoclonal antibodies, *CT* chemotherapy etiology of oral side effects difficult to distinguish. A 2006 phase III trial involving 400 patients compared patients treated with RT alone and RT plus cetuximab. The reported grade 3 and above adverse events (AEs) did not differ significantly between these two groups [8].

However, a review and meta-analysis reported EGFRI plus RT to a have higher reported prevalence of mucositis compared to RT alone (1.76 risk ratio) [99]. A small study of 13 patients reported exacerbated toxicity with cetuximab in HNC with grade 3 OM in ten patients (77%), while the remaining three patients developed grade 2 OM [100]. Numerous studies about cetuximab do not describe the oral AEs which limits the understanding about the role of cetuximab in OM [101–109].

Panitumumab is a fully humanized IgG2 mAb EGFRI, approved for treatment of wild-type RAS mCRC (in both KRAS and NRAS) [110, 111]. Several studies reported stomatitis as "mild to moderate" [112] and to develop in 7–23% of patients [113–115].

Erlotinib is a small molecule tyrosine kinase inhibitor (TKI) of EGFR, approved for metastatic non-small cell lung cancer (NSCLC), locally advanced, unresectable, or metastatic pancreatic cancer, and malignant gliomas [116–120]. A study of previously treated NSCLC patients found 19% of patients experienced OM—compared to 3% in the placebo group, 1% had above grade 3 [119]. A meta-analysis reported an increased risk of all-grade OM (3.2 adjusted relative risk), with no significant risk for high-grade OM [121].

Afatinib blocks signaling from the EGFR (erbB1), EGFR2 (HER2/erbB2), and erbB4, which has been approved for mNSCLC with nonresistant EGFR mutations. Higher rates of stomatitis (72% all-grade, 9% grade 3 or worse) are reported with afatinib, compared to combination of cisplatin and pemetrexed [122].

mTOR inhibitors (mTORI) are drugs that inhibit the mammalian target of rapamycin and are used in the treatment of RCC and various other indications and demonstrate high level of efficacy with acceptable tolerability [123]. In a meta-analysis of randomized controlled clinical trials (RCTs) of patients receiving mTORI, the incidence of all-grade (grade 1–4) stomatitis was 33.5%, and the incidence of high-grade stomatitis (grade 3–4) was 4.1% [124]. The incidence of high-grade stomatitis significantly varied with tumor types (increased risk in breast cancer (RR: 11.18) and progressive neuroendocrine tumor (RR: 28.52)). In comparison with controls, mTORI significantly increased the risk for developing all-grade stomatitis (RR: 4.04) and high-grade stomatitis (RR: 8.84) [124].

The mTORI that were reported to cause oral mucosal injury include everolimus, sirolimus, temsirolimus, and deforolimus.

Stomatitis with **everolimus** was reported in 30–44% of patients vs. 8% in the placebo group, with 2.2–5% experiencing grade 3 reactions [103, 125–127]. Mucosal inflammation of grade 2 or less was reported in 14% of patients (vs. 2% in placebo), with 1% of patients reporting grade 3 events [103]. In a phase III RCT evaluating everolimus in patients with metastatic RCC, the incidence of stomatitis was approximately 39% with the majority of cases resolving within 3 days [128, 129]. Out of 277 patients, 13 required dose modification or interruption, 49 patients required supportive therapy, and everolimus was permanently discontinued in one patient [128, 129].

A phase I study of **sirolimus** as a major metabolite reported 71% with grade 2 and below stomatitis and only 4% with grade 3 mucositis. These oral ulcers were dose dependent and resolved despite continued drug therapy [130, 131].

Among patients on **temsirolimus**, 19–20% reported stomatitis/mucositis, with 1% grade 3 mucositis, 4% aphthous stomatitis, and 3% mouth ulceration [132]. Another study reported stomatitis/mucositis in 41% of patient, with 3% grade 3 mucositis [133]. Almost all mucositis-type AEs were low grade and manageable with supportive measures.

A phase I trial of **deforolimus**, currently investigated for use/treatment in solid tumors, sarcoma, cancer/tumors (unspecified), endometrial cancer, prostate cancer, and bone metastases, with 32 patients, reported mouth sores, including mouth pain, mucosal inflammation, and stomatitis in 79% of patients, with 16% grades 3–4. Ulcers were more frequent at high doses. Three dose-limiting toxicity events of grade 3 mouth sores were reported. The patients were treated symptomatically and usually achieved complete recovery. These reactions appear less frequent and severe at subsequent administration [134].

Stomatitis or OM is also reported due to multikinase inhibitors, including imatinib, sorafenib, sunitinib, bevacizumab, and lapatinib. Among patients treated with VEGFR-directed multi-targeted TKI, the most commonly reported oral AE was oral mucosal sensitivity or pain, occurring in 12% of patients [135]. Approximately one-quarter resulted in at least one dose alteration in part attributable to the oral AE. Among these alterations, 16.2% led to dose interruption, 11.0% led to dose modifications, and 6.3% resulted in drug discontinuation. The majority (65.9%) of dose alterations were associated with sunitinib or sorafenib [135].

Imatinib mesylate is a TKI that selectively targets the abl-bcr fusion gene, platelet-derived growth factor receptor (PDGF-R), and c-kit kinases [136, 137]. Stomatitis was reported in 10.6% of patients [138]. Mouth ulcers were reported in 2.8% and mucosal sensitivity in 0.7% [135].

Sorafenib tosylate is a multikinase which inhibits VEGF, PDGF, and TK. Stomatitis was reported in 11–38% of cases [96, 139–150], with 2–9% grade 2 or more [151–154]. Mucosal sensitivity was reported in 14.5% of cases [135]. In 7% and 18% of cases, dose was interrupted or reduced due to oral AEs, respectively [150, 155]. A meta-analysis reported an increased risk of all-grade OM (3.3 adjusted relative risk), with no significant risk for high-grade OM [121].

For **sunitinib malate**, grade 1 or 2 stomatitis has been reported in 17–38% and grade 3 stomatitis in 1–4% [150, 156–159]. Mucosal sensitivity was reported in 23% of cases [135]. Others report oral ulcers in 8.7% [135]. Aphthous-like ulcers are reported in 33–43% of cases [150]. In 9% and 26% of cases, dose was interrupted or reduced due to oral AEs, respectively [150]. For sunitinib, an increased risk for all-grade OM was reported in a meta-analysis (7.7 adjusted relative risk), with no increased risk for high-grade OM [121].

Bevacizumab is an anti-VEGF mAbs that inhibits angiogenesis used for various indications [160, 161]. Mucosal sensitivity was reported in 6.3% of cases [135], with ulcers reported in 5.7% [135]. A meta-analysis showed that bevacizumab led to an increased risk of all-grade OM (1.8 adjusted relative risk), but no significant difference was found for high-grade OM [121].

Stomatitis in patients treated with **lapatinib**, a TKI of EGFR and HER2, was reported to reach 13% grade 1 [162, 163] and 21% grade 2 [164].

5.3 Risk Factors

Patient-related variables that may influence the risk for OM include age, gender, body mass index, smoking, genetic factors, the tumor itself, oral environment related factors and comorbidities [14, 50]. Risk factors for OM are outlined in Table 5.4.

5.3.1 Age

Conflicting data exist regarding the effect of patient age on development of OM. One study reported younger age as a risk factor for overall oral complications, without referring specifically to OM [165]. A prospective cohort study in 63 patients reported a trend for increased prevalence and severity of OM in older patients [166]. Likewise, a phase III study in 439 patients treated with 5-FU identified a significant correlation of moderate and severe OM with advancing age [167]. A small study of 50 patients receiving high-dose antineoplastic therapy found that increasing age was a risk factor for developing OM [168]. Possible interpretation of these results could be that in the very young age, there is increased cell turnover rate, and in the old age there is decreased rate of healing [169, 170].

Table 5.4 Risk factors for OM

Age	Trends for increased risk in older age
Gender	Trends for increased risk in females
Body Mass Index	Lower BMI
Smoking	Mixed reports
Genetic factors	MTHFR polymorphism TSMT polymorphism TNF-alpha polymorphism DPYD polymorphism GST polymorphism
Oral environment	Poor oral hygiene Hyposalivation
Comorbidities	Addison's disease increases risk Poor renal function increases risk Psoriasis lowers risk

BMI body mass index, *MTHFR* methylenetetrahydrofolate reductase, *TSMT* thiopurine *S*-methyltransferase, *TNF* tumor necrosis factor, *DPYD* dihydropyrimidine dehydrogenase, *GST* glutathione *S*-transferase

5.3.2 Gender

There are inconsistent reports on gender as a risk factor for OM. A study reporting 1074 patients treated with 5-FU for colorectal carcinoma found that female gender confers increased toxicity in terms of number of different types of toxicity experienced, average maximum toxicity grade, and incidence of severe toxicities. Females had 1.59 OR for developing OM, 1.8 OR for hematologic toxicities, and 1.92 OR for GI toxicities [171]. Other clinical trials also found that female patients have approximately a 2–2.37-fold higher risk for severe FU-related OM as compared with male patients, after adjusting for dose, body mass index, and age [39, 167, 172]. Other studies found no gender-related difference [77, 166].

5.3.3 BMI

Some studies have reported low body mass to be associated with an increased risk of OM [34, 173, 174]. It is postulated that poorly nourished individuals are more likely to experience increased breakdown and delayed healing [169]. However, another study reported no association of OM with patients' body surface area [166, 175].

5.3.4 Smoking

Smoking was reported to be associated with an increased risk of OM in radiation-induced OM for HNC patients [174, 176] and in CT for solid tumors [36]. Smoking affects microcirculation and can potentially delay healing. Conversely, nonsmokers were found to have a 2.70-fold increase in risk for severe OM, in oropharyngeal SCC patients undergoing concurrent CT and RT [26]. Another study showed a protective effect of smoking in patients undergoing HSCT [177]. Some evidence shows that smoking was associated with reduced pain due to OM, presumably due to loss of nociceptive receptors [36]. Other studies found no association between smoking and risk for OM [166, 178].

5.3.5 Genetic Factors

It becomes clear that genetic factors play a role in toxicity risk [19]. Differences in drug metabolism, absorption, distribution, and excretion, due to the genetic variants of several families of enzymes, seem to have pronounced effects [179].

Genetic determinants of OM risk include genes that regulate the availability of active CT drug metabolites. It seems that enzyme deficiencies may be relatively rare, and rather polymorphism and differences in the expression of genes associated with biological pathways that drive OM are more common.

For example, evaluation of genetic variation in folate-metabolizing enzymes may help to identify patients at greater risk for methotrexate toxicity [178]. The administration of methotrexate, a highly mucotoxic agent, was associated with different rates of OM in patients undergoing allo-BMT according to patient's genotype of a polymorphism in the 5,10-methylenetetrahydrofolate reductase (MTHFR) gene; patients with the *MTHFR* TT genotype have lower MTHFR activity and were noted to have more severe OM than patients with wild-type enzymes [180].

Moreover, genetic polymorphisms for thiopurine *S*-methyltransferase (TSMT) are a major factor responsible for large individual variations in both the toxicity and therapeutic effect of thiopurine [181].

Similar findings of genetic polymorphisms associated with the expression of inflammatory mediators such as TNF-alpha have been implicated in severe toxicities in patients undergoing allo-BMT [182]. Curiously, TNF-alpha polymorphism influenced significantly toxicity risk more than aggressive conditioning regimens (17.2 vs. 6.9 OR) [182].

A clinical trial that included 683 patients with cancer, treated with 5-FU monotherapy, showed patients with the dihydropyrimidine dehydrogenase (DPYD) polymorphism had a 5.8 fold higher risk of OM [39]. It is unclear if this study included OM exclusively or combined OM and gastrointestinal mucositis.

Glutathione *S*-transferase (GST) protects against oxidative stress, a key component in the initiation of OM. In a study of 699 patients undergoing BMT, a deletion polymorphism in one or two GST genes (GSTM1 and GSTT1) was significantly associated with increased occurrence of overall toxicity (71% versus 56%) and OM (74% versus 55%).

5.3.6 The Tumor

The site and stage of HNC determine the radiation plan and the addition of chemotherapy, which influence on the risk for OM [184]. Several studies aimed at the role of the tumor itself on the response to RT and CT. Additionally, the tumor itself is biologically active and might contribute to OM risk [185, 186]. Both tumor parenchyma and stroma are sources of molecules (peptides, MMPs), which influence cell behavior, and could directly modify normal cell response and enhance the breakdown of the local tissue environment [51]. Studies about the interaction between the tumor and the host are warranted.

5.3.7 Oral Environment

The oral cavity is a complex environment, which includes a wide range of microbiota comprised of bacteria, fungi, and viruses and saliva on all its components. Many studies have shown that local environmental factors might influence the course of OM but are not considered as the primary etiology of OM [50, 51].

The oral microflora has been conceptually linked to severity of OM for many years. As a result, several studies have addressed oral decontamination as a prophylactic or therapeutic intervention for OM; however, these studies presented conflicting results [187–194].

It is recognized that mucosal injury precedes increase in bacterial load [51]. During OM ulceration phase, there is an increase in gram-negative organisms, indicating that an increase in bacterial load is insufficient to hold the healing phase. Moreover, reestablishment of normal bacterial flora seems to be necessary for spontaneous ulcer resolution, irrespective of bacterial numbers [195]. The ulcerated mucosa represents a desirable colonization site, possibly contributing to increased severity and delayed healing at highly corroded areas. Thus, the oral microflora is currently considered to play a secondary role in the pathogenesis of OM.

This is also the case for other oral microorganisms, with purely correlative findings linking certain infections and OM. For example, candidiasis is a common finding in patients receiving H&N RT or myeloablative CT; however, candida has not been substantiated as a risk factor for OM and is therefore considered a coinciding condition rather than causal. Correspondingly, antifungals as interventions for RT-associated OM in HNC patients have not been effective in preventing OM [196].

Similarly, the role of HSV in OM remains unclear, despite increasing evidence of higher HSV rates in OM. For example, HSV was found in higher rates among cancer patients treated with CT who developed clinically evident mucositis, compared to patients who did not develop clinical lesions [197]. Other studies showed that OM development was unrelated to HSV antibody status or positive viral cultures, that acyclovir prophylaxis was ineffective in preventing OM, and that there was no relationship between the rate of viral reactivation and the presence or absence of OM [198, 199]. Furthermore, poor overall predictive value (both positive and negative) was reported for surveillance cultures of the oral microflora, and it was concluded that their significant expense does not support their routine use [200].

Regarding salivary flow, xerostomia was reported to be one of the two best predictors for development of OM in 5-FU-treated patients [166]; however, therapeutic approaches directed at stimulating salivary flow have not been successful. Pilocarpine was ineffective in modifying the incidence or course of OM in HNC patients and HSCT patients [201, 202]. Moreover, two studies reported that propantheline, an anticholinergic drug, protected patients from etoposide-induced OM [48, 49]. The authors indicated that propantheline may have protected oral mucosa from salivary-excreted etoposide and thus reduced prevalence of OM.

5.3.8 Comorbidities

Preexisting conditions may also impact OM risk and disease course. In a study of patients receiving induction therapy for leukemia, OM risk was compared among individuals who had precancer diagnoses of psoriasis and Addison's disease [51]. The authors found that psoriasis patients had a significantly lower risk of OM and Addison's disease patients had significantly higher risk for OM, compared to controls. These results could be interpreted due to inherent effect of psoriasis on epithelial proliferation and due to the fact that Addison's disease patients present with high preexisting pro-inflammatory cytokine levels. In addition, decreased renal function with elevated blood urea nitrogen and creatinine was associated with increased risk for OM [168].

These data indicate the potential importance of the patient's underlying condition on OM risk.

5.4 Pathogenesis

The pathogenesis of OM was conceptually defined in 2004 [30, 203, 204], in which a series of independent yet overlapping phases were used to describe the complex interactions underpinning mucositis development. This has undoubtedly been the gold standard model for OM for over a decade, shaping approaches to intervention design and guiding its clinical management [178, 205]. Introduction of this model saw a greater appreciation placed on non-epithelial mechanisms, a great leap forward in our understanding, with mucositis typically considered a strictly epithelial phenomenon. Over the years, our understanding of mucositis development has grown exponentially, particularly with regard to the oral microbiome, and has learned to adapt to the ever-changing landscape of cancer medicine in which the idiosyncrasies of newer targeted and immune therapies present supportive care experts with new challenges.

Although the clinical symptoms of mucositis are primarily driven by epithelial injury, the condition itself is the consequence of a dynamic series of biological events that take place throughout the different cellular and tissue compartments of the mucosa and submucosa. These biological stages are defined as initiation, upregulation (primary damage response), signal amplification, ulceration, and healing [206].

5.4.1 Five-Phase Model

DNA and non-DNA damage, caused by traditional anticancer agents (CT and radiotherapy), **initiates** direct cellular damage in highly proliferative basal epithelial and submucosal stem cells resulting in p53-dependent apoptosis [207, 208]. Simultaneously, reactive oxygen species (ROS) production drives a cascade of secondary signals which indirectly contribute to mucosal injury and biological dysfunction [209]. Critical to the transduction of this response is the activation of nuclear factor kappa B (NFκB), widely considered the gatekeeper of mucositis development, regulating over 200 downstream genes associated with mucosal injury [210, 211]. NFκB defines the **primary damage response,** in which an intense inflammatory response is observed, characterized by increased local and systemic levels of interleukin 1β (IL-1β), tumor necrosis factor-α

(TNFα), and IL-6 [212]. These cytokines are suggested to drive endothelial injury, connective tissue dysfunction, and mesenchymal signaling resulting in reduced epithelial oxygenation, confounding the initial direct injury to basal epithelial cells. Furthermore, it is well demonstrated that a number of downstream molecules produced in the primary damage response phase exert a positive feedback effect on NFκB, thus exacerbating the primary insult initiated by CT and radiotherapy [30]. This **signal amplification** is coupled with additional downstream activation of mitogen-activated protein kinase (MAPK) signaling and the activation of JNK, which in turn regulates the transcriptional activity of AP1 [213]. This pathway ultimately results in the activation of caspase 3, resulting in a second wave of NFκB-dependent apoptosis. NFκB is also a potent activator of cyclooxygenase (COX) 2 resulting in the production of matrix metalloproteinases (MMPs) [214]. Despite this tsunami of pro-inflammatory signaling occurring on a biological level, it is important to note that the clinical scenario remains quiescent. The oral mucosa may show signs of erythema during these phases; however, tissue integrity remains unaffected, and there are negligible oral symptoms.

The **ulcerative** stage is universally recognized as the most clinically relevant for the patient, caregivers, and oncology support staff. It represents the cumulative effect of direct cell death caused by the anticancer therapy, coupled with a cascade of potentially lethal cytokines, chemokines, kinases, and proteinases that ultimately destroy the integrity of the oral mucosa [30], although the true mechanisms underpinning tissue injury remain poorly defined. Patients present with painful, ulcerative lesions affecting almost all regions of the oral mucosa. Symptoms such as pain, xerostomia, and dysphagia severely impact on the ability of the patient to perform daily tasks, with eating, drinking, and speaking commonly affected [215]. Oral lesions are prone to superficial colonization with the many microorganisms that inhabit the oral cavity, increasing the risk of infection and sepsis particularly in neutropenic patients [216, 217]. Even in the absence of microbial translocation, bacterial products easily penetrate into the submucosa, aided by frank ulceration and compromised epithelial barrier function, activating innate immune responses and the further release of proapoptotic genes [218]. This promotes the migration of immune cells to the area of insult and the subsequent production of inflammatory signals.

In many cases, mucositis is a self-limiting condition, with **healing** evident after the cessation of anticancer treatment. However, healing is thought to be more complex than purely the removal of the initial insult, with submucosal and extracellular matrix (ECM) remodeling critical in governing the rate of repopulation and differentiation of the oral epithelium [178].

5.4.2 Emerging Evidence

The five-phase model of mucositis has instrumentally enhanced our understanding of mucositis development, with the appreciation for non-epithelial mechanisms seeing it maintained as the gold standard model for almost two decades. However, with greater research efforts and an increasing awareness for the importance of supportive oncology, it is becoming increasingly clear that the mechanisms of mucositis extend far beyond the mucosa. Advances in our understanding have undoubtedly centered on the role of the ECM, in both the initiation and healing phases, the importance of maintaining epithelial barrier function, and the role of resident microflora.

Cellular Kinetics: Disruption to homeostatic mechanisms that regulate cellular kinetics has always been central to our understanding of mucositis development. In 2013, emerging evidence on the pathobiology of mucositis suggested that maintenance of the ECM was critical across all phases of the model [178]. For example, it was demonstrated that augmented cellular kinetics during the initiation of mucositis were not only characterized by apoptosis but also cellular cytostasis, fibronectin loss, and collagen deposition during the ulcerative phase [36]. This understanding was also complimented by comprehensive characterization of MMP changes throughout the mucosa and submucosa following CT [26]. Mechanistically, the causal relationship between MMPs and symptoms remains unclear; however, it has been suggested that MMPs contribute to mucositis development via regulation of the mesenchymal-epithelial communication, epithelial proliferation/differentiation, and destruction of epithelial barrier function [30, 178, 219, 220].

Epithelial Barrier Function: Epithelial barrier integrity is critical for any epithelium, particularly those of the alimentary tract. Tight junctions maintain barrier integrity, ensuring strict control of paracellular transport [221]. A variety of physiological and pharmacological stimuli can modulate the integrity of tight junctions, including MMPs, pro-inflammatory cytokines, and bacterial byproducts (e.g., lipopolysaccharide), leading to hyperpermeability and compromised barrier integrity.

Despite a wealth of preclinical and clinical data indicating alterations in *intestinal* barrier function following a variety of anticancer therapies [222], translation of this mechanisms to the *oral* cavity is scarce. This likely reflects the challenges in quantifying barrier function in a stratified oral mucosa and the relative magnitude of clinical consequences that arise from altered barrier dysfunction in the gut. To date, only morphological changes in oral barrier function have been identified, with proteolysis and translocation of key tight junction proteins in the buccal epithelium of patients undergoing standard dose CT for a range of solid malignancies [223]. Importantly, correlations between peak barrier dysfunction, pro-inflammatory cytokine production, and MMP signaling were evident, supporting the mechanistic hypothesis that barrier dysfunction occurs secondarily to the initiation of mucositis. These findings also compliment previous research demonstrating the efficacy of antrum mucosal protein (AMP)-18 in mitigating OM via regulation of tight junction assembly [224]. As such, epithelial barrier dysfunction is considered central to the pathogenesis of mucositis; however, the clinical consequences are considered more profound in the gastrointestinal tract given the abundance of luminal microbes and its contribution to diarrhea.

Host-Microbe Interactions: The historical paradigm of OM, which was predicated on indiscriminate clonogenic cell death of highly proliferative cell populations, has clearly been overturned in favor of a more complex cascade of biological events [225]. The appreciation of the oral microbiome has certainly been a clear driver of this new biological approach to mucositis, with increasingly sophisticated genomic technology enabling in-depth analysis of the complex ecosystem that resides throughout the alimentary tract (mouth to anus). A growing body of evidence supports microbial interference with key mechanisms of *gastrointestinal* mucositis such as intestinal barrier function, mucin production, ROS activation, and inflammatory signaling. Unfortunately, the same mechanistic appreciation for the microbiome in the development of OM is lacking, with conclusions clouded by variations in patient populations, sample collection, culturing/processing, and bioinformatic approaches [226]. Nonetheless, it can be concluded that the oral microbiome shifts in its composition with a gram-negative dominant phenotype [227–229]. An interesting finding from some studies is the elevation in species diversity following anticancer therapy, due to the emergence of opportunistic strains. This is in stark contrast to the significant drop in species diversity seen in the fecal microbiome, suggesting that although dysbiosis is a common trait of oral and gastrointestinal mucositis, the complexities of these changes are region-specific.

Mechanistically, the understanding of the causal relationship between oral dysbiosis and mucositis symptomology is unclear, and the "chicken or the egg" puzzle is frequently raised [225]. However, it has been suggested that certain microbial subtypes are critical in the local activation of certain anticancer drugs, in turn regulating their efficacy and toxicity [177]. Furthermore, it is also likely that these shifts in the oral microbiome drive innate immune signaling, thus enhancing chemotactic recruitment of immune cells and initiating local innate immune responses [230]. Of particular interest is the interaction between resident microbes and Toll-like receptors (TLRs), with bacterial signals (e.g., PAMPs/DAMPs) potent activators of TLR subtypes, many of which have been implicated in the pathobiology of mucositis [231]. Similarly, evidence also suggests that some bacterial subtypes linked with mucositis, as well as oxidative stress, can elicit robust inflammasome assembly characterized by caspapse-1 activation and the proteolytic cleavage of pro-inflammatory cytokines [232]. Although this mechanism has been studied in greater detail in the gastrointestinal tract [233], it is likely that core mechanisms translate to the oral cavity.

5.4.3 A New Era of Oral Complications

The emergence of newer targeted and immune-based anticancer therapies has drastically altered the current supportive care landscape, with newly defined adverse toxicities underpinned by largely unclear mechanisms. This is certainly the case for OM among the most common side effects of these new wave anticancer therapies [206, 228]. There remains no pathobiological model for oral complication of non-cytotoxic therapy, despite their increasing prevalence. Current evidence suggests that "off-target" tyrosine kinase inhibition mediated through endothelial growth factor receptor (EGFR) and HER2 is central to the oral complications associated with targeted therapies [206], while monoclonal antibody targeting of programmed cell death ligand-1 (PD-L1) contributes to oral complications of immune checkpoint inhibitors [234].

5.5 Clinical Presentation

OM typically manifests as erythema, swelling, atrophy, ulceration, and pseudomembranous formations (Fig. 5.1) [14]. The ulcerative phase of OM presents clinically with irregular and often confluent ulceration that is typically preceded by regional erythema. The nonkeratinized mucosae of the cheeks, lips, soft palate, ventral surface of the tongue, and the floor of the mouth are frequently affected [14, 46, 173].

Figure 5.2 illustrates the expected time course of OM caused by various anticancer therapies. CT may be delivered over a short time, in which case the injury to mucosal tissues tends to be immediate and acute. CT-induced OM usually develops within 4–7 days after initiation of cytotoxics and peaks within 2 weeks, usually resolving within 3 weeks of treatment [15, 51, 173]. RT has a more gradual clinical course since it is most often administered in small fractions given over weeks. Thus, RT-induced OM takes longer both to develop and to heal, with clinical manifestations typically beginning at cumulative doses of about 15 Gy (after about 10–14 days), typically reaching full severity at 30 Gy. RT-induced OM usually resolves in 3–4 weeks but may last months after treatment has ended [51, 173].

Historically, OM caused by allo-HSCT was reported to last up to day +21; however, with the shift to RIC-HSCT, OM tends to be shorter [86]. In allo-HSCT cohorts, clinical evidence of oral injury begins 2–5 days following transplant, lasting approximately 6–9 days and resolving by 12–15 days post-HSCT [40, 44, 45, 64, 235, 236]. In actuality, injury begins with the initiation of the conditioning

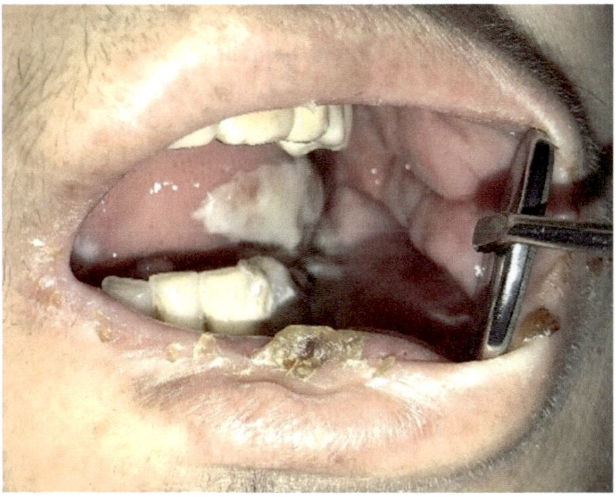

Fig. 5.1 Oral mucositis. Chemotherapy-related oral mucositis, presenting as confluent ulcerations covered with yellowish pseudomembrane

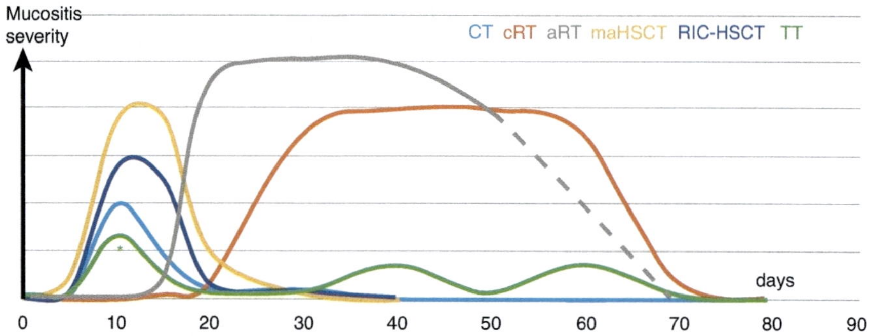

Fig. 5.2 Dynamics over time of OM severity due to various cancer therapies. *CT* chemotherapy, *cRT* conventional radiotherapy, *aRT* accelerated radiotherapy, *maHSCT* myeloablative hematopoietic stem cell transplantation, *RIC-HSCT* reduced intensity conditioning for hematopoietic stem cell transplantation, *TT* targeted therapy. In RT, the onset of OM is later than CT. Severity of OM in RIC-HSCT is usually lower than in maHSCT. Estimated course of aRT (dashed line). Following adjustment of dose (asterisk) of TT, an improvement in OM severity occurs. Thereafter, lesions may wax and wane as long as the patient receives the medication

regimen, with subclinical changes occurring in the oral cavity [12]. In some cases, oral ulcers may persist beyond day 15 post-HSCT and after recovery of the neutrophil count particularly in patients who initially develop more severe ulcerations [46]. While the regeneration of the oral mucosa begins 9–14 days after injury, the resolution of the OM usually coincides with the time of neutrophil engraftment following HSCT, when granulocyte counts exceeded 500/mm^3 [46, 237]. Epithelial cell regeneration is also associated with the return of a normal oral bacterial flora [12].

A chronic form of OM was described [238], in patients, who underwent C-RT for squamous cell carcinoma in the oral cavity. The chronic OM was defined as appearing more than 3 months following the completion of the C-RT. Two patients presented with long-lasting ulcers persisting from unresolved acute lesions, named *persistent form*. Two patients presented with new discrete ulcers that were episodic in nature, named *recurrent form*. Prior to diagnosing the oral mucosal injury as chronic OM, other etiologies need to be ruled out. It was suggested that the persistent form stems from delayed wound healing, and the lesions of the recurrent form are due to the friability of the postradiation mucosae. A prospective multi-central study reported chronic OM to have an incidence of 8.1% in post-RT patients [239].

Pain associated with OM is a also major concern for clinicians and patients due to its impact on daily tasks such as eating, swallowing, and talking [1]. Other symptoms are dysphagia, which may be mild or severe, drooling, and infections. Although pain is the hallmark of OM, the issue of pain related to OM has been poorly addressed. The incidence of OM-related pain is 40–70% among patients treated with CT, 100% in those receiving RT for HNC, and 60–89% in the setting of allo-BMT [64, 240]. Pain in allo-BMT, on average, begins 4–4.5 days posttransplant, although it may begin several days prior to transplant, lasts 6.5–9.5 days, and resolves by 11–13 days posttransplant [46, 64, 241]. Pain is described as "tender," "irritating," and "sore" [46]. The pain can range from a sense of burning in the initial phases up to severe pain and are caused by a mixture of different types of pain [15].

In a model adopted from oral mucosal injury, it was suggested that the main components are nociceptive pain, mediated by C fibers and relievable by opioids, and incidental pain, caused by movement and contact with the mucosal surface, mediated by the fast-conducting A-δ fibers [242]. The latter component is insensitive to analgesics, and the only effective pain treatment is the functional exclusion of the anatomic parts involved until the resolution of the ulcers and full recovery of the mouth's functionality.

Oral AEs due to targeted therapy have been reported to include OM or stomatitis, dysphagia, taste alterations and dysgeusia, xerostomia, lichenoid reactions, mucosal inflammation, and nonspecific mucosal sensitivity and pain [10]. These AEs can result in significant clinical impact affecting function and quality of life (QOL) and are consequently a negative impact on patient treatment adherence [243, 244]. In many cases, lesions are less severe than those induced by CT and radiotherapy; however, given the chronicity of treatment, the long-term impact of these oral complications warrants further investigation.

Clinical characteristics of targeted therapy-induced stomatitis are mainly reported in mTORI. Targeted therapy-induced mucosal lesions are characterized by repeated episodes of ulcerations [238]. The episode may include a single or multiple sites of mucosal ulcerations affecting primarily nonkeratinized oral tissues such as labial and buccal mucosa and the ventral surface of the tongue and floor of the mouth [10, 245].

Specifically, mTORI-associated stomatitis is classically characterized to be well-circumscribed single or multiple ovoid ulcerations less than 1 cm with central gray area surrounded by erythema [245–248] that closely resemble aphthous stomatitis [130, 246]. Mouth pain, dysgeusia, and dysphagia may be reported without clinical signs of ulceration [246], possibly indicative of early or low-grade mTORI-related stomatitis. The onset of mTORI-associated stomatitis usually occurs during the first 2 weeks of therapy with the majority of cases grades 1–2 in severity, with a median of 10 days (4–25 days) [246, 249].

Stomatitis secondary to mTORI usually resolves with dose reductions; however, recurrence of the oral ulcers has also been documented [247]. An observational study of mTORI in a variety of solid tumors noted that the majority of stomatitis cases resolved spontaneously without scarring in 4–5 days [245].

With the mTORI sirolimus, lesions are dose dependent and resolve following dose adjustment [130]. Generally, stomatitis is considered low-to-moderate grade and manageable with supportive therapy; however, optimal management remains unclear due to the lack of uniform measurement scales and terminology [125].

In a similarly undefined area, VEGFR multikinase inhibitors sunitinib and sorafenib had a median time to stomatitis of 1.1 months (range: 0.2–6.7 months) and 1.4 months (range: 0.2–15.7 months), respectively [135].

Cetuximab-associated mucositis appears to present with a general erythema and sensitivity of nonkeratinized mucosa that may be less ulcerative than typically seen with conventional cytotoxic CT and RT [250]. Combination therapy with cytotoxic agents may lead to combined presentation of more classical ulcerative mucositis. A small study of 13 patients under concurrent cetuximab and RT for HNC reported OM frequently involved areas that had received less than 10–15 Gy, most commonly the mucocutaneous junction of the lips [100]. It should be noted that, in these patients, HSV was not ruled out.

5.6 Clinical and Economic Consequences

The impact of OM extends far beyond the oral cavity, predisposing to systemic complications and impacting the delivery of optimal cancer therapy. In fact, several studies report that OM is associated with significantly worse outcomes in various patient populations. For example, in HSCT recipients, it was found that OM was associated with additional day with fever, increase in risk of significant infection, additional days of total parenteral nutrition (TPN), and additional days of injectable narcotic therapy [84, 251].

Similarly, the breakage of the mucosal barrier in neutropenic patients predisposes to septicemia or bacteremia, in particular viridans streptococci [252, 253]. A study reported a 47-fold increase in the incidence of these infections during a 17-year period and described a significant risk for septic shock (26% of cases with viridans streptococci septicemia vs. 4% of cases of septicemia involving other gram-positive bacteria) [253]. These complications can be life-threatening in many cases, particularly in immunocompromised patients. In fact, data indicate a significant increase in 100-day mortality risk in HSCT patients with OM. An increase of 3.9-fold in mortality rate was associated with each one-point increase in peak OMAS score [251].

OM may also predict the onset of hepatic veno-occlusive disease [254]. The sensitivity, specificity, and predictive value was high to suggest that in patients with hepatic abnormalities but without OM, other causes of the hepatic dysfunction should be investigated. It was suggested that this correlation reflects a similar cytotoxic-induced pathogenesis [254].

In terms of economic outcomes, HSCT patients with OM had significantly longer hospital stays, and the hospital-associated expenses increased by US$ 25,405 for each one-point increase in peak OMAS score [251]. When comparing low-grade OM (no ulceration) to high-grade OM (ulcerations), the difference in mean hospital charges reached 42,749$ [251]. Importantly, these data are based on fee schedules in the early 2000s, and the absolute numbers are likely higher now. Furthermore, these figures did not adequately capture additional economic burdens including lost or lowered employment income and the use of complimentary medicines, and as such the economic burden associated with OM is expected to be much greater.

In patients with H&N cancer treated with RT, OM-associated pain is associated with weight loss or ≥5% and requires feeding tube insertion [255]. In patients with

H&N cancer treated with RT, the rate of hospitalization due to OM was 16% for all RT protocols and 32% for altered fractionation RT [28]. The functional status decreased by 33%, and QOL decreased by 20% by the sixth week of the RT [256], indicating that opioid analgesia provides inadequate relief. In 11% of patients, OM resulted in RT regimen interruption or medication [256], thus impacting on local tumor control and patient survival.

RT-related OM is also associated with increased utilization of resources, such as ED visits, admission, consultations with dietician, opioid analgesics, and gastrostomy. It results in an incremental cost of US$ 1700–6000, depending on the grade, as of cost data in 2006 [255].

Targeted therapy-induced OM has a relatively variable presentation and is a relatively new entity within the scope of OM. Nevertheless, reports consistently presented pain-associated functional limitations, such as limited diet, difficulty eating, difficulty swallowing, or difficulty speaking. These unsurprisingly predispose to dose reduction or discontinuation of the treatment, with an incidence of 47% in patients treated with mTORI [246].

5.6.1 Outcome Assessment Measures

OM assessment scales should be able to describe precisely, classify objectively, and measure reproducibly the severity of the mucosal damage [31]. Ideally, an OM scoring system should be validated and will require minimal training to produce systematic, accurate results characterized by intra-rater and inter-rater reliability. Unfortunately, no scale currently meets all these criteria or is accepted universally. As such, the assessment and clinical evaluation of OM still pose significant challenges in clinical practice and research [30, 31].

A number of instruments to evaluate the observable and functional dimensions of OM are available [31, 257, 258]. These OM scales range considerably in their complexity and have undergone varying degrees of validation. In addition, patient-reported outcome measures have been developed based on purely subjective criteria; however, they hold great importance in illustrating the impact of OM [69, 256, 259].

5.6.1.1 Clinician-Reported Outcome Measures

A series of scales have been developed by international societies and organizations for the assessment and diagnosis of OM (Table 5.5). These scales combine elements such as symptoms, signs, and function, usually comprising of four-point or five-point scales, that rate the overall status of oral mucosal, severity of oral pain, and, in some instances, the patient's functional capabilities relative to his or her oral status (e.g., the ability to swallow). Historically, many of these scales are based on the World Health Organization (WHO) developed in 1979 [260]. The National Cancer Institute published the fifth version for Common Toxicity Criteria (NCI-CTC) scales [261], and the Radiation Therapy Oncology Group (RTOG) scale is popular for assessment of RT-induced OM. These scales are used frequently by cooperative oncology groups and oncology researchers [262].

Table 5.5 OM scales assessing both objective and subjective variables: WHO, NCI-CTC, and RTOG

Scale	Cancer treatment	Grade 0	Grade 1 (mild)	Grade 2 (moderate)	Grade 3 (severe)	Grade 4 (life-threatening)	Grade 5 (death)
WHO [260]	All types	None	Oral soreness, erythema	Oral erythema, ulcers, solid diet tolerated	Oral ulcers, liquid diet only	Oral alimentation impossible	N/A
NCI-CTC [261]	All types		Asymptomatic or mild symptoms; intervention not indicate	Moderate pain or ulcer that does not interfere with oral intake; modified diet indicated	Severe pain; interfering with oral intake	Life-threatening consequences; urgent intervention indicated	Death related to toxicity
RTOG [262]	Radiotherapy		Irritation/may experience mild pain not requiring analgesic	Patchy mucositis that may produce an inflammatory serosanguinous discharge/may experience moderate pain requiring analgesia	Confluent fibrinous mucositis/ may include severe pain requiring narcotic	Ulceration, hemorrhage, or necrosis	N/A

WHO World Health Organization, *NCI-CTC* National Cancer Institute-Common Toxicity Criteria, *RTOG* Radiation Therapy Oncology Group

Table 5.6 Selected OM scales assessing objective variables

Scale	Grade 0	Grade 1	Grade 2	Grade 3
WCCNR [266]	Lesions: none Color: pink Bleeding: none	Lesions: 1–4 Color: slight red Bleeding: N/A	Lesions: >4 Color: moderate red Bleeding: with eating and oral hygiene	Lesions: coalescing Color: very red Bleeding: spontaneous
OMI [264]	Included 34 items: various oral locations assessed for 11 atrophy items, 11 pseudomembrane items, ten erythema items, and two edema items; all are scored from 0 (normal) to 3 (severe), with overall scale ranging from 0 to 102			
20 item OMI [263]	Modified to include 20 items: Various oral locations assessed for nine erythema items, nine ulceration items, one atrophy item, and one edema item; all are scored from 0 (normal) to 3 (severe), summed for a total possible score of 0–60			
OMAS [265]	Nine oral locations assessed for erythema (0 = none, 2 = severe) and ulcers or pseudomembranes in the oral cavity (0 = no ulcer, 1 = <1 cm^2, 2 = 1–3 cm^2, 3 = >3 cm^2)			

WCCNR Western Consortium for Cancer Nursing Research, *OMI* Oral Mucositis Index, *OMAS* Oral Mucositis Assessment Scale

Additional OM scales have also been developed, and several examples are listed (Table 5.6). These scales use objective descriptors and apply them to specific anatomic areas, adding greater specificity with various aspects of oral function and subjective patient responses, and more accurately represent the anatomic severity of OM. These scales include, among others, Oral Mucositis Index (OMI) [263, 264], Oral Mucositis Assessment Scale (OMAS) [265], and Western Consortium for Cancer Nursing Research (WCCNR) [266]. The OMI and the OMAS have been found to correlate closely with OM pain scores [241, 264].

Another clinician-rated instrument is the Performance Status Scale for Head and Neck Cancer (PSS-HN) [267], which was designed to evaluate performance in areas of functioning most likely affected by HNC and its treatment. The PSS-HN is determined through the use of an unstructured interview with the patient. It consists of three subscales: normalcy of diet, understandability of speech, and eating in public. Each is rated from 0 to 100, with higher scores indicating better performance. The PSS-HN has been shown to have adequate inter-rater reliability and to be sensitive to differences in performance and change over time [268–270].

In addition to these commonly used approaches, there are a number of detailed objective and combined scoring scales, which are designed for clinical and research purposes, as well as various study-specific scales, such as Oral Assessment Guide [271], Southwest Oncology Group Criteria [272], Eastern Cooperative Oncology Group Scale [273], Spijkervet Radiation Mucositis Scale [274], Walsh Quantitative Scoring System for Oral Mucositis [275], Tardieu Quantitative Scale of Oral Mucositis for HSCT [276], Daily Mucositis Scale for HSCT [277], MacDibbs Mouth Assessment [278], and more.

The most relevant scales for routine clinical management, which are also most widely used, appear to be those based on NCI (43–63%) or WHO (31–38%) design [31, 38, 215]. Briefly, the WHO scale measures anatomical, symptomatic, and functional components of OM. The severity of the condition is graded by a scale from 0 (no OM) to 4 (patient requiring TPN). The NCI-CTC scale also combines variables of symptoms, signs, and function. Severity is graded from 0 (no OM) to 5 (death related to toxicity). It is noteworthy to mention that NCI-CTC v3 scored separately clinical and functional variables. This was merged into one scale in the NCI-CTC v4 and stayed this way for the NCI-CTC v5. RTOG scale to address OM due to radiotherapy, graded 0 (no change over baseline) to 4 (ulceration, hemorrhage, or necrosis).

The most noticeable drawbacks of the OM scales include the fact that assessment potentially is confounded by a combination of symptoms, signs, and functional changes. Scoring of functional variables may not be correlated directly with oral mucosal events. For example, OM assessed with a scale such as the NCI-CTC scale may be rated grade 4, which describes the patient as requiring "parenteral or enteral nutrition or support." However, in the HSCT setting, many patients are placed on TPN because of intestinal toxicity. Moreover, the symptoms that the WHO scale measures may not be due to OM at all but to local infection, hemorrhage, or the presence of an underlying malignancy. The WHO scale can be assigned without even examining the patient and thus can potentially reflect etiologies other than clinical OM. Despite these drawbacks, the WHO scale is considered most accurate in measuring the clinical consequences of OM (i.e., pain and the requirement of parenteral medication and nutrition).

A major disadvantage of the more detailed and complex clinician-reported scales (Table 5.6) is that they are best delivered and performed by an experienced/trained examiner and are often more laborious. Furthermore, only some have been validated for their accuracy with many only validated in narrow clinical cohorts. The OMAS scale is the most technically challenging as it measures lesion size and erythema at nine different sites in the oral cavity. Obviously, this scale is very difficult to use in patients with severe pain who are unable to open their mouths for an adequate oral examination. Similar challenges are also faced in children affected by cancer, in which communication and cooperation may be difficult.

The frequency with which the scales are applied relates to the objective of the examination. Whereas daily evaluations are of value for a nursing care plan, an intense, twice-weekly examination may be effective for an interventional study [31].

The sensitivity and accuracy of each scale are often a function of the conditions under which the examination takes place, including adequate illumination and inspection of oral tissues, depending on the place where the patient is being evaluated—a hospital bed, dental chair, etc. Regardless of the scale used, increasing evidence confirms the importance of training and standardization in improving the accuracy and consistency of OM assessment [31].

5.6.1.2 Patient-Related Outcome Measures

Quality-of-life instruments are needed in order to estimate OM severity and patients' experiences during therapy, thus guiding patient care and assessing the efficacy of therapeutic interventions targeted against OM. These patient-related outcome measures are used in clinical investigations and research settings.

The OM Daily Questionnaire (OMDQ) [69, 279] contains ten items and was developed originally for use of palifermin in HSCT patients' clinical trials. Items included questions regarding degree of mouth soreness and degree of limitation of functioning (swallowing, eating, drinking, talking, and sleeping) due to mouth soreness. Mouth and throat soreness (MTS) scores were highly correlated with functioning limitation items and also with the WHO scale. Interestingly, patients reported changes 1–3 days earlier than clinicians [69, 279].

The OMDQ has also been used and validated in HNC patients undergoing radiotherapy, with or without CT [256]. Mean QOL scores decreased significantly during RT, corresponding with the peak of OM severity. Symptomatic management of OM was insufficient to avoid negative patient-reported outcomes.

The Oral Mucositis Weekly Questionnaire-Head and Neck Cancer (OMWQ-HN) is another validated, reliable, and feasible patient-reported outcome instrument for assessing the impact of OM [259]. It consists of 12 items that assess patient well-being and function. The time frame for reference is the past week. The first two questions assess overall health and QOL, rated on a seven-point scale. The third question quantifies MTS the patient is experiencing on a five-point scale. The remaining three questions assess the degree of mouth, throat, and overall mouth and throat pain and soreness using an 11-point scale [259].

The Functional Assessment of Cancer Therapy-Head and Neck Cancer (FACT-HN) includes the FACT-General (FACT-G) and an HNC-specific additional-concerns subscale (HNCS) [280]. The FACT-G is a general cancer QOL scale for evaluating patients receiving cancer treatment [281]. The FACT-G can be supplemented by site- and/or treatment-specific subscales, including HNCS. The FACT-G has four subscales: physical well-being (PWB) (seven items), social/family well-being (SWB) (seven items), emotional well-being (EWB) (six items), and functional well-being (FWB) (seven items). The HNCS has additional 9–12 HNC specific items, each rated on a 1 to 4 Likert-type response format (ranging from 0 [not at all] to 4 [very much]). Items are then combined to describe patient functioning in these six areas. Higher subscale scores represent better QOL. The FACT-HN was found to be reliable and valid when applied to HNC patients [269, 270, 280].

The FACT-HN Symptom Index (FHNSI) is comprised of ten items from the FACT-HN that have been selected by expert clinicians from 17 National Comprehensive Cancer Network (NCCN) institutions, as the most important symptom targets when treating patients with advanced HNC [282].

Another questionnaire developed to assess the QOL of cancer patients is the European Organization for Research and Treatment of Cancer Quality of Life questionnaire (EORTC QLQ-C30) [283]. The questionnaire is composed of five multi-item scales (physical, role, social, emotional, and cognitive functioning) and nine single items (pain, fatigue, financial impact, appetite loss, nausea/vomiting, diarrhea, constipation, sleep disturbance, and QOL). It is supplemented by disease-specific modules, e.g., HN. It includes 28 questions rated on a Likert-type scale (1–4) and other two questions rated on a 1–7 scale, regarding overall health and

QOL. All items relate to the past week. The QLQ-C30 is a well-validated instrument providing a broad view of the patients' QOL [284, 285]. This has evolved into the EORTC H&N35 module—a lengthy but well-validated questionnaire—general to all HNCs and all modalities of treatment, assessing seven scales: pain, swallowing, senses, speech, social eating, social contact, and sexuality [286].

Other patient-reported outcome measures exist and are beyond the scope of this section.

5.7 Treatment and Prevention

There is extensive literature about the management of OM, which indicates the great need for an effective treatment. However, as of today, there is only a single drug that the FDA has cleared for the prevention of OM. This fact represents the numerous challenges in identifying an effective and safe treatment and to successfully complete the regulatory phases.

In attempt to identify the interventions for OM which have the strongest evidence, the Multinational Association of Supportive Care in Cancer/International Society of Oral Oncology (MASCC/ISOO) conduct periodically a systematic review. The results of the systematic review are presented as three types of guidelines: recommendation, suggestion, and no guideline possible (NGP). Additionally, the guidelines specify the aim of the intervention: prevention, treatment, or management of OM-associated pain [287].

The current version of the MASCC/ISOO clinical practice guidelines for the management of OM was published in 2019–2020 (Tables 5.7 and 5.8). The details of the systematic review appear in the set of guideline publications [288–295] and are summarized in formal guidelines summary paper [296]. Guidelines for the management of gastrointestinal mucositis were developed as well (Table 5.9) [291].

Targeted therapy-related mucositis requires a dedicated clinical approach as the pathogenesis of this oral lesions is different than the pathogenesis of the conventional OM. Furthermore, from the current data, it seems that steroids, which are effective for targeted therapy-related mucositis, are reported to be ineffective for conventional OM. A key element in the management of targeted therapy-related mucositis is the dose reduction of the drug [246]. Dose reduction reduces the severity and frequency of the oral eruptions; however, this approach clearly compromises the efficacy of cancer therapy and thus affects prognosis. Among the interventions studied for targeted therapy-related mucositis are topical steroids, such as clobetasol gel 0.05% and dexamethasone solution 0.01% [246]. Systemic steroids were also reported to be effective, for example, intralesional injections of triamcinolone 40 mg/mL or prednisone 5 mg/day [246, 297]. Interestingly, a case report of steroid-resistant temsirolimus mucositis suggested that colchicine may be effective in healing of existing lesions and reduce frequency of new lesions [298]. These therapeutic interventions are enhanced by palliative treatments with local anesthetics or topical antihistamines [297].

Table 5.7 MASCC/ISOO clinical practice guidelines for the management of oral mucositis [288–290, 292–296]

Section	Intervention		LoE	Category	Guideline statement
Guidelines that were determined in 2019–2020 based on new evidence					
BOC	Multi-agent combination	1	III	Suggestion	The panel suggests that implementation of **multi-agent combination** oral care protocols is beneficial for the prevention of OM during CT
		2	III	Suggestion	The panel suggests that implementation of **multi-agent combination** oral care protocols is beneficial for the prevention of OM during H&N RT
		3	III	Suggestion	The panel suggests that implementation of **multi-agent combination** oral care protocols is beneficial for the prevention of OM during HSCT
	Professional oral care	4	III	NGP/expert opinion	No guideline was possible regarding the use of **professional oral care** for the prevention of OM for patients with hematologic, solid, or H&N cancers due to limited and inconsistent data An expert opinion complements this guideline. Although there was insufficient evidence to support the use of professional oral care for OM prevention, the panel is of the opinion that dental evaluation and treatment as indicated prior to cancer therapy is desirable to reduce risk for local and systemic infections from odontogenic sources
	Patient education	5	III	NGP/expert opinion	No guideline was possible regarding the use of **patient education** for the prevention of OM in hematologic cancer patients during HSCT or CT due to limited and inconsistent data An expert opinion complements this guideline. The panel is of the opinion that educating patients about the benefits of BOC strategies is still appropriate as this may improve self-management and adherence to the recommended oral care protocol during cancer treatment
	Saline or sodium bicarbonate	6	III	NGP/expert opinion	No guideline was possible regarding the use **of saline or sodium bicarbonate** rinses in the prevention or treatment of OM in patients undergoing cancer therapy due to limited data An expert opinion complements this guideline. Despite the limited data available for both saline and sodium bicarbonate, the panel recognizes that these are inert bland rinses that increase oral clearance which may be helpful for maintaining oral hygiene and improving patient comfort
	CHX	7	III	Suggestion against	The panel suggests that **CHX** not be used in the prevention of OM in patients undergoing H&N RT
Anti-inflammatory agents	Benzydamine	8	I	Recommendation	The panel recommends **benzydamine** mouthwash for the prevention of OM in patients with H&N cancer receiving a moderate-dose RT (<50 Gy)
		9	II	Suggestion	The panel suggests the use of **benzydamine** mouthwash for the prevention of OM in patients with H&N cancer receiving RT-CT

(continued)

Table 5.7 (continued)

Section	Intervention		LoE	Category	Guideline statement
PBM (laser/ light therapy)	PBM	10	I	Recommendation	The panel recommends the use of intraoral **PBM** therapy using low-level laser therapy for the prevention of OM in adult patients receiving HSCT conditioned with high-dose CT, with or without total body irradiation using one of the selected protocols[a]; it is recommended that the specific PTPs of the selected protocol will be followed for optimal therapy
		11	II	Recommendation	The panel recommends the use of intraoral **PBM** therapy using low-level laser therapy for prevention of OM in adults receiving RT to the H&N (without CT)[a]; the specific PTPs of the selected protocol should be followed for optimal therapy Safety considerations unique to patients with oral cancer should be considered
		12	I	Recommendation	The panel recommends the use of intraoral **PBM** therapy using low-level laser therapy for the prevention of OM in adults receiving RT-CT for H&N cancer (LoE I)[a]; the specific PTPs of the selected protocol should be followed for optimal therapy Safety considerations unique to patients with oral cancer should be considered
Cryotherapy	Cryotherapy	13	II	Recommendation	The panel recommends using oral **cryotherapy** to prevent oral mucositis in patients undergoing autologous HSCT when the conditioning includes high-dose melphalan
		14	II	Recommendation	The panel recommends using 30 min of oral **cryotherapy** to prevent oral mucositis in patients receiving bolus 5-FU CT during the infusion of the CT
Antimicrobials, coating agents, anesthetics, analgesics	Morphine rinse	15	III	Suggestion	Topical **morphine** 0.2% mouthwash is suggested for the treatment of OM-associated pain in H&N cancer patients treated with RT-CT
	Sucralfate	16	II	Recommendation against	**Sucralfate** (combined topical and systemic) is not recommended for the prevention of OM-associated pain in H&N cancer patients treated with RT
		17	II	Recommendation against	**Sucralfate** (combined topical and systemic) is not recommended for the treatment of OM-associated pain in H&N cancer patients treated with RT
		18	II	Recommendation against	**Sucralfate** (combined topical and systemic) is not recommended for the treatment of OM-associated pain in solid cancer patients treated with CT
Growth factors and cytokines	KGF-1	19	I	Recommendation	The use of **KGF-1** intravenously is recommended for prevention of OM in patients with hematological cancer undergoing autologous HSCT with a conditioning regimen that includes high-dose chemotherapy and TBI
	GM-CSF	20	II	Suggestion against	The evidence suggests that topical **GM-CSF** should not be used for the prevention of OM in patients undergoing HSCT

Natural and misc.	Glutamine	21	I	Recommendation against	The panel recommends against the use of **glutamine** (parenteral) for the prevention of OM in patients undergoing HSCT
		22	II	Suggestion	The panel suggests **glutamine** (per os) for the prevention of OM in patients with H&N cancer receiving RT-CT The suggestion is with caution due to the higher mortality rate seen in HSCT patients treated with parenteral glutamine
	Honey	23	II	Suggestion	**Honey** is suggested for the prevention of OM in H&N cancer patients treated with either RT or RT-CT
	Chewing gum	24	III	Suggestion against	**Chewing gum** is not suggested for the prevention of OM in pediatric patients with hematological or solid cancer treated with CT
Guidelines that were determined in 2014 and no new evidence for these agents was published since					
Antimicrobials, coating agents, anesthetics, analgesics	Patient-controlled analgesia with morphine	1	II	Recommendation	The panel recommends that **patient-controlled analgesia with morphine** be used to treat pain due to oral mucositis in patients undergoing HSCT
	PTA or BCoG	2	III	Recommendation against	The panel recommends that **PTA** and **BCoG** antimicrobial lozenges and PTA paste not be used to prevent OM in patients receiving RT for H&N cancer
	Iseganan	3	II	Recommendation against	The panel recommends that **iseganan** antimicrobial mouthwash not be used to prevent OM in patients receiving high-dose chemotherapy, with or without total body irradiation, for HSCT
		4	II	Recommendation against	The panel recommends that **iseganan** antimicrobial mouthwash not be used to prevent OM in patients receiving RT or RT-CT for H&N cancer
	Pentoxifylline	5	III	Suggestion against	The panel suggests that **systemic pentoxifylline**, administered orally, not be used to prevent OM in patients undergoing bone marrow transplantation
Natural and miscellaneous	Pilocarpine	6	III	Suggestion against	The panel suggests that **systemic pilocarpine**, administered orally, not be used to prevent OM in patients receiving RT for H&N cancer
		7	II	Suggestion against	The panel suggests that **systemic pilocarpine**, administered orally, not be used to prevent OM in patients receiving high-dose CT, with or without total body irradiation, for HSCT

[a]These guidelines refer to specific PBM protocols. For the detailed protocols, see the full text in the 2019 guidelines paper [288]

OM oral mucositis, *BOC* basic oral care, *NPG* no guideline possible, *CHX* chlorhexidine, *PBM* photobiomodulation, *PTP* physical therapy parameters, *KGF-1* keratinocyte growth factor 1, *GM-CSF* granulocyte macrophage colony-stimulating factor, *PTA* polymyxin, tobramycin, and amphotericin B (as a lozenge or a paste), *BCoG* bacitracin, clotrimazole, and gentamicin (as a lozenge), *HSCT* hematopoietic stem cell transplantation, *CT* chemotherapy, *RT* radiotherapy, *RT-CT* radiochemotherapy, *H&N* head and neck, *TBI* total body irradiation

Table 5.8 Recommended intraoral photobiomodulation therapy protocols for the prevention of oral mucositis (details in Zadik 2019) [288]

Cancer treatment modality	Wavelength (nm)	Power density (irradiance; mW/cm²)	Time per spot (s)	Energy density (fluence; J/cm²)	Spot size (cm²)	Number of sites	Duration
HSCT	632.8	31.25	40	1.0	0.8	18	From day after cessation of conditioning for 5 days
	650	1000[a]	2	2.0	0.04	54–70	From the first day of conditioning till day +2 post-HSCT (for 7–13 days)
RT	632.8	24	125	3.0	1	12	Entire RT course
RT-CT	660	417[a]	10	4.2	0.24	72	Entire RT course
	660	625[a]	10	6.2	0.04	69	Entire RT course

[a]Potential thermal effect; the clinician is advised to pay attention to the combination of specific parameters

CT chemotherapy, *HSCT* hematopoietic stem cell transplantation, *IO* intraoral, *NR* not reported, *PBM* photobiomodulation, *RT* radiotherapy, *wk* week

Patient education is also an important, yet commonly overlooked, part of the overall supportive treatment approach. Although there is currently no proof that patient-targeted education leads to significantly reduced OM prevalence, it is assumed that patient education encourages the patient to maintain adequate oral hygiene, which in turn reduces the risk for oral infections and systemic spread of the infections through the ulcerated oral mucosa.

Lastly, OM should be differentiated from oral infections that often develop while patient is administered the anticancer therapy and may coincide with OM. These infections are typically bacterial, viral, or fungal. While the symptoms may be similar (e.g., OM and candidiasis may cause burning pain), or the signs may be similar (e.g., OM, bacterial infection, and HSV reactivation during neutropenia may cause oral ulcerations on nonkeratinized mucosa), the coinfection amplifies the clinical presentation and hinders the diagnosis of OM. The clinical presentation and laboratory tests are critical in confirming a diagnosis. Empiric antimicrobial treatment may be initiated based on the clinical presentation but must then be reevaluated once laboratory results are available.

5.8 Summary

OM is a clinical entity with a significant impact on the patient, clinicians, and health-care system. The understanding of the pathogenesis has improved markedly over the last few decades; however, this has not yet led to universally adopted

Table 5.9 MASCC/ISOO clinical practice guidelines for the management of gastrointestinal mucositis [291]

Intervention		LoE	Guideline category	Guideline statement
Guidelines that were determined in 2019–2020 based on new evidence				
Probiotics	1	II	Suggestion	The panel suggests that **probiotics containing *Lactobacillus*** spp. may be beneficial for prevention of RT or RT-CT-induced diarrhea in patients with pelvic malignancy
HBO	2	II	Suggestion	The panel suggests that **hyperbaric oxygen** is an effective way to treat RT-induced proctitis in patients with pelvic malignancy
Guidelines that were determined in 2014 and no new evidence for these agents was published since				
Amifostine	1	II	Recommendation	The panel recommends that intravenous **amifostine** be used, at a dose of ≥340 mg/m², to prevent radiation proctitis in patients receiving RT
	2	III	Suggestion	The panel suggests that intravenous **amifostine** be used to prevent esophagitis induced by RT-CT in patients with non-small cell lung carcinoma
Octreotide	3	II	Recommendation	The panel recommends that **octreotide**, at a dose of ≥100 µg subcutaneously twice daily, be used to treat diarrhea induced by standard- or high-dose CT associated with HSCT, if loperamide is ineffective
Sucralfate	4	III	Suggestion	The panel suggests that **sucralfate** enemas be used to treat chronic radiation-induced proctitis in patients with rectal bleeding
	5	I	Recommendation against	The panel recommends that systemic **sucralfate**, administered orally, not be used to treat gastrointestinal mucositis in patients receiving RT for a solid tumor
Sulfasalazine	6	II	Suggestion	The panel suggests that systemic **sulfasalazine**, at a dose of 500 mg administered orally twice a day, be used to prevent radiation-induced enteropathy in patients receiving RT to the pelvis
ASA, mesalazine, olsalazine	7	I	Recommendation against	The panel recommends that **ASA, and the related compounds mesalazine and olsalazine**, administered orally, not be used to prevent acute radiation-induced diarrhea in patients receiving RT for a pelvic malignancy
Misoprostol	8	I	Recommendation against	The panel recommends that **misoprostol** suppositories not be used to prevent acute radiation-induced proctitis in patients receiving RT for prostate cancer

OM oral mucositis, *GM-CSF* granulocyte macrophage colony-stimulating factor, *PTA* polymyxin, tobramycin, and amphotericin B (as a lozenge or a paste), *CT* chemotherapy, *RT* radiotherapy, *RT-CT* radiochemotherapy, *HBO* hyperbaric oxygen, *ASA* 5-acetylsalicylic acid preventative or therapeutic approaches. As such, there remains a great need for effective prophylactic therapies to mitigate OM prevalence and severity without compromising treatment efficacy. The clinical practice guidelines for the management of OM provide the current evidence-based summary of the best practice for OM.

Bibliography

1. Scully C, Sonis S, Diz PD. Oral mucositis. Oral Dis. 2006;12(3):229–41.
2. Basu B, Eisen T. Perspectives in drug development for metastatic renal cell cancer. Target Oncol. 2010;5(2):139–56.
3. Harris M. Monoclonal antibodies as therapeutic agents for cancer. Lancet Oncol. 2004;5(5):292–302.
4. Herbst RS, Shin DM. Monoclonal antibodies to target epidermal growth factor receptor-positive tumors: a new paradigm for cancer therapy. Cancer. 2002;94(5):1593–611.
5. John AM, Thomas NS, Mufti GJ, Padua RA. Targeted therapies in myeloid leukemia. Semin Cancer Biol. 2004;14(1):41–62.
6. Moon C, Chae YK, Lee J. Targeting epidermal growth factor receptor in head and neck cancer: lessons learned from cetuximab. Exp Biol Med. 2010;235(8):907–20.
7. Mukai H. Targeted therapy in breast cancer: current status and future directions. Jpn J Clin Oncol. 2010;40(8):711–6.
8. Bonner JA, Harari PM, Giralt J, Azarnia N, Shin DM, Cohen RB, et al. Radiotherapy plus cetuximab for squamous-cell carcinoma of the head and neck. N Engl J Med. 2006;354(6):567–78.
9. Hansel TT, Kropshofer H, Singer T, Mitchell JA, George AJ. The safety and side effects of monoclonal antibodies. Nat Rev Drug Discov. 2010;9(4):325–38.
10. Watters AL, Epstein JB, Agulnik M. Oral complications of targeted cancer therapies: a narrative literature review. Oral Oncol. 2011;47(6):441–8.
11. Bellm LA, Epstein JB, Rose-Ped A, Martin P, Fuchs HJ. Patient reports of complications of bone marrow transplantation. Support Care Cancer. 2000;8(1):33–9.
12. Stiff P. Mucositis associated with stem cell transplantation: current status and innovative approaches to management. Bone Marrow Transplant. 2001;27(2):S3–S11.
13. Al-Dasooqi N, Sonis ST, Bowen JM, Bateman E, Blijlevens N, Gibson RJ, et al. Emerging evidence on the pathobiology of mucositis. Support Care Cancer. 2013;21(11):3233–41.
14. Raber-Durlacher JE, Elad S, Barasch A. Oral mucositis. Oral Oncol. 2010;46(6):452–6.
15. Niscola P, Romani C, Cupelli L, Scaramucci L, Tendas A, Dentamaro T, et al. Mucositis in patients with hematologic malignancies: an overview. Haematologica. 2007;92(2):222–31.
16. Peterson DE, Lalla RV. Oral mucositis: the new paradigms. Curr Opin Oncol. 2010;22(4):318–22.
17. Peterson DE, Srivastava R, Lalla RV. Oral mucosal injury in oncology patients: perspectives on maturation of a field. Oral Dis. 2015;21(2):133–41.
18. Logan RM. Advances in understanding of toxicities of treatment for head and neck cancer. Oral Oncol. 2009;45(10):844–8.
19. Sonis ST. Regimen-related gastrointestinal toxicities in cancer patients. Curr Opin Support Palliat Care. 2010;4(1):26–30.
20. Romesser PB, Cahlon O, Scher ED, Hug EB, Sine K, DeSelm C, et al. Proton beam reirradiation for recurrent head and neck cancer: multi-institutional report on feasibility and early outcomes. Int J Radiat Oncol Biol Phys. 2016;95(1):386–95.
21. Bonner JA, Giralt J, Harari PM, Baselga J, Spencer S, Bell D, et al. Association of human papillomavirus and p16 status with mucositis and dysphagia for head and neck cancer patients treated with radiotherapy with or without cetuximab: assessment from a phase 3 registration trial. Eur J Cancer. 2016;64:1–11.

22. Guo R, Tang LL, Mao YP, Zhou GQ, Qi ZY, Liu LZ, et al. Clinical outcomes of volume-modulated arc therapy in 205 patients with nasopharyngeal carcinoma: an analysis of survival and treatment toxicities. PLoS One. 2015;10(7):e0129679.
23. Hu MH, Wang LW, Lu HJ, Chu PY, Tai SK, Lee TL, et al. Cisplatin-based chemotherapy versus cetuximab in concurrent chemoradiotherapy for locally advanced head and neck cancer treatment. Biomed Res Int. 2014;904341(10):6.
24. Lin L, Yao JJ, Zhou GQ, Guo R, Zhang F, Zhang Y, et al. The efficacy and toxicity of individualized intensity-modulated radiotherapy based on the tumor extension patterns of nasopharyngeal carcinoma. Oncotarget. 2016;7(15):20680–90.
25. Manas A, Palacios A, Contreras J, Sanchez-Magro I, Blanco P, Fernandez-Perez C. Incidence of oral mucositis, its treatment and pain management in patients receiving cancer treatment at Radiation Oncology Departments in Spanish hospitals (MUCODOL Study). Clin Transl Oncol. 2009;11(10):669–76.
26. Vatca M, Lucas JT Jr, Laudadio J, D'Agostino RB, Waltonen JD, Sullivan CA, et al. Retrospective analysis of the impact of HPV status and smoking on mucositis in patients with oropharyngeal squamous cell carcinoma treated with concurrent chemotherapy and radiotherapy. Oral Oncol. 2014;50(9):869–76.
27. Peterson DE, Bensadoun RJ, Roila F. Management of oral and gastrointestinal mucositis: ESMO Clinical Practice Guidelines. Ann Oncol. 2011;22(6):vi78–84.
28. Trotti A, Bellm LA, Epstein JB, Frame D, Fuchs HJ, Gwede CK, et al. Mucositis incidence, severity and associated outcomes in patients with head and neck cancer receiving radiotherapy with or without chemotherapy: a systematic literature review. Radiother Oncol. 2003;66(3):253–62.
29. Lalla RV, Bowen J, Barasch A, Elting L, Epstein J, Keefe DM, et al. MASCC/ISOO clinical practice guidelines for the management of mucositis secondary to cancer therapy. Cancer. 2014;120(10):1453–61.
30. Sonis ST. The pathobiology of mucositis. Nat Rev Cancer. 2004;4(4):277–84.
31. Sonis ST, Elting LS, Keefe D, Peterson DE, Schubert M, Hauer-Jensen M, et al. Perspectives on cancer therapy-induced mucosal injury: pathogenesis, measurement, epidemiology, and consequences for patients. Cancer. 2004;100(9 Suppl):1995–2025.
32. Scully C, Epstein J, Sonis S. Oral mucositis: a challenging complication of radiotherapy, chemotherapy, and radiochemotherapy: Part 1, Pathogenesis and prophylaxis of mucositis. Head Neck. 2003;25(12):1057–70.
33. Nishimura N, Nakano K, Ueda K, Kodaira M, Yamada S, Mishima Y, et al. Prospective evaluation of incidence and severity of oral mucositis induced by conventional chemotherapy in solid tumors and malignant lymphomas. Support Care Cancer. 2012;20(9):2053–9.
34. Raber-Durlacher JE, Weijl NI, Abu Saris M, de Koning B, Zwinderman AH, Osanto S. Oral mucositis in patients treated with chemotherapy for solid tumors: a retrospective analysis of 150 cases. Support Care Cancer. 2000;8(5):366–71.
35. Tachi T, Teramachi H, Tanaka K, Asano S, Osawa T, Kawashima A, et al. The impact of outpatient chemotherapy-related adverse events on the quality of life of breast cancer patients. PLoS One. 2015;10(4):e0124169.
36. Wuketich S, Hienz SA, Marosi C. Prevalence of clinically relevant oral mucositis in outpatients receiving myelosuppressive chemotherapy for solid tumors. Support Care Cancer. 2012;20(1):175–83.
37. Mercadante S, Aielli F, Adile C, Ferrera P, Valle A, Fusco F, et al. Prevalence of oral mucositis, dry mouth, and dysphagia in advanced cancer patients. Support Care Cancer. 2015;23(11):3249–55.
38. Jones JA, Avritscher EB, Cooksley CD, Michelet M, Bekele BN, Elting LS. Epidemiology of treatment-associated mucosal injury after treatment with newer regimens for lymphoma, breast, lung, or colorectal cancer. Support Care Cancer. 2006;14(6):505–15.
39. Schwab M, Zanger UM, Marx C, Schaeffeler E, Klein K, Dippon J, et al. Role of genetic and nongenetic factors for fluorouracil treatment-related severe toxicity: a prospective clinical trial by the German 5-FU Toxicity Study Group. J Clin Oncol. 2008;26(13):2131–8.

40. Wilkes JD. Prevention and treatment of oral mucositis following cancer chemotherapy. Semin Oncol. 1998;25(5):538–51.
41. Peterson DE. Oral toxicity of chemotherapeutic agents. Semin Oncol. 1992;19(5):478–91.
42. Seto BG, Kim M, Wolinsky L, Mito RS, Champlin R. Oral mucositis in patients undergoing bone marrow transplantation. Oral Surg Oral Med Oral Pathol. 1985;60(5):493–7.
43. Zerbe MB, Parkerson SG, Ortlieb ML, Spitzer T. Relationships between oral mucositis and treatment variables in bone marrow transplant patients. Cancer Nurs. 1992;15(3):196–205.
44. Barasch A, Peterson DE, Tanzer JM, D'Ambrosio JA, Nuki K, Schubert MM, et al. Helium-neon laser effects on conditioning-induced oral mucositis in bone marrow transplantation patients. Cancer. 1995;76(12):2550–6.
45. Mattsson T, Heimdahl A, Dahllof G, Nilsson B, Lonnqvist B, Ringden O. Variables predicting oral mucosal lesions in allogenic bone marrow recipients. Head Neck. 1991;13(3):224–9.
46. Woo SB, Sonis ST, Monopoli MM, Sonis AL. A longitudinal study of oral ulcerative mucositis in bone marrow transplant recipients. Cancer. 1993;72(5):1612–7.
47. Peterson DE, Schubert MM. Oral toxicity. In: Perry MC, editor. The chemotherapy source book. 3rd ed. Baltimore: Williams and Wilkins; 2001.
48. Ahmed T, Engelking C, Szalyga J, Helson L, Coombe N, Cook P, et al. Propantheline prevention of mucositis from etoposide. Bone Marrow Transplant. 1993;12(2):131–2.
49. Oblon DJ, Paul SR, Oblon MB, Malik S. Propantheline protects the oral mucosa after high-dose ifosfamide, carboplatin, etoposide and autologous stem cell transplantation. Bone Marrow Transplant. 1997;20(11):961–3.
50. Barasch A, Peterson DE. Risk factors for ulcerative oral mucositis in cancer patients: unanswered questions. Oral Oncol. 2003;39(2):91–100.
51. Sonis ST. Mucositis: the impact, biology and therapeutic opportunities of oral mucositis. Oral Oncol. 2009;45(12):1015–20.
52. Martinez JM, Pereira D, Chacim S, Mesquita E, Sousa I, Martins A, et al. Mucositis care in acute leukemia and non-Hodgkin lymphoma patients undergoing high-dose chemotherapy. Support Care Cancer. 2014;22(9):2563–9.
53. Friedenberg WR, Miller HJ, Marx JJ Jr, Schloesser LL, Reding DJ, Mazza JJ, et al. The treatment of older adult patients with acute myeloid leukemia by triple infusion chemotherapy. Am J Clin Oncol. 1995;18(2):105–10.
54. Pea F, Russo D, Michieli M, Damiani D, Fanin R, Michelutti A, et al. Disposition of liposomal daunorubicin during cotreatment with cytarabine in patients with leukaemia. Clin Pharmacokinet. 2003;42(9):851–62.
55. Ferrara F, Palmieri S, Pocali B, Pollio F, Viola A, Annunziata S, et al. De novo acute myeloid leukemia with multilineage dysplasia: treatment results and prognostic evaluation from a series of 44 patients treated with fludarabine, cytarabine and G-CSF (FLAG). Eur J Haematol. 2002;68(4):203–9.
56. Pastore D, Specchia G, Carluccio P, Liso A, Mestice A, Rizzi R, et al. FLAG-IDA in the treatment of refractory/relapsed acute myeloid leukemia: single-center experience. Ann Hematol. 2003;82(4):231–5.
57. Girmenia C, Lo Coco F, Breccia M, Latagliata R, Spadea A, D'Andrea M, et al. Infectious complications in patients with acute promyelocytic leukaemia treated with the AIDA regimen. Leukemia. 2003;17(5):925–30.
58. Testi AM, Biondi A, Lo Coco F, Moleti ML, Giona F, Vignetti M, et al. GIMEMA-AIEOPAIDA protocol for the treatment of newly diagnosed acute promyelocytic leukemia (APL) in children. Blood. 2005;106(2):447–53.
59. Mazza P, Zinzani PL, Martelli M, Fiacchini M, Bocchia M, Pileri S, et al. MACOP-B vs F-MACHOP regimen in the treatment of high-grade non-Hodgkin's lymphomas. Leuk Lymphoma. 1995;16(5–6):457–63.
60. Milone G, Di Raimondo F, Gioi FL, Palumbo GA, Manenti GO, Pafumi M, et al. Alternation of epirubicin and mitoxantrone in CHOP-like regimens retains efficacy and reduces overall toxicity in elderly patients with high and intermediate grade non-Hodgkin lymphomas. Leuk Lymphoma. 2002;43(12):2319–24.

61. Osby E, Hagberg H, Kvaloy S, Teerenhovi L, Anderson H, Cavallin-Stahl E, et al. CHOP is superior to CNOP in elderly patients with aggressive lymphoma while outcome is unaffected by filgrastim treatment: results of a Nordic Lymphoma Group randomized trial. Blood. 2003;101(10):3840–8.
62. Johnson PW, Radford JA, Cullen MH, Sydes MR, Walewski J, Jack AS, et al. Comparison of ABVD and alternating or hybrid multidrug regimens for the treatment of advanced Hodgkin's lymphoma: results of the United Kingdom Lymphoma Group LY09 Trial (ISRCTN97144519). J Clin Oncol. 2005;23(36):9208–18.
63. Bearman SI, Appelbaum FR, Buckner CD, Petersen FB, Fisher LD, Clift RA, et al. Regimen-related toxicity in patients undergoing bone marrow transplantation. J Clin Oncol. 1988;6(10):1562–8.
64. McGuire DB, Altomonte V, Peterson DE, Wingard JR, Jones RJ, Grochow LB. Patterns of mucositis and pain in patients receiving preparative chemotherapy and bone marrow transplantation. Oncol Nurs Forum. 1993;20(10):1493–502.
65. Pico JL, Avila-Garavito A, Naccache P. Mucositis: its occurrence, consequences, and treatment in the oncology setting. Oncologist. 1998;3(6):446–51.
66. Chaudhry HM, Bruce AJ, Wolf RC, Litzow MR, Hogan WJ, Patnaik MS, et al. The incidence and severity of oral mucositis among allogeneic hematopoietic stem cell transplantation patients: a systematic review. Biol Blood Marrow Transplant. 2016;22(4):605–16.
67. McCann S, Schwenkglenks M, Bacon P, Einsele H, D'Addio A, Maertens J, et al. The Prospective Oral Mucositis Audit: relationship of severe oral mucositis with clinical and medical resource use outcomes in patients receiving high-dose melphalan or BEAM-conditioning chemotherapy and autologous SCT. Bone Marrow Transplant. 2009;43(2):141–7.
68. Vagliano L, Feraut C, Gobetto G, Trunfio A, Errico A, Campani V, et al. Incidence and severity of oral mucositis in patients undergoing haematopoietic SCT—results of a multicentre study. Bone Marrow Transplant. 2011;46(5):727–32.
69. Stiff PJ, Erder H, Bensinger WI, Emmanouilides C, Gentile T, Isitt J, et al. Reliability and validity of a patient self-administered daily questionnaire to assess impact of oral mucositis (OM) on pain and daily functioning in patients undergoing autologous hematopoietic stem cell transplantation (HSCT). Bone Marrow Transplant. 2006;37(4):393–401.
70. Bolwell BJ, Kalaycio M, Sobecks R, Andresen S, Kuczkowski E, Bernhard L, et al. A multivariable analysis of factors influencing mucositis after autologous progenitor cell transplantation. Bone Marrow Transplant. 2002;30(9):587–91.
71. Wardley AM, Jayson GC, Swindell R, Morgenstern GR, Chang J, Bloor R, et al. Prospective evaluation of oral mucositis in patients receiving myeloablative conditioning regimens and haemopoietic progenitor rescue. Br J Haematol. 2000;110(2):292–9.
72. Cutler C, Li S, Kim HT, Laglenne P, Szeto KC, Hoffmeister L, et al. Mucositis after allogeneic hematopoietic stem cell transplantation: a cohort study of methotrexate- and non-methotrexate-containing graft-versus-host disease prophylaxis regimens. Biol Blood Marrow Transplant. 2005;11(5):383–8.
73. Ferrara F, Palmieri S, De Simone M, Sagristani M, Viola A, Pocali B, et al. High-dose idarubicin and busulphan as conditioning to autologous stem cell transplantation in adult patients with acute myeloid leukaemia. Br J Haematol. 2005;128(2):234–41.
74. Moreau P, Facon T, Attal M, Hulin C, Michallet M, Maloisel F, et al. Comparison of 200 mg/m(2) melphalan and 8 Gy total body irradiation plus 140 mg/m(2) melphalan as conditioning regimens for peripheral blood stem cell transplantation in patients with newly diagnosed multiple myeloma: final analysis of the Intergroupe Francophone du Myelome 9502 randomized trial. Blood. 2002;99(3):731–5.
75. Palumbo A, Bringhen S, Petrucci MT, Musto P, Rossini F, Nunzi M, et al. Intermediate-dose melphalan improves survival of myeloma patients aged 50 to 70: results of a randomized controlled trial. Blood. 2004;104(10):3052–7.
76. Wang EH, Chen YA, Corringham S, Bashey A, Holman P, Ball ED, et al. High-dose CEB vs BEAM with autologous stem cell transplant in lymphoma. Bone Marrow Transplant. 2004;34(7):581–7.

77. Rapoport AP, Miller Watelet LF, Linder T, Eberly S, Raubertas RF, Lipp J, et al. Analysis of factors that correlate with mucositis in recipients of autologous and allogeneic stem-cell transplants. J Clin Oncol. 1999;17(8):2446–53.
78. Grazziutti ML, Dong L, Miceli MH, Krishna SG, Kiwan E, Syed N, et al. Oral mucositis in myeloma patients undergoing melphalan-based autologous stem cell transplantation: incidence, risk factors and a severity predictive model. Bone Marrow Transplant. 2006;38(7):501–6.
79. Jones JA, Qazilbash MH, Shih YC, Cantor SB, Cooksley CD, Elting LS. In-hospital complications of autologous hematopoietic stem cell transplantation for lymphoid malignancies: clinical and economic outcomes from the Nationwide Inpatient Sample. Cancer. 2008;112(5):1096–105.
80. Martino M, Montanari M, Ferrara F, Ciceri F, Scortechini I, Palmieri S, et al. Very low rate of readmission after an early discharge outpatient model for autografting in multiple myeloma patients: an Italian multicenter retrospective study. Biol Blood Marrow Transplant. 2014;20(7):1026–32.
81. Gupta V, Panzarella T, Li L, Khan J, Sharma A, Lipton JH, et al. A prospective study comparing the outcomes and health-related quality of life in adult patients with myeloid malignancies undergoing allogeneic transplantation using myeloablative or reduced-intensity conditioning. Biol Blood Marrow Transplant. 2012;18(1):113–24.
82. Kashiwazaki H, Matsushita T, Sugita J, Shigematsu A, Kasashi K, Yamazaki Y, et al. A comparison of oral mucositis in allogeneic hematopoietic stem cell transplantation between conventional and reduced-intensity regimens. Support Care Cancer. 2012;20(5):933–9.
83. Urbain P, Raynor A, Bertz H, Lambert C, Biesalski HK. Role of antioxidants in buccal mucosa cells and plasma on the incidence and severity of oral mucositis after allogeneic haematopoietic cell transplantation. Support Care Cancer. 2012;20(8):1831–8.
84. Vera-Llonch M, Oster G, Ford CM, Lu J, Sonis S. Oral mucositis and outcomes of allogeneic hematopoietic stem-cell transplantation in patients with hematologic malignancies. Support Care Cancer. 2007;15(5):491–6.
85. Johansson JE, Brune M, Ekman T. The gut mucosa barrier is preserved during allogeneic, haemopoietic stem cell transplantation with reduced intensity conditioning. Bone Marrow Transplant. 2001;28(8):737–42.
86. Legert KG, Remberger M, Ringden O, Heimdahl A, Dahllof G. Reduced intensity conditioning and oral care measures prevent oral mucositis and reduces days of hospitalization in allogeneic stem cell transplantation recipients. Support Care Cancer. 2014;22(8):2133–40.
87. Anand A, Anandi P, Jain NA, Lu K, Dunavin N, Hourigan CS, et al. CD34+ selection and the severity of oropharyngeal mucositis in total body irradiation-based allogeneic stem cell transplantation. Support Care Cancer. 2016;24(2):815–22.
88. Takahashi K, Soga Y, Murayama Y, Udagawa M, Nishimoto H, Sugiura Y, et al. Oral mucositis in patients receiving reduced-intensity regimens for allogeneic hematopoietic cell transplantation: comparison with conventional regimen. Support Care Cancer. 2010;18(1):115–9.
89. Baselga J, Arteaga CL. Critical update and emerging trends in epidermal growth factor receptor targeting in cancer. J Clin Oncol. 2005;23(11):2445–59.
90. Chan KC, Knox WF, Gee JM, Morris J, Nicholson RI, Potten CS, et al. Effect of epidermal growth factor receptor tyrosine kinase inhibition on epithelial proliferation in normal and premalignant breast. Cancer Res. 2002;62(1):122–8.
91. Haddad RI, Shin DM. Recent advances in head and neck cancer. N Engl J Med. 2008;359(11):1143–54.
92. Kris MG, Natale RB, Herbst RS, Lynch TJ Jr, Prager D, Belani CP, et al. Efficacy of gefitinib, an inhibitor of the epidermal growth factor receptor tyrosine kinase, in symptomatic patients with non-small cell lung cancer: a randomized trial. JAMA. 2003;290(16):2149–58.
93. Stadler WM. Targeted agents for the treatment of advanced renal cell carcinoma. Cancer. 2005;104(11):2323–33.
94. Wong SF. Cetuximab: an epidermal growth factor receptor monoclonal antibody for the treatment of colorectal cancer. Clin Ther. 2005;27(6):684–94.

95. Gold KA, Lee HY, Kim ES. Targeted therapies in squamous cell carcinoma of the head and neck. Cancer. 2009;115(5):922–35.
96. Adjei AA, Molina JR, Mandrekar SJ, Marks R, Reid JR, Croghan G, et al. Phase I trial of sorafenib in combination with gefitinib in patients with refractory or recurrent non-small cell lung cancer. Clin Cancer Res. 2007;13(9):2684–91.
97. Cunningham D, Humblet Y, Siena S, Khayat D, Bleiberg H, Santoro A, et al. Cetuximab monotherapy and cetuximab plus irinotecan in irinotecan-refractory metastatic colorectal cancer. N Engl J Med. 2004;351(4):337–45.
98. Blick SK, Scott LJ. Cetuximab: a review of its use in squamous cell carcinoma of the head and neck and metastatic colorectal cancer. Drugs. 2007;67(17):2585–607.
99. Tejwani A, Wu S, Jia Y, Agulnik M, Millender L, Lacouture ME. Increased risk of high-grade dermatologic toxicities with radiation plus epidermal growth factor receptor inhibitor therapy. Cancer. 2009;115(6):1286–99.
100. Pryor DI, Porceddu SV, Burmeister BH, Guminski A, Thomson DB, Shepherdson K, et al. Enhanced toxicity with concurrent cetuximab and radiotherapy in head and neck cancer. Radiother Oncol. 2009;90(2):172–6.
101. Belani CP, Schreeder MT, Steis RG, Guidice RA, Marsland TA, Butler EH, et al. Cetuximab in combination with carboplatin and docetaxel for patients with metastatic or advanced-stage nonsmall cell lung cancer: a multicenter phase 2 study. Cancer. 2008;113(9):2512–7.
102. Lenz HJ. Anti-EGFR mechanism of action: antitumor effect and underlying cause of adverse events. Oncology. 2006;20(5 Suppl 2):5–13.
103. Motzer RJ, Amato R, Todd M, Hwu WJ, Cohen R, Baselga J, et al. Phase II trial of antiepidermal growth factor receptor antibody C225 in patients with advanced renal cell carcinoma. Investig New Drugs. 2003;21(1):99–101.
104. Reynolds NA, Wagstaff AJ. Cetuximab: in the treatment of metastatic colorectal cancer. Drugs. 2004;64(1):109–18.
105. Saltz LB, Meropol NJ, Loehrer PJ Sr, Needle MN, Kopit J, Mayer RJ. Phase II trial of cetuximab in patients with refractory colorectal cancer that expresses the epidermal growth factor receptor. J Clin Oncol. 2004;22(7):1201–8.
106. Thomas M. Cetuximab: adverse event profile and recommendations for toxicity management. Clin J Oncol Nurs. 2005;9(3):332–8.
107. Vermorken JB, Mesia R, Rivera F, Remenar E, Kawecki A, Rottey S, et al. Platinum-based chemotherapy plus cetuximab in head and neck cancer. N Engl J Med. 2008;359(11):1116–27.
108. Vermorken JB, Trigo J, Hitt R, Koralewski P, Diaz-Rubio E, Rolland F, et al. Open-label, uncontrolled, multicenter phase II study to evaluate the efficacy and toxicity of cetuximab as a single agent in patients with recurrent and/or metastatic squamous cell carcinoma of the head and neck who failed to respond to platinum-based therapy. J Clin Oncol. 2007;25(16):2171–7.
109. Xiong HQ, Rosenberg A, LoBuglio A, Schmidt W, Wolff RA, Deutsch J, et al. Cetuximab, a monoclonal antibody targeting the epidermal growth factor receptor, in combination with gemcitabine for advanced pancreatic cancer: a multicenter phase II Trial. J Clin Oncol. 2004;22(13):2610–6.
110. Van Cutsem E, Peeters M, Siena S, Humblet Y, Hendlisz A, Neyns B, et al. Open-label phase III trial of panitumumab plus best supportive care compared with best supportive care alone in patients with chemotherapy-refractory metastatic colorectal cancer. J Clin Oncol. 2007;25(13):1658–64.
111. Van Cutsem E, Siena S, Humblet Y, Canon JL, Maurel J, Bajetta E, et al. An open-label, single-arm study assessing safety and efficacy of panitumumab in patients with metastatic colorectal cancer refractory to standard chemotherapy. Ann Oncol. 2008;19(1):92–8.
112. Rowinsky EK, Schwartz GH, Gollob JA, Thompson JA, Vogelzang NJ, Figlin R, et al. Safety, pharmacokinetics, and activity of ABX-EGF, a fully human anti-epidermal growth factor receptor monoclonal antibody in patients with metastatic renal cell cancer. J Clin Oncol. 2004;22(15):3003–15.
113. Giusti RM, Shastri KA, Cohen MH, Keegan P, Pazdur R. FDA drug approval summary: panitumumab (Vectibix). Oncologist. 2007;12(5):577–83.

114. Muro K, Yoshino T, Doi T, Shirao K, Takiuchi H, Hamamoto Y, et al. A phase 2 clinical trial of panitumumab monotherapy in Japanese patients with metastatic colorectal cancer. Jpn J Clin Oncol. 2009;39(5):321–6.
115. Weiner LM, Belldegrun AS, Crawford J, Tolcher AW, Lockbaum P, Arends RH, et al. Dose and schedule study of panitumumab monotherapy in patients with advanced solid malignancies. Clin Cancer Res. 2008;14(2):502–8.
116. Kinnings SL, Jackson RM. Binding site similarity analysis for the functional classification of the protein kinase family. J Chem Inf Model. 2009;49(2):318–29.
117. Wang LX, Agulnik M. Promising newer molecular-targeted therapies in head and neck cancer. Drugs. 2008;68(12):1609–19.
118. Laurent-Puig P, Taieb J. Lessons from Tarceva in pancreatic cancer: where are we now, and how should future trials be designed in pancreatic cancer? Curr Opin Oncol. 2008;20(4):454–8.
119. Shepherd FA, Rodrigues Pereira J, Ciuleanu T, Tan EH, Hirsh V, Thongprasert S, et al. Erlotinib in previously treated non-small-cell lung cancer. N Engl J Med. 2005;353(2):123–32.
120. Sandler AB. Nondermatologic adverse events associated with anti-EGFR therapy. Oncology. 2006;20(5 Suppl 2):35–40.
121. Elting LS, Chang YC, Parelkar P, Boers-Doets CB, Michelet M, Hita G, et al. Risk of oral and gastrointestinal mucosal injury among patients receiving selected targeted agents: a meta-analysis. Support Care Cancer. 2013;21(11):3243–54.
122. Sequist LV, Yang JC, Yamamoto N, O'Byrne K, Hirsh V, Mok T, et al. Phase III study of afatinib or cisplatin plus pemetrexed in patients with metastatic lung adenocarcinoma with EGFR mutations. J Clin Oncol. 2013;31(27):3327–34.
123. Bukowski RM. Systemic therapy for metastatic renal cell carcinoma in treatment naive patients: a risk-based approach. Expert Opin Pharmacother. 2010;11(14):2351–62.
124. Shameem R, Lacouture M, Wu S. Incidence and risk of high-grade stomatitis with mTOR inhibitors in cancer patients. Cancer Investig. 2015;33(3):70–7.
125. Boers-Doets CB, Raber-Durlacher JE, Treister NS, Epstein JB, Arends AB, Wiersma DR, et al. Mammalian target of rapamycin inhibitor-associated stomatitis. Future Oncol. 2013;9(12):1883–92.
126. Amato RJ, Jac J, Giessinger S, Saxena S, Willis JP. A phase 2 study with a daily regimen of the oral mTOR inhibitor RAD001 (everolimus) in patients with metastatic clear cell renal cell cancer. Cancer. 2009;115(11):2438–46.
127. Wolpin BM, Hezel AF, Abrams T, Blaszkowsky LS, Meyerhardt JA, Chan JA, et al. Oral mTOR inhibitor everolimus in patients with gemcitabine-refractory metastatic pancreatic cancer. J Clin Oncol. 2009;27(2):193–8.
128. Motzer RJ, Escudier B, Oudard S, Hutson TE, Porta C, Bracarda S, et al. Phase 3 trial of everolimus for metastatic renal cell carcinoma: final results and analysis of prognostic factors. Cancer. 2010;116(18):4256–65.
129. Porta C, Osanto S, Ravaud A, Climent MA, Vaishampayan U, White DA, et al. Management of adverse events associated with the use of everolimus in patients with advanced renal cell carcinoma. Eur J Cancer. 2011;47(9):1287–98.
130. Raymond E, Alexandre J, Faivre S, Vera K, Materman E, Boni J, et al. Safety and pharmacokinetics of escalated doses of weekly intravenous infusion of CCI-779, a novel mTOR inhibitor, in patients with cancer. J Clin Oncol. 2004;22(12):2336–47.
131. Gridelli C, Maione P, Rossi A. The potential role of mTOR inhibitors in non-small cell lung cancer. Oncologist. 2008;13(2):139–47.
132. Bellmunt J, Szczylik C, Feingold J, Strahs A, Berkenblit A. Temsirolimus safety profile and management of toxic effects in patients with advanced renal cell carcinoma and poor prognostic features. Ann Oncol. 2008;19(8):1387–92.
133. Kwitkowski VE, Prowell TM, Ibrahim A, Farrell AT, Justice R, Mitchell SS, et al. FDA approval summary: temsirolimus as treatment for advanced renal cell carcinoma. Oncologist. 2010;15(4):428–35.
134. Mita MM, Mita AC, Chu QS, Rowinsky EK, Fetterly GJ, Goldston M, et al. Phase I trial of the novel mammalian target of rapamycin inhibitor deforolimus (AP23573; MK-8669)

administered intravenously daily for 5 days every 2 weeks to patients with advanced malignancies. J Clin Oncol. 2008;26(3):361–7.
135. Yuan A, Kurtz SL, Barysauskas CM, Pilotte AP, Wagner AJ, Treister NS. Oral adverse events in cancer patients treated with VEGFR-directed multitargeted tyrosine kinase inhibitors. Oral Oncol. 2015;51(11):1026–33.
136. Kennedy JA, Hobbs G. Tyrosine kinase inhibitors in the treatment of chronic-phase CML: strategies for frontline decision-making. Curr Hematol Malig Rep. 2018;13(3):202–11.
137. Watson GA, Kelly D, Melland-Smith M, Gleeson J, McEntee G, Kelly CM, et al. Get the GIST? An overview of gastrointestinal stromal tumours. Ir J Med Sci. 2016;185(2):319–26.
138. Ryu MH, Kang WK, Bang YJ, Lee KH, Shin DB, Ryoo BY, et al. A prospective, multicenter, phase 2 study of imatinib mesylate in Korean patients with metastatic or unresectable gastrointestinal stromal tumor. Oncology. 2009;76(5):326–32.
139. Kloos RT, Ringel MD, Knopp MV, Hall NC, King M, Stevens R, et al. Phase II trial of sorafenib in metastatic thyroid cancer. J Clin Oncol. 2009;27(10):1675–84.
140. da Motta Girardi D, Correa TS, Crosara Teixeira M, Dos Santos Fernandes G. Hepatocellular carcinoma: review of targeted and immune therapies. J Gastrointest Cancer. 2018;28(10):018–0121.
141. Coppin C, Kollmannsberger C, Le L, Porzsolt F, Wilt TJ. Targeted therapy for advanced renal cell cancer (RCC): a Cochrane systematic review of published randomised trials. BJU Int. 2011;108(10):1556–63.
142. Chi KN, Ellard SL, Hotte SJ, Czaykowski P, Moore M, Ruether JD, et al. A phase II study of sorafenib in patients with chemo-naive castration-resistant prostate cancer. Ann Oncol. 2008;19(4):746–51.
143. Duran I, Hotte SJ, Hirte H, Chen EX, MacLean M, Turner S, et al. Phase I targeted combination trial of sorafenib and erlotinib in patients with advanced solid tumors. Clin Cancer Res. 2007;13(16):4849–57.
144. Eisen T, Ahmad T, Flaherty KT, Gore M, Kaye S, Marais R, et al. Sorafenib in advanced melanoma: a phase II randomised discontinuation trial analysis. Br J Cancer. 2006;95(5):581–6.
145. Escudier B, Szczylik C, Hutson TE, Demkow T, Staehler M, Rolland F, et al. Randomized phase II trial of first-line treatment with sorafenib versus interferon Alfa-2a in patients with metastatic renal cell carcinoma. J Clin Oncol. 2009;27(8):1280–9.
146. Herrmann E, Bierer S, Gerss J, Kopke T, Hertle L, Wulfing C. Prospective comparison of sorafenib and sunitinib for second-line treatment of cytokine-refractory kidney cancer patients. Oncology. 2008;74(3–4):216–22.
147. Mross K, Steinbild S, Baas F, Gmehling D, Radtke M, Voliotis D, et al. Results from an in vitro and a clinical/pharmacological phase I study with the combination irinotecan and sorafenib. Eur J Cancer. 2007;43(1):55–63.
148. Richly H, Henning BF, Kupsch P, Passarge K, Grubert M, Hilger RA, et al. Results of a phase I trial of sorafenib (BAY 43-9006) in combination with doxorubicin in patients with refractory solid tumors. Ann Oncol. 2006;17(5):866–73.
149. Siu LL, Awada A, Takimoto CH, Piccart M, Schwartz B, Giannaris T, et al. Phase I trial of sorafenib and gemcitabine in advanced solid tumors with an expanded cohort in advanced pancreatic cancer. Clin Cancer Res. 2006;12(1):144–51.
150. Lee WJ, Lee JL, Chang SE, Lee MW, Kang YK, Choi JH, et al. Cutaneous adverse effects in patients treated with the multitargeted kinase inhibitors sorafenib and sunitinib. Br J Dermatol. 2009;161(5):1045–51.
151. Awada A, Hendlisz A, Gil T, Bartholomeus S, Mano M, de Valeriola D, et al. Phase I safety and pharmacokinetics of BAY 43-9006 administered for 21 days on/7 days off in patients with advanced, refractory solid tumours. Br J Cancer. 2005;92(10):1855–61.
152. Procopio G, Verzoni E, Gevorgyan A, Mancin M, Pusceddu S, Catena L, et al. Safety and activity of sorafenib in different histotypes of advanced renal cell carcinoma. Oncology. 2007;73(3–4):204–9.
153. Riechelmann RP, Chin S, Wang L, Tannock IF, Berthold DR, Moore MJ, et al. Sorafenib for metastatic renal cancer: the Princess Margaret experience. Am J Clin Oncol. 2008;31(2):182–7.

154. Strumberg D, Clark JW, Awada A, Moore MJ, Richly H, Hendlisz A, et al. Safety, pharmacokinetics, and preliminary antitumor activity of sorafenib: a review of four phase I trials in patients with advanced refractory solid tumors. Oncologist. 2007;12(4):426–37.
155. Llovet JM, Ricci S, Mazzaferro V, Hilgard P, Gane E, Blanc JF, et al. Sorafenib in advanced hepatocellular carcinoma. N Engl J Med. 2008;359(4):378–90.
156. George S, Blay JY, Casali PG, Le Cesne A, Stephenson P, Deprimo SE, et al. Clinical evaluation of continuous daily dosing of sunitinib malate in patients with advanced gastrointestinal stromal tumour after imatinib failure. Eur J Cancer. 2009;45(11):1959–68.
157. Motzer RJ, Hutson TE, Tomczak P, Michaelson MD, Bukowski RM, Rixe O, et al. Sunitinib versus interferon alfa in metastatic renal-cell carcinoma. N Engl J Med. 2007;356(2):115–24.
158. Uemura H, Shinohara N, Yuasa T, Tomita Y, Fujimoto H, Niwakawa M, et al. A phase II study of sunitinib in Japanese patients with metastatic renal cell carcinoma: insights into the treatment, efficacy and safety. Jpn J Clin Oncol. 2010;40(3):194–202.
159. Adams VR, Leggas M. Sunitinib malate for the treatment of metastatic renal cell carcinoma and gastrointestinal stromal tumors. Clin Ther. 2007;29(7):1338–53.
160. Ferrara N, Hillan KJ, Gerber HP, Novotny W. Discovery and development of bevacizumab, an anti-VEGF antibody for treating cancer. Nat Rev Drug Discov. 2004;3(5):391–400.
161. Herbst RS, Sandler A. Bevacizumab and erlotinib: a promising new approach to the treatment of advanced NSCLC. Oncologist. 2008;13(11):1166–76.
162. Agulnik M, Cohen EW, Cohen RB, Chen EX, Vokes EE, Hotte SJ, et al. Phase II study of lapatinib in recurrent or metastatic epidermal growth factor receptor and/or erbB2 expressing adenoid cystic carcinoma and non adenoid cystic carcinoma malignant tumors of the salivary glands. J Clin Oncol. 2007;25(25):3978–84.
163. Chu QS, Cianfrocca ME, Goldstein LJ, Gale M, Murray N, Loftiss J, et al. A phase I and pharmacokinetic study of lapatinib in combination with letrozole in patients with advanced cancer. Clin Cancer Res. 2008;14(14):4484–90.
164. Nakagawa K, Minami H, Kanezaki M, Mukaiyama A, Minamide Y, Uejima H, et al. Phase I dose-escalation and pharmacokinetic trial of lapatinib (GW572016), a selective oral dual inhibitor of ErbB-1 and -2 tyrosine kinases, in Japanese patients with solid tumors. Jpn J Clin Oncol. 2009;39(2):116–23.
165. Sonis ST, Sonis AL, Lieberman A. Oral complications in patients receiving treatment for malignancies other than of the head and neck. J Am Dent Assoc. 1978;97(3):468–72.
166. McCarthy GM, Awde JD, Ghandi H, Vincent M, Kocha WI. Risk factors associated with mucositis in cancer patients receiving 5-fluorouracil. Oral Oncol. 1998;34(6):484–90.
167. Zalcberg J, Kerr D, Seymour L, Palmer M. Haematological and non-haematological toxicity after 5-fluorouracil and leucovorin in patients with advanced colorectal cancer is significantly associated with gender, increasing age and cycle number. Tomudex International Study Group. Eur J Cancer. 1998;34(12):1871–5.
168. Berger AM, Eilers J. Factors influencing oral cavity status during high-dose antineoplastic therapy: a secondary data analysis. Oncol Nurs Forum. 1998;25(9):1623–6.
169. Eilers J, Million R. Prevention and management of oral mucositis in patients with cancer. Semin Oncol Nurs. 2007;23(3):201–12.
170. Maria OM, Eliopoulos N, Muanza T. Radiation-induced oral mucositis. Front Oncol. 2017;7:89.
171. Chansky K, Benedetti J, Macdonald JS. Differences in toxicity between men and women treated with 5-fluorouracil therapy for colorectal carcinoma. Cancer. 2005;103(6):1165–71.
172. Sloan JA, Goldberg RM, Sargent DJ, Vargas-Chanes D, Nair S, Cha SS, et al. Women experience greater toxicity with fluorouracil-based chemotherapy for colorectal cancer. J Clin Oncol. 2002;20(6):1491–8.
173. Raber-Durlacher JE. Current practices for management of oral mucositis in cancer patients. Support Care Cancer. 1999;7(2):71–4.
174. Chen SC, Lai YH, Huang BS, Lin CY, Fan KH, Chang JT. Changes and predictors of radiation-induced oral mucositis in patients with oral cavity cancer during active treatment. Eur J Oncol Nurs. 2015;19(3):214–9.

175. Yarom N, Hovan A, Bossi P, Ariyawardana A, Jensen SB, Gobbo M, et al. Systematic review of natural and miscellaneous agents for the management of oral mucositis in cancer patients and clinical practice guidelines-Part 1: Vitamins, minerals, and nutritional supplements. Support Care Cancer. 2019;27(10):3997–4010.
176. Luo DH, Hong MH, Guo L, Cao KJ, Deng MQ, Mo HY. Analysis of oral mucositis risk factors during radiotherapy for nasopharyngeal carcinoma patients and establishment of a discriminant model. Ai Zheng. 2005;24(7):850–4.
177. Patussi C, Sassi LM, Munhoz EC, Zanicotti RT, Schussel JL. Clinical assessment of oral mucositis and candidiasis compare to chemotherapic nadir in transplanted patients. Braz Oral Res. 2014;28:1–7.
178. Robien K, Schubert MM, Bruemmer B, Lloid ME, Potter JD, Ulrich CM. Predictors of oral mucositis in patients receiving hematopoietic cell transplants for chronic myelogenous leukemia. J Clin Oncol. 2004;22(7):1268–75.
179. Evans WE, McLeod HL. Pharmacogenomics—drug disposition, drug targets, and side effects. N Engl J Med. 2003;348(6):538–49.
180. Robien K, Schubert MM, Chay T, Bigler J, Storb R, Yasui Y, et al. Methylenetetrahydrofolate reductase and thymidylate synthase genotypes modify oral mucositis severity following hematopoietic stem cell transplantation. Bone Marrow Transplant. 2006;37(8):799–800. https://doi.org/10.1038/sj.bmt.1705330.
181. Salavaggione OE, Wang L, Wiepert M, Yee VC, Weinshilboum RM. Thiopurine S-methyltransferase pharmacogenetics: variant allele functional and comparative genomics. Pharmacogenet Genomics. 2005;15(11):801–15.
182. Bogunia-Kubik K, Polak M, Lange A. TNF polymorphisms are associated with toxic but not with aGVHD complications in the recipients of allogeneic sibling haematopoietic stem cell transplantation. Bone Marrow Transplant. 2003;32(6):617–22.
183. Hahn T, Zhelnova E, Sucheston L, Demidova I, Savchenko V, Battiwalla M, et al. A deletion polymorphism in glutathione-S-transferase mu (GSTM1) and/or theta (GSTT1) is associated with an increased risk of toxicity after autologous blood and marrow transplantation. Biol Blood Marrow Transplant. 2010;16(6):801–8.
184. Wardill HR, Sonis ST, Blijlevens NMA, et al. Prediction of mucositis risk secondary to cancer therapy: a systematic review of current evidence and call to action. Support Care Cancer. 2020;28:5059–73. https://doi.org/10.1007/s00520-020-05579-7.
185. Ostman A, Augsten M. Cancer-associated fibroblasts and tumor growth—bystanders turning into key players. Curr Opin Genet Dev. 2009;19(1):67–73.
186. Pries R, Wollenberg B. Cytokines in head and neck cancer. Cytokine Growth Factor Rev. 2006;17(3):141–6.
187. Bondi E, Baroni C, Prete A, Gatti M, Carrassi A, Lodi G, et al. Local antimicrobial therapy of oral mucositis in paediatric patients undergoing bone marrow transplantation. Oral Oncol. 1997;33(5):322–6.
188. Dodd MJ, Larson PJ, Dibble SL, Miaskowski C, Greenspan D, MacPhail L, et al. Randomized clinical trial of chlorhexidine versus placebo for prevention of oral mucositis in patients receiving chemotherapy. Oncol Nurs Forum. 1996;23(6):921–7.
189. Epstein JB, Vickars L, Spinelli J, Reece D. Efficacy of chlorhexidine and nystatin rinses in prevention of oral complications in leukemia and bone marrow transplantation. Oral Surg Oral Med Oral Pathol. 1992;73(6):682–9.
190. Ferretti GA, Raybould TP, Brown AT, Macdonald JS, Greenwood M, Maruyama Y, et al. Chlorhexidine prophylaxis for chemotherapy- and radiotherapy-induced stomatitis: a randomized double-blind trial. Oral Surg Oral Med Oral Pathol. 1990;69(3):331–8.
191. Foote RL, Loprinzi CL, Frank AR, O'Fallon JR, Gulavita S, Tewfik HH, et al. Randomized trial of a chlorhexidine mouthwash for alleviation of radiation-induced mucositis. J Clin Oncol. 1994;12(12):2630–3.
192. Loury D, Embree JR, Steinberg DA, Sonis ST, Fiddes JC. Effect of local application of the antimicrobial peptide IB-367 on the incidence and severity of oral mucositis in hamsters. Oral Surg Oral Med Oral Pathol Oral Radiol Endod. 1999;87(5):544–51.

193. Spijkervet FK, van Saene HK, Panders AK, Vermey A, van Saene JJ, Mehta DM, et al. Effect of chlorhexidine rinsing on the oropharyngeal ecology in patients with head and neck cancer who have irradiation mucositis. Oral Surg Oral Med Oral Pathol. 1989;67(2):154–61.
194. Wahlin YB. Effects of chlorhexidine mouthrinse on oral health in patients with acute leukemia. Oral Surg Oral Med Oral Pathol. 1989;68(3):279–87.
195. Bodey GP, Rodriguez V, Chang HY, Narboni. Fever and infection in leukemic patients: a study of 494 consecutive patients. Cancer. 1978;41(4):1610–22.
196. El-Sayed S, Nabid A, Shelley W, Hay J, Balogh J, Gelinas M, et al. Prophylaxis of radiation-associated mucositis in conventionally treated patients with head and neck cancer: a double-blind, phase III, randomized, controlled trial evaluating the clinical efficacy of an antimicrobial lozenge using a validated mucositis scoring system. J Clin Oncol. 2002;20(19):3956–63.
197. Rand KH, Kramer B, Johnson AC. Cancer chemotherapy associated symptomatic stomatitis: role of herpes simplex virus (HSV). Cancer. 1982;50(7):1262–5.
198. Djuric M, Jankovic L, Jovanovic T, Pavlica D, Brkic S, Knezevic A, et al. Prevalence of oral herpes simplex virus reactivation in cancer patients: a comparison of different techniques of viral detection. J Oral Pathol Med. 2009;38(2):167–73.
199. Woo SB, Sonis ST, Sonis AL. The role of herpes simplex virus in the development of oral mucositis in bone marrow transplant recipients. Cancer. 1990;66(11):2375–9.
200. Feld R. The role of surveillance cultures in patients likely to develop chemotherapy-induced mucositis. Support Care Cancer. 1997;5(5):371–5.
201. Lockhart PB, Brennan MT, Kent ML, Packman CH, Norton HJ, Fox PC, et al. Randomized controlled trial of pilocarpine hydrochloride for the moderation of oral mucositis during autologous blood stem cell transplantation. Bone Marrow Transplant. 2005;35(7):713–20.
202. Scarantino C, LeVeque F, Swann RS, White R, Schulsinger A, Hodson DI, et al. Effect of pilocarpine during radiation therapy: results of RTOG 97-09, a phase III randomized study in head and neck cancer patients. J Support Oncol. 2006;4(5):252–8.
203. Sonis ST. A biological approach to mucositis. J Support Oncol. 2004;2(1):21–32.
204. Sonis ST. Pathobiology of mucositis. Semin Oncol Nurs. 2004;20(1):11–5.
205. Song SJ, Han K, Lee SS, Park JB. Association between the number of natural teeth and diabetic retinopathy among type 2 diabetes mellitus: the Korea national health and nutrition examination survey. Medicine. 2017;96(47):0000000000008694.
206. Elad S, Yarom N, Zadik Y, Kuten-Shorrer M, Sonis ST. The broadening scope of oral mucositis and oral ulcerative mucosal toxicities of anticancer therapies. CA Cancer J Clin. 2021;29. https://doi.org/10.3322/caac.21704. Online ahead of print. PMID: 34714553.
207. Kojima I, Sakamoto M, Iikubo M, Kumamoto H, Muroi A, Sugawara Y, et al. Diagnostic performance of MR imaging of three major salivary glands for Sjogren's syndrome. Oral Dis. 2017;23(1):84–90.
208. Eslamipour F, Borzabadi-Farahani A, Asgari I. The relationship between aging and oral health inequalities assessed by the DMFT index. Eur J Paediatr Dent. 2010;11(4):193–9.
209. Zimmermann H, Hagenfeld D, Diercke K, El-Sayed N, Fricke J, Greiser KH, et al. Pocket depth and bleeding on probing and their associations with dental, lifestyle, socioeconomic and blood variables: a cross-sectional, multicenter feasibility study of the German National Cohort. BMC Oral Health. 2015;15(7):1472–6831.
210. Sonis ST. The biologic role for nuclear factor-kappaB in disease and its potential involvement in mucosal injury associated with anti-neoplastic therapy. Crit Rev Oral Biol Med. 2002;13(5):380–9.
211. Lee HK, Lee KD, Merchant AT, Lee SK, Song KB, Lee SG, et al. More missing teeth are associated with poorer general health in the rural Korean elderly. Arch Gerontol Geriatr. 2010;50(1):30–3.
212. Aoyama N, Suzuki JI, Kobayashi N, Hanatani T, Ashigaki N, Yoshida A, et al. Japanese cardiovascular disease patients with diabetes mellitus suffer increased tooth loss in comparison to those without diabetes mellitus—a cross-sectional study. Intern Med. 2018;57(6):777–82.

213. Nakamura T, Oshiumi Y, Yonetsu K, Muranaka T, Sakai K, Kanda S. Salivary SPECT and factor analysis in Sjogren's syndrome. Acta Radiol. 1991;32(5):406–10.
214. Pimentel EL, Azevedo VM, Castro Rde A, Reis LC, De Lorenzo A. Caries experience in young children with congenital heart disease in a developing country. Braz Oral Res. 2013;27(2):103–8.
215. Berger K, Schopohl D, Bollig A, Strobach D, Rieger C, Rublee D, et al. Burden of oral mucositis: a systematic review and implications for future research. Oncol Res Treat. 2018;41(6):399–405.
216. Sikka M, Sequeira PS, Acharya S, Bhat M, Rao A, Nagaraj A. Poor oral health in patients with coronary heart disease: a case-control study of Indian adults. N Z Med J. 2011;124(1347):53–62.
217. Shin HS. Association between the number of teeth and hypertension in a study based on 13,561 participants. J Periodontol. 2018;89(4):397–406.
218. Musskopf ML, Daudt LD, Weidlich P, Gerchman F, Gross JL, Oppermann RV. Metabolic syndrome as a risk indicator for periodontal disease and tooth loss. Clin Oral Investig. 2017;21(2):675–83.
219. Sharda AJ, Shetty S. Relationship of periodontal status and dental caries status with oral health knowledge, attitude and behavior among professional students in India. Int J Oral Sci. 2009;1(4):196–206.
220. Shin HS. The number of teeth is inversely associated with metabolic syndrome: a Korean nationwide population-based study. J Periodontol. 2017;88(9):830–8.
221. Cao X, Wang D, Zhou J, Yuan H, Chen Z. Relationship between dental caries and metabolic syndrome among 13,998 middle-aged urban Chinese. J Diabetes. 2017;9(4):378–85.
222. Tonami H, Ogawa Y, Matoba M, Kuginuki Y, Yokota H, Higashi K, et al. MR sialography in patients with Sjogren syndrome. AJNR Am J Neuroradiol. 1998;19(7):1199–203.
223. de Clerck LS, Corthouts R, Francx L, Brussaard C, de Schepper A, Vercruysse HA, et al. Ultrasonography and computer tomography of the salivary glands in the evaluation of Sjogren's syndrome. Comparison with parotid sialography. J Rheumatol. 1988;15(12):1777–81.
224. Eke PI, Dye BA, Wei L, Slade GD, Thornton-Evans GO, Borgnakke WS, et al. Update on prevalence of periodontitis in adults in the United States: NHANES 2009 to 2012. J Periodontol. 2015;86(5):611–22.
225. DeStefano F, Anda RF, Kahn HS, Williamson DF, Russell CM. Dental disease and risk of coronary heart disease and mortality. BMJ. 1993;306(6879):688–91.
226. Najafipour H, Malek Mohammadi T, Rahim F, Haghdoost AA, Shadkam M, Afshari M. Association of oral health and cardiovascular disease risk factors "results from a community based study on 5900 adult subjects". ISRN Cardiol. 2013;9:782126.
227. Jadu FM, Hill ML, Yaffe MJ, Lam EW. Optimization of exposure parameters for cone beam computed tomography sialography. Dentomaxillofac Radiol. 2011;40(6):362–8.
228. Joshipura KJ, Rimm EB, Douglass CW, Trichopoulos D, Ascherio A, Willett WC. Poor oral health and coronary heart disease. J Dent Res. 1996;75(9):1631–6.
229. Song GG, Lee YH. Diagnostic accuracies of sialography and salivary ultrasonography in Sjogren's syndrome patients: a meta-analysis. Clin Exp Rheumatol. 2014;32(4):516–22.
230. Ali HM, Mustafa M, Hasabalrasol S, Elshazali OH, Nasir EF, Ali RW, et al. Presence of plaque, gingivitis and caries in Sudanese children with congenital heart defects. Clin Oral Investig. 2017;21(4):1299–307.
231. Bernabe E, Sheiham A. Age, period and cohort trends in caries of permanent teeth in four developed countries. Am J Public Health. 2014;104(7):15.
232. Franco E, Saunders CP, Roberts GJ, Suwanprasit A. Dental disease, caries related microflora and salivary IgA of children with severe congenital cardiac disease: an epidemiological and oral microbial survey. Pediatr Dent. 1996;18(3):228–35.
233. Delgado-Perez VJ, De La Rosa-Santillana R, Marquez-Corona ML, Avila-Burgos L, Islas-Granillo H, Minaya-Sanchez M, et al. Diabetes or hypertension as risk indicators for missing teeth experience: an exploratory study in a sample of Mexican adults. Niger J Clin Pract. 2017;20(10):1335–41.

234. Jansson L, Lavstedt S, Frithiof L, Theobald H. Relationship between oral health and mortality in cardiovascular diseases. J Clin Periodontol. 2001;28(8):762–8.
235. Peterson DE. Research advances in oral mucositis. Curr Opin Oncol. 1999;11(4):261–6.
236. Sonis ST. Mucositis as a biological process: a new hypothesis for the development of chemotherapy-induced stomatotoxicity. Oral Oncol. 1998;34(1):39–43.
237. Blijlevens N, Schwenkglenks M, Bacon P, D'Addio A, Einsele H, Maertens J, et al. Prospective oral mucositis audit: oral mucositis in patients receiving high-dose melphalan or BEAM conditioning chemotherapy—European Blood and Marrow Transplantation Mucositis Advisory Group. J Clin Oncol. 2008;26(9):1519–25.
238. Elad S, Zadik Y. Chronic oral mucositis after radiotherapy to the head and neck: a new insight. Support Care Cancer. 2016;24(11):4825–30.
239. Lalla RV, Treister N, Sollecito T, Schmidt B, Patton LL, Mohammadi K, et al. Oral complications at 6 months after radiation therapy for head and neck cancer. Oral Dis. 2017;23(8):1134–43.
240. McGuire DB, Yeager KA, Dudley WN, Peterson DE, Owen DC, Lin LS, et al. Acute oral pain and mucositis in bone marrow transplant and leukemia patients: data from a pilot study. Cancer Nurs. 1998;21(6):385–93.
241. Chapko MK, Syrjala KL, Schilter L, Cummings C, Sullivan KM. Chemoradiotherapy toxicity during bone marrow transplantation: time course and variation in pain and nausea. Bone Marrow Transplant. 1989;4(2):181–6.
242. Miaskowski C. Biology of mucosal pain. J Natl Cancer Inst Monogr. 2001;29:37–40.
243. Harris DJ, Eilers J, Harriman A, Cashavelly BJ, Maxwell C. Putting evidence into practice: evidence-based interventions for the management of oral mucositis. Clin J Oncol Nurs. 2008;12(1):141–52.
244. Lalla RV, Sonis ST, Peterson DE. Management of oral mucositis in patients who have cancer. Dent Clin N Am. 2008;52(1):61–77.
245. Sonis S, Treister N, Chawla S, Demetri G, Haluska F. Preliminary characterization of oral lesions associated with inhibitors of mammalian target of rapamycin in cancer patients. Cancer. 2010;116(1):210–5.
246. de Oliveira MA, Martins EMF, Wang Q, Sonis S, Demetri G, George S, et al. Clinical presentation and management of mTOR inhibitor-associated stomatitis. Oral Oncol. 2011;47(10):998–1003.
247. Martins F, de Oliveira MA, Wang Q, Sonis S, Gallottini M, George S, et al. A review of oral toxicity associated with mTOR inhibitor therapy in cancer patients. Oral Oncol. 2013;49(4):293–8.
248. Yuan R, Kay A, Berg WJ, Lebwohl D. Targeting tumorigenesis: development and use of mTOR inhibitors in cancer therapy. J Hematol Oncol. 2009;2(45):1756–8722.
249. Pavel ME, Hainsworth JD, Baudin E, Peeters M, Horsch D, Winkler RE, et al. Everolimus plus octreotide long-acting repeatable for the treatment of advanced neuroendocrine tumours associated with carcinoid syndrome (RADIANT-2): a randomised, placebo-controlled, phase 3 study. Lancet. 2011;378(9808):2005–12.
250. Lacouture ME, Maitland ML, Segaert S, Setser A, Baran R, Fox LP, et al. A proposed EGFR inhibitor dermatologic adverse event-specific grading scale from the MASCC skin toxicity study group. Support Care Cancer. 2010;18(4):509–22.
251. Sonis ST, Oster G, Fuchs H, Bellm L, Bradford WZ, Edelsberg J, et al. Oral mucositis and the clinical and economic outcomes of hematopoietic stem-cell transplantation. J Clin Oncol. 2001;19(8):2201–5.
252. Cohen J, Donnelly JP, Worsley AM, Catovsky D, Goldman JM, Galton DA. Septicaemia caused by viridans streptococci in neutropenic patients with leukaemia. Lancet. 1983;2(8365–66):1452–4.
253. Elting LS, Bodey GP, Keefe BH. Septicemia and shock syndrome due to viridans streptococci: a case-control study of predisposing factors. Clin Infect Dis. 1992;14(6):1201–7.
254. Wingard JR, Niehaus CS, Peterson DE, Jones RJ, Piantadosi S, Levin LS, et al. Oral mucositis after bone marrow transplantation. A marker of treatment toxicity and predictor of hepatic veno-occlusive disease. Oral Surg Oral Med Oral Pathol. 1991;72(4):419–24.

255. Elting LS, Cooksley CD, Chambers MS, Garden AS. Risk, outcomes, and costs of radiation-induced oral mucositis among patients with head-and-neck malignancies. Int J Radiat Oncol Biol Phys. 2007;68(4):1110–20.
256. Elting LS, Keefe DM, Sonis ST, Garden AS, Spijkervet FK, Barasch A, et al. Patient-reported measurements of oral mucositis in head and neck cancer patients treated with radiotherapy with or without chemotherapy: demonstration of increased frequency, severity, resistance to palliation, and impact on quality of life. Cancer. 2008;113(10):2704–13.
257. Parulekar W, Mackenzie R, Bjarnason G, Jordan RC. Scoring oral mucositis. Oral Oncol. 1998;34(1):63–71.
258. Squier CA. Oral complications of cancer therapies. Mucosal alterations. NCI Monogr. 1990;9:169–72.
259. Epstein JB, Beaumont JL, Gwede CK, Murphy B, Garden AS, Meredith R, et al. Longitudinal evaluation of the oral mucositis weekly questionnaire-head and neck cancer, a patient-reported outcomes questionnaire. Cancer. 2007;109(9):1914–22.
260. World Health Organization. WHO handbook for reporting results of cancer treatment. Geneva: World Health Organization; 1979.
261. https://ctep.cancer.gov/protocoldevelopment/electronic_applications/docs/CTCAE_v5_Quick_Reference_8.5x11.pdf.
262. Cox JD, Stetz J, Pajak TF. Toxicity criteria of the Radiation Therapy Oncology Group (RTOG) and the European Organization for Research and Treatment of Cancer (EORTC). Int J Radiat Oncol Biol Phys. 1995;31(5):1341–6. https://doi.org/10.1016/0360-3016(95)00060-C.
263. McGuire DB, Peterson DE, Muller S, Owen DC, Slemmons MF, Schubert MM. The 20 item oral mucositis index: reliability and validity in bone marrow and stem cell transplant patients. Cancer Investig. 2002;20(7–8):893–903.
264. Schubert MM, Williams BE, Lloid ME, Donaldson G, Chapko MK. Clinical assessment scale for the rating of oral mucosal changes associated with bone marrow transplantation. Development of an oral mucositis index. Cancer. 1992;69(10):2469–77.
265. Sonis ST, Eilers JP, Epstein JB, LeVeque FG, Liggett WH Jr, Mulagha MT, et al. Validation of a new scoring system for the assessment of clinical trial research of oral mucositis induced by radiation or chemotherapy. Mucositis Study Group. Cancer. 1999;85(10):2103–13.
266. Development of a staging system for chemotherapy-induced stomatitis. Western Consortium for Cancer Nursing Research. Cancer Nurs. 1991;14(1):6–12.
267. List MA, Ritter-Sterr C, Lansky SB. A performance status scale for head and neck cancer patients. Cancer. 1990;66(3):564–9.
268. List MA, Ritter-Sterr CA, Baker TM, Colangelo LA, Matz G, Pauloski BR, et al. Longitudinal assessment of quality of life in laryngeal cancer patients. Head Neck. 1996;18(1):1–10.
269. List MA, Mumby P, Haraf D, Siston A, Mick R, MacCracken E, et al. Performance and quality of life outcome in patients completing concomitant chemoradiotherapy protocols for head and neck cancer. Qual Life Res. 1997;6(3):274–84.
270. List MA, Siston A, Haraf D, Schumm P, Kies M, Stenson K, et al. Quality of life and performance in advanced head and neck cancer patients on concomitant chemoradiotherapy: a prospective examination. J Clin Oncol. 1999;17(3):1020–8.
271. Eilers J, Berger AM, Petersen MC. Development, testing, and application of the oral assessment guide. Oncol Nurs Forum. 1988;15(3):325–30.
272. Green S, Weiss GR. Southwest Oncology Group standard response criteria, endpoint definitions and toxicity criteria. Investig New Drugs. 1992;10(4):239–53.
273. Oken MM, Creech RH, Tormey DC, Horton J, Davis TE, McFadden ET, et al. Toxicity and response criteria of the Eastern Cooperative Oncology Group. Am J Clin Oncol. 1982;5(6):649–55.
274. Spijkervet FK, van Saene HK, Panders AK, Vermey A, Mehta DM. Scoring irradiation mucositis in head and neck cancer patients. J Oral Pathol Med. 1989;18(3):167–71.
275. Walsh LJ, Hill G, Seymour G, Roberts A. A scoring system for the quantitative evaluation of oral mucositis during bone marrow transplantation. Spec Care Dentist. 1990;10(6):190–5.

276. Tardieu C, Cowen D, Thirion X, Franquin JC. Quantitative scale of oral mucositis associated with autologous bone marrow transplantation. Eur J Cancer B Oral Oncol. 1996;6:381–7.
277. Donnelly JP, Muus P, Schattenberg A, De Witte T, Horrevorts A, DePauw BE. A scheme for daily monitoring of oral mucositis in allogeneic BMT recipients. Bone Marrow Transplant. 1992;9(6):409–13.
278. Dibble SL, Shiba G, MacPhail L, Dodd MJ. MacDibbs Mouth Assessment. A new tool to evaluate mucositis in the radiation therapy patient. Cancer Pract. 1996;4(3):135–40.
279. Stiff PJ, Emmanouilides C, Bensinger WI, Gentile T, Blazar B, Shea TC, et al. Palifermin reduces patient-reported mouth and throat soreness and improves patient functioning in the hematopoietic stem-cell transplantation setting. J Clin Oncol. 2006;24(33):5186–93.
280. List MA, D'Antonio LL, Cella DF, Siston A, Mumby P, Haraf D, et al. The performance status scale for head and neck cancer patients and the functional assessment of cancer therapy-head and neck scale. A study of utility and validity. Cancer. 1996;77(11):2294–301.
281. Cella DF, Tulsky DS, Gray G, Sarafian B, Linn E, Bonomi A, et al. The Functional Assessment of Cancer Therapy scale: development and validation of the general measure. J Clin Oncol. 1993;11(3):570–9.
282. Cella D, Paul D, Yount S, Winn R, Chang CH, Banik D, et al. What are the most important symptom targets when treating advanced cancer? A survey of providers in the National Comprehensive Cancer Network (NCCN). Cancer Investig. 2003;21(4):526–35.
283. Aaronson NK, Ahmedzai S, Bergman B, Bullinger M, Cull A, Duez NJ, et al. The European Organization for Research and Treatment of Cancer QLQ-C30: a quality-of-life instrument for use in international clinical trials in oncology. J Natl Cancer Inst. 1993;85(5):365–76.
284. Duncan GG, Epstein JB, Tu D, El Sayed S, Bezjak A, Ottaway J, et al. Quality of life, mucositis, and xerostomia from radiotherapy for head and neck cancers: a report from the NCIC CTG HN2 randomized trial of an antimicrobial lozenge to prevent mucositis. Head Neck. 2005;27(5):421–8.
285. Kyriaki M, Eleni T, Efi P, Ourania K, Vassilios S, Lambros V. The EORTC core quality of life questionnaire (QLQ-C30, version 3.0) in terminally ill cancer patients under palliative care: validity and reliability in a Hellenic sample. Int J Cancer. 2001;94(1):135–9.
286. Bjordal K, Hammerlid E, Ahlner-Elmqvist M, de Graeff A, Boysen M, Evensen JF, et al. Quality of life in head and neck cancer patients: validation of the European Organization for Research and Treatment of Cancer Quality of Life Questionnaire-H&N35. J Clin Oncol. 1999;17(3):1008–19.
287. Ranna V, Cheng KKF, Castillo DA, Porcello L, Vaddi A, Lalla RV, et al. Development of the MASCC/ISOO clinical practice guidelines for mucositis: an overview of the methods. Support Care Cancer. 2019;27(10):3933–48.
288. Zadik Y, Arany PR, Fregnani ER, Bossi P, Antunes HS, Bensadoun RJ, et al. Systematic review of photobiomodulation for the management of oral mucositis in cancer patients and clinical practice guidelines. Support Care Cancer. 2019;27(10):3969–83.
289. Ariyawardana A, Cheng KKF, Kandwal A, Tilly V, Al-Azri AR, Galiti D, et al. Systematic review of anti-inflammatory agents for the management of oral mucositis in cancer patients and clinical practice guidelines. Support Care Cancer. 2019;27(10):3985–95.
290. Hong CHL, Gueiros LA, Fulton JS, Cheng KKF, Kandwal A, Galiti D, et al. Systematic review of basic oral care for the management of oral mucositis in cancer patients and clinical practice guidelines. Support Care Cancer. 2019;27(10):3949–67.
291. Bowen JM, Gibson RJ, Coller JK, Blijlevens N, Bossi P, Al-Dasooqi N, et al. Systematic review of agents for the management of cancer treatment-related gastrointestinal mucositis and clinical practice guidelines. Support Care Cancer. 2019;27(10):4011–22.
292. Correa MEP, Cheng KKF, Chiang K, Kandwal A, Loprinzi CL, Mori T, et al. Systematic review of oral cryotherapy for the management of oral mucositis in cancer patients and clinical practice guidelines. Support Care Cancer. 2020;28(5):2449–56.
293. Saunders DP, Rouleau T, Cheng K, Yarom N, Kandwal A, Joy J, et al. Systematic review of antimicrobials, mucosal coating agents, anesthetics, and analgesics for the management

of oral mucositis in cancer patients and clinical practice guidelines. Support Care Cancer. 2020;28(5):2473–84.

294. Yarom N, Hovan A, Bossi P, Ariyawardana A, Jensen SB, Gobbo M, et al. Systematic review of natural and miscellaneous agents, for the management of oral mucositis in cancer patients and clinical practice guidelines—Part 2: Honey, herbal compounds, saliva stimulants, probiotics, and miscellaneous agents. Support Care Cancer. 2020;28(5):2457–72.
295. Logan RM, Al-Azri AR, Bossi P, Stringer AM, Joy JK, Soga Y, et al. Systematic review of growth factors and cytokines for the management of oral mucositis in cancer patients and clinical practice guidelines. Support Care Cancer. 2020;28(5):2485–98.
296. Elad S, Cheng KKF, Lalla RV, Yarom N, Hong C, Logan RM, Bowen J, Gibson R, Saunders DP, Zadik Y, Ariyawardana A, Correa ME, Ranna V, Bossi P; MASCC/ISOO clinical practice guidelines for the management of mucositis secondary to cancer therapy. Mucositis guidelines leadership group of the multinational association of supportive care in cancer and international society of oral oncology (MASCC/ISOO). Cancer. 2020;126(19):4423–4431. https://doi.org/10.1002/cncr.33100. Epub 2020 Jul 28. PMID: 32786044.
297. Peterson DE, O'Shaughnessy JA, Rugo HS, Elad S, Schubert MM, Viet CT, et al. Oral mucosal injury caused by mammalian target of rapamycin inhibitors: emerging perspectives on pathobiology and impact on clinical practice. Cancer Med. 2016;5(8):1897–907.
298. De Masson A, Fouchard N, Mery-Bossard L, Dauendorffer JN. Cutaneous and mucosal aphthosis during temsirolimus therapy for advanced renal cell carcinoma: review of cutaneous and mucosal side effects of mTOR inhibitors. Dermatology. 2011;223(1):4–8.
299. Busemann C, Wilfert H, Neumann T, Kiefer T, Dolken G, Kruger WH. Mucositis after reduced intensity conditioning and allogeneic stem cell transplantation. Onkologie. 2011;34(10):518–24.

Oral Bacterial, Viral, and Fungal Infections

6

Yuanming Xu and Alessandro Villa

6.1 Introduction

Patients receiving cancer therapy are at higher risk of developing treatment-related complications. Oral infections (bacterial, fungal, and viral) are among the most common oral complications and may develop during or after cancer treatment. Compared to relatively healthy individuals, oral infections in cancer patients present with unusual clinical patterns and different disease progression. Reasons for the higher risk of oral infections in cancer patients include immunosuppression, changes in the oral microbiota, and loss of epithelium integrity.

Oral infections in cancer patients often require a multidisciplinary effort with the dentist and the patient's oncology team. This chapter aims to highlight the most common oral infections encountered in patients who receive cancer therapy. Diagnostic methods and management strategies for these infections are also discussed.

6.2 Bacterial Infections

Chemotherapeutic regimen-induced myelosuppression results in neutropenia and impaired cellular and humoral immunity response, with an increased risk for opportunistic infections. Neutropenic patients are more susceptible to bacterial infections

Y. Xu (✉)
Division of Oral Medicine and Dentistry, Brigham and Women's Hospital and Dana Farber Cancer Institute, Boston, MA, USA

Department of Oral Medicine Infection and Immunity, Harvard School of Dental Medicine, Boston, MA, USA
e-mail: yuanming_xu@hsdm.harvard.edu

A. Villa (✉)
Department of Orofacial Sciences, University of California San Francisco, San Francisco, CA, USA
e-mail: Alessandro.villa@ucsf.edu

R. Nair (ed.), *Orofacial Supportive Care in Cancer*,
https://doi.org/10.1007/978-3-030-86510-8_6

in general, and in the oral cavity, these may present as acute or chronic infections. Bacterial infections are typically seen during the early phases of neutropenia.

Radiation therapy to the head and neck causes salivary gland damage with hyposalivation and xerostomia. A change of the oral microbial flora due to hyposalivation is associated with rampant radiation caries and may predispose to infections and periodontal disease in head and neck cancer patients.

Mucositis is another common side effect of radiotherapy in head and neck cancer patients and of high-dose chemotherapy prior to hematopoietic cell transplantation. Ulcerative lesions of oral mucositis in periods of immunosuppression may increase the risk for local and systemic infection.

6.2.1 Odontogenic Infections

Odontogenic (originating from tooth) infections are the most common bacterial infections in the oral cavity and can be secondary to a pulpal infection or of periodontal origins. Odontogenic infections can spread to the adjacent hard and soft tissues (Fig. 6.1). If left untreated, odontogenic infections may lead to severe complications such as cellulitis, cavernous sinus thrombosis, and mediastinitis. Clinical symptoms and signs of odontogenic infections depend on the sources and phase of the infection.

During the initial phase, pulpal infections present as acute pulpitis with hypersensitivity to stimuli and spontaneous, prolonged dental (tooth) pain. The increased inflammation in the periapical (apex of the tooth) area may generate purulence discharge with local destruction of the alveolar bone and formation of a fistula. Typical radiographic characteristics of periapical lesion include an enlarged periodontal space and periapical radiolucency.

Untreated periapical infections arising from the mandibular teeth may result in osteomyelitis of the jaw. Patients may present with fever, pain, swelling, suppuration, sinus tract formation, and bone sequestration. For the infection arising from the posterior maxillary teeth, paranasal sinus can be infected when the infection perforates the Schneiderian membrane. Symptoms may include headache, maxillary tenderness, and pain. Intraoral radiographs and CT of the maxillary sinuses may be necessary for a correct diagnosis.

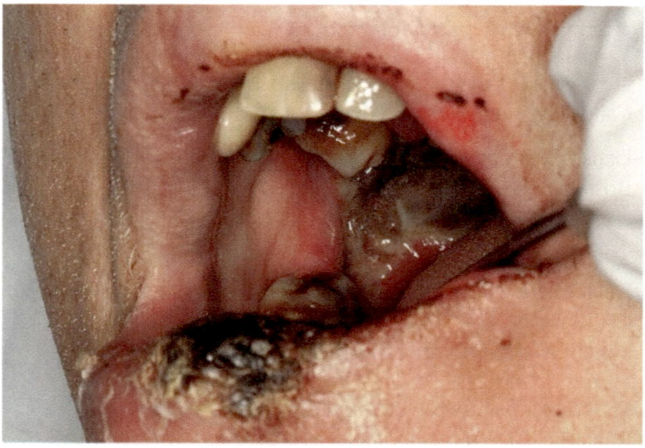

Fig. 6.1 Necrotizing ulcerative stomatitis with bacterial colonization

6.2.2 Pericoronitis

Pericoronitis is related to impacted partially erupted third molars with the deep periodontal pockets, which provide an ideal space for food debris accumulation as well as bacteria growth (Fig. 6.2). Pericoronitis (around the crown of the tooth) presents with pain and swelling; in severe cases, the infection can spread through the fascial space and cause cellulitis of adjacent tissues.

The most common fascial spaces involved in odontogenic infections include the buccal space, masticatory space, submandibular space, and sublingual space. Patients with cellulitis often present with fever, severe pain, swelling, limited mouth opening, and difficulty in swallowing. Ludwig angina is a type of severe bacterial infection characterized by severe swelling of the sublingual, submental, and submandibular space, bilaterally. The swelling may lead to airway obstruction and require rapid intervention.

6.2.3 Periodontitis

Periodontitis is an infectious and inflammatory disease leading to alveolar bone loss with a high prevalence in the general population. Clinical presentation includes teeth mobility, gingival swelling, gingival recession, erythema, bleeding, and deep periodontal pockets. In cancer patients, the presence of periodontal disease is a unique risk factor for mucositis and osteoradionecrosis. In myelosuppressed patients, the periodontal disease tends to be more aggressive and resistant to conventional therapy. An association of poor periodontal condition with increased bacteremia has also been found.

6.2.4 Prevention

Prevention plays an essential role in the management of oral bacterial infections in cancer patients. All potential sources of infection should be minimized before the

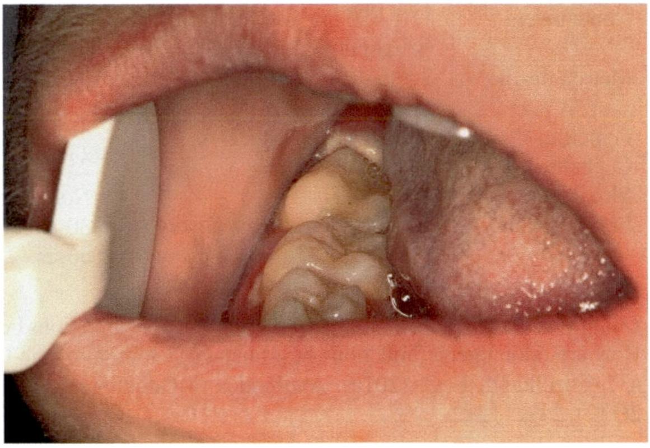

Fig. 6.2 Neutropenic ulcers and pericoronitis area tooth #31 in a 37-year-old patient with a history of breast carcinoma undergoing neoadjuvant chemotherapy with recurrent febrile neutropenia

initiation of cancer therapy. Patients awaiting chemotherapy, radiotherapy, or hematopoietic stem cell transplantation (HSCT) should undergo a complete dental examination with a full mouth series of radiographs. Dental prophylaxis and periodontal treatment should be provided to all patients. Caries should be restored, and unrestorable teeth and teeth with poor prognosis should be extracted. High-concentration fluoride products should be prescribed for caries prevention. Patients should be followed up for routine dental examinations.

6.2.5 Treatment

The treatment plan for an active odontogenic infection in cancer patients is based on the source and severity of the infection as well as the patient's immune function. For localized odontogenic infection, removal of the primary source is essential and includes the extraction of the affected tooth or endodontic therapy and/or incision and drainage for fluctuant swellings. The complete blood count should be reviewed before any invasive dental procedures to avoid the risk of bleeding or additional infections. Empiric treatment with amoxicillin combined with clavulanic acid or clindamycin should be used for small periapical infections. Other commonly prescribed antibiotics for odontogenic infections are listed in Table 6.1.

Acute periodontal infections in cancer patients are managed with scaling and curettage, root planing, and extraction of hopeless teeth. Penicillin, clindamycin, and metronidazole along with antimicrobial rinses (e.g., chlorhexidine) are used for periodontitis management. Immunosuppressed patients with severe odontogenic infections and associated systemic symptoms should be hospitalized for close monitoring, IV antibiotics, possible surgical drainage, and multidisciplinary care.

Table 6.1 Commonly used antibiotics in odontogenic infections

	Dosage of common use	
Antibiotics	Adults	Children
Amoxicillin with clavulanic acid	500–875 mg every 12 h	25–45 mg/kg/day in two divided doses
Amoxicillin	250–500 mg every 8 h	20–40 mg/kg/day in three divided doses
Clindamycin	150–450 mg every 6 h (maximum 1.8 g/day)	8–20 mg/kg/day in three to four divided doses
Metronidazole	7.5 mg/kg every 6 h (maximum 4 g/24 h)	30/mg/kg/day in four divided doses
Penicillin V	600 mg every 6 h	25–50 mg/kg/day in four divided doses
Cephalexin	500 mg every 6 h	25–50 mg/kg/day in four divided doses
Moxifloxacin	400 mg daily	Not established
Erythromycin	500 mg enteric coated every 8 h 333 mg enteric coated every 6 h 250 mg (base) every 6 h	30–50 mg/kg/day in two to four divided doses

Data from: Davis, B. J. (2010). How are odontogenic infections best managed? Gregoire, C. (2010). How are odontogenic infections best managed? Journal of the Canadian Dental Association. 76, a37. Peedikayil, F. C. (2016). Antibiotics in Odontogenic Infections-An Update. J Antimicro, 2(117), 2472–1212

Aerobic and anaerobic cultures should be obtained following drainage of abscesses, in cases of poor clinical response to empiric antibiotic therapy and suspected streptococcal pharyngitis; culture and sensitivity testing should also be requested.

6.3 Fungal Infections

Compromised lymphocytic function places patients at higher risk of acquiring fungal infections. Fungal infections occur more often in patients with a longer neutropenic state.

Based on the depth of invasion, fungal infections can be divided into superficial and deep. *Candida* species are the main source of superficial oral mucosal infection. Deep fungal infections include mucormycosis, histoplasmosis, blastomycosis, and aspergillosis.

6.3.1 Oropharyngeal Candidiasis (OPC)

Oropharyngeal candidiasis (OPC) is the most frequent fungal infection in cancer patients. Approximately 30% of the patients receiving cancer treatment develop an oral fungal infection. *Candida albicans* is a commensal organism of the oral cavity present in about 20% of individuals and represents the most common causative agent. Other pathogens include *C. parapsilosis*, *C. glabrata*, *C. krusei*, *C. tropicalis*, *C. guilliermondii*, and *C. lusitaniae*. *Candida albicans* can penetrate the epithelium by epithelial cell receptor-mediated endocytosis, active hyphus elongation, and proteolytic degradation of the intercellular junction. Candidalysin, a toxin secreted by *C. albicans*, can directly damage the epithelial membranes and trigger a local inflammation response, causing pain, erythema, and other symptoms. The coinfection with other microorganisms such as *C. glabrata*, *C. tropicalis*, and some other bacteria can augment the virulence and damage caused by *C. albicans*.

6.3.1.1 Risk Factors

In cancer patients, *Candida* colonization is influenced by the underlying condition, immune status, and salivary gland function. In cancer patients, chemotherapy-induced myelosuppression decreases both the innate and adaptive responses against fungi. Head and neck radiotherapy causes hyposalivation and decreases antimicrobial peptide secretion, leading to *Candida* accumulation. The use of antibiotics interrupts the homeostasis of the oral microbiome and increases the risk of fungal infection.

6.3.1.2 Classification and Clinical Presentations

OPC has variable symptoms which may range from none to generalized discomfort, burning sensation, and pain. Patients may also complain of xerostomia and dysgeusia (often reported as a "metallic" taste). OPC may also involve the esophagus and interfere with the ability to swallow and lead to malnutrition.

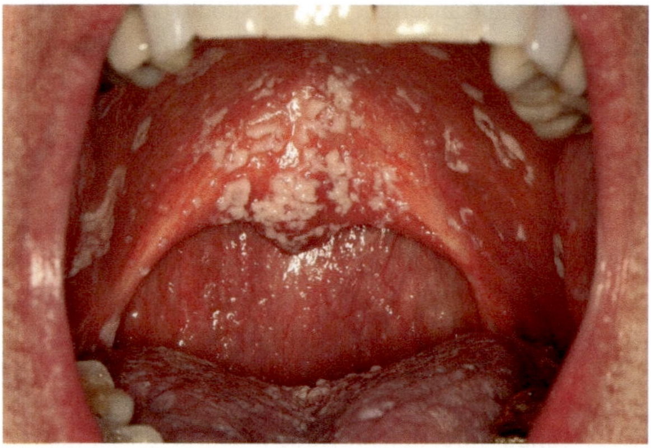

Fig. 6.3 A 64-year-old patient presented with classic oral pseudomembranous candidiasis. Discrete white papules and irregular plaques with underlying erythema presented on the hard palate, soft palate, dorsal tongue, buccal mucosa, and other mucosal surfaces

There are four main clinical presentations of OPC: pseudomembranous candidiasis (the so-called "thrush"), erythematous candidiasis, angular cheilitis, and hyperplastic candidiasis. Pseudomembranous candidiasis is characterized by white thick papules and plaques that appear on any surface of the mucosa in either confluent or discrete way (Fig. 6.3). The white papules or plaques represent a *Candida* overgrowth and an accumulation of desquamated epithelial cells, bacteria, keratin, and necrotic tissue. These lesions can be easily removed with a gauze, leaving in some cases an erythematous surface.

Erythematous candidiasis presents as diffuse erythema of any mucosal surface with a palatal and tongue predilection. Dorsal tongue lesions show depapillation with a smooth surface, and patients usually complain of a localized burning sensation. Denture-associated stomatitis is a specific clinical presentation of erythematous candidiasis with a classic erythematous patch that follows the shape of the denture base. The porosity of the acrylic-based denture isolates the underneath space from the oral cavity and provides an ideal microenvironment for *Candida* growth.

Hyperplastic candidiasis presents as white plaques that cannot be readily wiped off. The buccal commissures, tongue, palatal mucosa, and oropharynx are the most commonly affected sites. Hyperplastic candidiasis is a chronic *Candida* infection with epithelial hyperplasia, which raises a concern of potential dysplastic changes within the lesion. A biopsy of the suspected lesion should be performed to differentiate this lesion from a true leukoplakia (a potentially malignant disorder).

Angular cheilitis is characterized by erythematous fissuring and cracking at the commissures of the lips, which can present with one of the other intraoral forms mentioned above. Bacterial species such as staphylococci and streptococci are also found in association with angular cheilitis.

6.3.1.3 Diagnosis

The diagnosis of OPC is usually clinical. Patients' immuno-status and medical history should also be considered. Empirical treatment can be used for classic OPC without any additional diagnostic test. However, the diagnosis of OPC can be challenging in cancer patients undergoing chemo- or radiotherapy. The symptoms and signs of erythema may overlap with those of oral mucositis. Further diagnostic tests may be necessary and include exfoliative cytology, oral culture, and tissue biopsy (especially for hyperplastic candidiasis and resistant lesions with white and erythematous changes).

6.3.1.4 Prevention

Antifungal prophylaxis is recommended in immunosuppressed cancer patients. The IDSA guidelines recommend fluconazole prophylaxis for patients undergoing HSCT. Chlorhexidine or nystatin rinse has been widely used for antifungal prophylaxis in patients with long-term use of topical steroid.

Prevention of OPC should address both local and systemic factors that promote candidiasis. Good oral hygiene is fundamental to maintain a balanced oral microenvironment and decrease the fungal biofilm formation. Dentures should be cleaned daily and soaked in chlorhexidine or diluted sodium hypochlorite solution.

In patients with hyposalivation, local saliva stimulation with sugar-free chewing gum or lozenges may be beneficial. Systemic sialagogues can be prescribed for selected patients.

6.3.1.5 Treatment

Azoles and polyenes are the two main antifungal agents prescribed for fungal infections. They both target ergosterol, which plays a critical role in regulating the stability and integrity of the cell membrane, and promote fungal growth. Azoles block the synthesis of ergosterol, resulting in the inhibition of fungal growth, while polyenes form a complex with ergosterol and disrupt the fungal membrane, leading to plasmatic leakage and ultimately cell death.

Common azoles include two categories: imidazoles (clotrimazole, ketoconazole, and miconazole) and triazoles (itraconazole, fluconazole, posaconazole, and voriconazole). Amphotericin B and nystatin are polyene antibiotics widely used as broad-spectrum antifungal agents. Echinocandins, including anidulafungin, caspofungin, and micafungin, inhibit (1,3)-β-D-glucan synthase interfering with the cell wall formation. Pyrimidine analogs such as flucytosine interfere with pyrimidine metabolism and disrupt RNA/DNA and protein synthesis. Flucytosine has been used as an adjuvant antifungal agent with amphotericin B.

Both topical and systemic antifungal agents are available for OPC management. Topical applications usually have fewer drug interactions and side effects but may not be as effective in moderate or severe cases. A combination of both topical and systemic antifungal treatments may accelerate the infection eradication and benefit the patient with lower doses and a shorter course.

The Infectious Disease Society of America (IDSA) has published detailed guidelines for the management of OPC (Table 6.2).

For cases of mild oral candidiasis, topical clotrimazole troches (10 mg, five times/day) or miconazole mucoadhesive tablet (50 mg, once daily) for 7–14 days is recommended. Alternatively, nystatin suspension (100,000 U/ml, 4–6 ml, four times/day or 1–2 200,000 U pastilles, four times/day) may be prescribed. Dentures

Table 6.2 IDSA 2016 updated clinical guideline for oropharyngeal candidiasis

Severity of OPC	Medication	Dosage and duration
Mild	Clotrimazole (troches)	10 mg, 5×/day, 7–14 days
	Miconazole (buccal tablet)	50 mg, qd, 7–14 days
	Nystatin (suspension rinse, 100,000 U/mL)	4–6 mL, qid, 7–14 days
	Nystatin (pastilles, 200,000 U each)	1–2 pastilles, qid, 7–14 days
Moderate to severe	Fluconazole	100–200 mg, qd, 7–14 days
Moderate to severe (fluconazole-refractory)	Itraconazole (solution)	200 mg, qd, 7–14 days
	Posaconazole (suspension)	400 mg, bid for the first 3 days and then qd up to 28 days
	Voriconazole	200 mg, bid
	AmB deoxycholate (oral suspension, 100 mg/ml)	Qid
Moderate to severe (refractory, intravenous)	Caspofungin	70 mg loading dose and then 50 mg daily
	Micafungin	100 mg daily
	Anidulafungin	200 mg loading dose and then 100 mg daily
	AmB deoxycholate	0.3 mg/kg daily
Chronic suppressive therapy	Fluconazole	100 mg, 3×/week

Data from: Pappas, P. G., Kauffman, C. A., Andes, D. R., Clancy, C. J., Marr, K. A., Ostrosky-Zeichner, L., et al. (2016). Clinical Practice Guideline for the Management of Candidiasis: 2016 Update by the Infectious Diseases Society of America. Clin Infect Dis, 62(4), e1–50. https://doi.org/10.1093/cid/civ933

IDSA Infectious Diseases Society of America, *OPC* oropharyngeal candidiasis, *AmB* Amphotericin B

should be soaked in 2% chlorhexidine digluconate or 3% sodium hypochlorite during nighttime and rinsed under water before use. For patients with hyposalivation or diabetes mellitus, nystatin mouth rinse or clotrimazole troches should be dispensed with caution as they may contain sugar.

For moderate to severe disease, IDSA recommends fluconazole (100–200 mg, daily) for 7–14 days. In fluconazole-refractory cases, itraconazole solution (200 mg once daily) or posaconazole suspension (400 mg twice/day for the first 3 days and then 400 mg once daily) is recommended. Itraconazole and posaconazole, voriconazole (200 mg, twice daily), or amphotericin B deoxycholate oral suspension (100 mg/ml, four times/day) can also be used as alternatives (Table 6.2).

6.3.2 Deep Fungal Infections

Deep fungal infections usually present with oral necrotic ulcers, and systemic dissemination is frequent. Mucormycosis is caused by the class of Zygomycetes which includes the Mucorales and Entomophthorales. Mucorales are the primary etiological agents for mucormycosis (zygomycosis) in immunocompromised patients. Oral lesions appear as necrotic and black and resemble malignancies. Mucormycosis involves multiple organs including lung, skin, and gastrointestinal and neural system, leading to high morbidity and mortality. Patients with diabetes mellitus (especially if ketoacidosis), malignancy, neutropenia, and post-organ transplantation may develop rhinocerebral mucormycosis with a mortality rate of 60–90%.

Aspergillosis is the second most common fungal opportunistic infection. *Aspergillus* species are ubiquitous in the natural environment, and their spores infect humans through airways. Aspergillosis (caused by *A. flavus* or *A. fumigatus*) is characterized by an invasive and noninvasive form. Invasive aspergillosis tends to affect immunocompromised patients such as those with hematologic malignancies, and the clinical presentation is similar to the one of mucormycosis. Vascular involvement leads to necrosis. Noninvasive infections typically present as a "fungus ball" (mycetoma) within the maxillary sinuses or as a hypersensitivity reaction to the fungus leading to allergic fungal sinusitis. Serum galactomannan detection may be helpful for the diagnosis, and monitoring of galactomannan may allow the beginning of preemptive antifungal treatment before life-threatening infection occurs.

Histoplasmosis is an endemic disease in the Mississippi and the Ohio River Valleys. *Histoplasma capsulatum* is a saprophytic and dimorphic fungus that infects the lung by aerosolization and inhalation, causing pulmonary disease and multiorgan involvement. Primary infection is usually a self-limiting pulmonary infection. Immunosuppressed patients may have multiple organs involved (lung, spleen, liver, meninges, and adrenal glands). Oral manifestation resembles squamous cell carcinomas with granulomatous-appearing ulceration and erythema. A biopsy is needed to confirm the diagnosis.

Blastomycosis is caused by saprophytic *Blastomyces dermatitidis* which most commonly affects the lungs. Immunocompromised patients may experience severe complications. Skin lesions commonly present as a verrucous mass with a raised border and with a crusted appearance or as indurated ulcerations. The orofacial region can also be involved. Oral manifestation is rare but can present as an ulcerative, verrucous, or granulomatous lesion with radiolucent bone lesions.

The diagnosis is made with a biopsy and histopathological examination. Culture, serological, and PCR studies can also be used. A chest radiograph or computed tomography (CT) scan may be helpful to rule out any lung involvement. Treatment for deep fungal infection requires aggressive systemic antifungal therapy and surgical debridement. The detailed treatment plan for specific deep fungal infections is reported in Table 6.3.

6.4 Viral Infections

Cancer patients are often immunosuppressed and become more susceptible to oral viral infections and associated life-threatening complications. The most common viral infections in the oral and maxillofacial region are caused by two viral families: human herpesvirus and human papillomavirus.

Table 6.3 Primary treatment for invasive fungal infections

	Medication	Dosage and duration
Candidemia in neutropenic patients	Echinocandin	Caspofungin: 70 mg/day for 1 day and then 50 mg daily Micafungin: 100 mg/day qd Anidulafungin: 200 mg/day for 1 day and then 100 mg daily
	Lipid formulation AmB	3–5 mg/kg/day
	Fluconazole	800 mg (12 mg/kg)/day for 1 day and then 400 mg (6 mg/kg) daily
	Voriconazole[a]	400 mg (6 mg/kg) bid for two doses and then 200–300 mg (3–4 mg/kg) bid
Aspergillosis	Voriconazole	IV: 6 mg/kg, 2×/day for 1 day, followed by 4 mg/kg 2×/day PO: 200–300 mg bid or weight based
	Liposomal AmB	IV 3–5 mg/kg/day
	Isavuconazole	200 mg 3–4×/day for six doses and then 200 mg daily
Mucormycosis	Liposomal AmB	IV 5–10 mg/kg/day
	ABLC	5–7.5 mg/kg
	Posaconazole	400 mg, bid, 300 mg, bid for 1 day and then 300 mg daily[b]
	Isavuconazole[b]	200 mg, tid for six doses and then 200 mg daily

Data from: Pappas, P. G., Kauffman, C. A., Andes, D. R., Clancy, C. J., Marr, K. A., Ostrosky-Zeichner, L., et al. (2016). Clinical Practice Guideline for the Management of Candidiasis: 2016 Update by the Infectious Diseases Society of America. Clin Infect Dis, 62(4), e1–50. https://doi.org/10.1093/cid/civ933. Ullmann, A. J., Schmidt-Hieber, M., Bertz, H., Heinz, W. J., Kiehl, M., Kruger, W., et al. (2016). Infectious diseases in allogeneic haematopoietic stem cell transplantation: prevention and prophylaxis strategy guidelines 2016. Ann Hematol, 95(9), 1435–1455. https://doi.org/10.1007/s00277-016-2711-1. Skiada, A., Lanternier, F., Groll, A. H., Pagano, L., Zimmerli, S., Herbrecht, R., et al., European Conference on Infections in, L. (2013). Diagnosis and treatment of mucormycosis in patients with hematological malignancies: guidelines from the 3rd European Conference on Infections in Leukemia (ECIL 3). Haematologica, 98(4), 492–504. https://doi.org/10.3324/haematol.2012.065110

AmB: amphotericin B

[a]Can be used in situations in which additional mold coverage is desired

[b]Salvage therapy for patients who cannot tolerate or do not respond to AmB

6.4.1 Human Herpesvirus (HHV)

6.4.1.1 Herpes Simplex Virus (HSV)

Herpes simplex viruses (HSV-1 and HSV-2) are the most common herpetic infections with oral mucosal involvement. Traditionally, HSV-1 is considered more likely to infect the oral cavity and pharyngeal area, while HSV-2 mainly affects the genitalia. HSV-1 infection is common with 60–90% of the population being exposed to the virus by age 70. However, only 1% of the exposed individuals present with herpetic gingivostomatitis. Herpetic gingivostomatitis is characterized by multiple diffuse oral ulcers, gingival bleeding, fever, malaise, nausea, and lymphadenopathy. The virus can remain latent in the trigeminal ganglion and causes recrudescent infection (in 20–40% of the immunocompetent individuals), especially when patients are exposed to sunlight, trauma, stress, or during hormonal changes. Recrudescent orofacial HSV-1 infections in relatively healthy patients mainly present as recurrent herpes labialis with classic prodromal symptoms (tingling of the lower lip). Intraoral lesions are rare and usually appear as small vesicles and become shallow ulcers of the keratinized mucosa.

Recrudescent HSV infection in immunocompromised patients is severe and present with large painful ulcerations of both the keratinized and nonkeratinized mucosae (Fig. 6.4). Because of pain, patients may become dehydrated and malnourished. In addition, recrudescent HSV may lead to disseminated life-threatening disease (e.g., pneumonitis and encephalitis). In immunosuppressed patients, the clinical features of recrudescent HSV infection can be atypical and difficult to differentiate from other oral conditions (such as mucositis). Therefore, patients with acute painful oral ulcers with atypical appearance should be tested to rule out HSV infection. Viral culture of active ulcers may be helpful in diagnosis but does not distinguish between asymptomatic viral shedding and actual recrudescence. Exfoliative cytology with direct fluorescent antibody testing may be performed when a diagnosis is needed within hours. Biopsy of the lesion is indicated in those cases that do not respond to therapy or in patients where the clinical diagnosis is not definitive.

6.4.1.2 Varicella-Zoster Virus (VZV)

Varicella-zoster virus (HHV-3) is responsible for primary varicella (chickenpox) and the recurrent infection, zosters (shingles), in 20–30% of cases. Chickenpox primarily affects children with a characteristic pruritic sensation and maculopapular lesions, followed by vesicles. Oral lesions may also be presented as vesicle or ulcers but are rare. Primary infections are now uncommon, thanks to the VZV vaccine which has been available since the 1990s.

After the primary infection, VZV becomes latent in the cranial nerve ganglia, dorsal root ganglia, and autonomic ganglia along the entire neuraxis and may be reactivated in older patients. Environmental changes, altered immunity, malignancy, and cytotoxic drug use are other risk factors that may trigger herpes zoster (HZ). HZ patients may present with prodromal pain before the onset of the skin lesion. Unilateral skin blisters and ulcers, usually on the trunk, are classic for HZ, which follow the distribution of the thoracic or lumbar dermatomes. Trigeminal nerve can also be affected by 2% of all cases. Ophthalmic nerve is the most commonly involved branch which may lead to severe complications that affected the eyes. Oral HZ is characterized by painful erythema or ulceration with vesicles and bullae on oral mucosa. The lesions may present similarly to the ones caused by HSV but usually unilateral. Pain and paresthesia can present as preceded symptoms. In severely immunosuppressed patients, HZ can present on both sides with multifocal lesions, which may also be associated with bacterial superinfection, encephalitis, pneumonitis, myocarditis, and hepatitis. Peripheral facial palsy and post-herpetic neuralgia (PHN) can occur in HZ patients. The incidence of PHN is

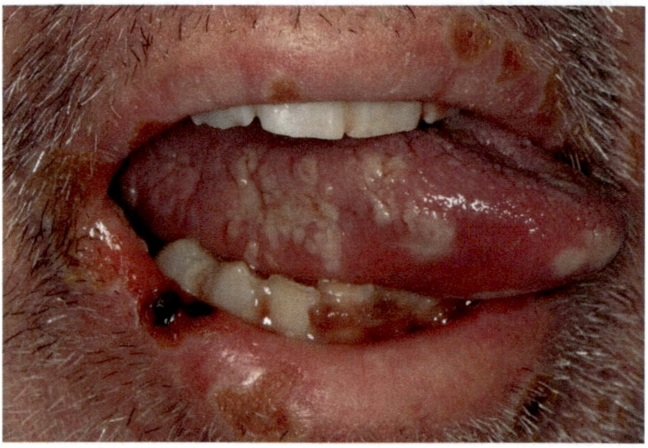

Fig. 6.4 Recrudescent HSV infection in a patient status post peripheral blood stem cell transplantation, with multiple ulcers on both ventral and lateral sides of the tongue and multifocal crusting of the lips

significantly higher in HSCT patients when compared to the immunocompetent population.

Approximately one-third of HSCT patients may experience HZ as VZV reactivation. Severe complications such as dissemination, superinfection, scarring, and mortality can occur in these immune suppressed patients. Diagnosis of HZ is usually based on clinical characteristics but may require other diagnostic tests such as an antibody titer test, viral culture, or PCR.

6.4.1.3 Epstein-Barr Virus (EBV)

EBV transmits through saliva and has a preference for infecting B lymphocytes. It replicates in the epithelial cells of the oropharynx and has been associated with several conditions, including infectious mononucleosis, nasopharyngeal carcinoma, lymphoproliferative malignancies, and oral hairy leukoplakia. Mononucleosis presents with classic symptoms of fever, lymphadenopathy, and pharyngitis. Oral manifestation may include ulcers and palatal petechiae.

Oral hairy leukoplakia is a benign plaque-like lesion with vertical lines of the lateral or ventral tongue. It occurs predominantly in patients with HIV infection and has also been reported in immunosuppressed patients following HSCT. Diagnosis of OHL is usually clinical although tissue biopsy may be helpful for challenging cases. OHL is a self-limited lesion in most of the cases.

Latent EBV infection is also associated with several malignancies such as Burkitt lymphoma, a subset of Hodgkin lymphoma, posttransplant lymphoproliferative disorders (PTLDs), and HIV-associated lymphoma. PTLDs typically present with fever and lymphadenopathy, with extra-nodal involvement occurring in more than two-thirds of cases. Diagnosis is made with an excisional biopsy or multiple core needle biopsies for flow cytometry/immunophenotyping and evaluation of EBV status.

6.4.1.4 Cytomegalovirus (CMV)

CMV infection is highly prevalent in the general population without overt symptoms. The virus can remain latent in leukocytes, salivary glands, and endothelial cells. Active infection can transmit through the placenta and cause congenital infection of the fetus. In immunocompromised patients such as recipients of bone marrow transplant, pneumonia is the most common complication. Retinitis, gastrointestinal disease, and encephalitis have also been reported.

CMV-related oral lesions are mostly seen in immunocompromised patients and present as painful, large deep ulcers (>1 cm). The ulceration can last for weeks to months. A biopsy with immunohistochemistry and in situ hybridization is the most useful technique for the diagnosis of CMV. The virus can also be detected in serum with polymerase chain reaction (PCR) to detect CMV DNA or by testing for CMV antigen on white blood cells.

6.4.1.5 Management of HHV Infections

Hydration, nutritional support, and topical and systemic pain control are important for the management of oral viral infections. Acyclovir, famciclovir, and valacyclovir are common antivirals used as systemic agents for the treatment of HSV, VZV, and CMV infections. Foscarnet has been shown effective in treating acyclovir-resistant cases. The different dosages for specific viral infection are reviewed in Table 6.4. According to the IDSA guideline in 2014, in immunocompromised patients, recipients of HSCT should take acyclovir (800 mg bid) or valacyclovir (500 mg bid) for 1 year routinely. For CMV infection, intravenous ganciclovir, foscarnet, and cidofovir have been shown to be effective; in addition, active treatment of HIV also improves the immune status in patients with both HIV and CMV infection.

Table 6.4 Systemic antiviral treatment

Viral infections	Agents used	Dosage and duration
Recurrent HSV (immunocompetent patients)	Acyclovir Famciclovir Valacyclovir	400 mg/day tid for 5–7 days 500 mg 2–3×/day for 2–3 days 500–2000 mg bid for 1 day
Recurrent HSV (immunocompromised patients)	Acyclovir Famciclovir Valacyclovir	400 mg/day tid for 10 days or longer 500 mg bid for 1 year 500–1000 mg bid for 10 days or longer
Recurrent HSV (acyclovir-resistant patients)	Foscarnet Cidofovir	40 mg/kg 2–3×/day for 14–21 days 5 mg/kg/week for 3 weeks and then 5 mg/kg/3 weeks for three doses (w/ probenecid)
Herpes zoster	Acyclovir Famciclovir Valacyclovir	800 mg 5×/day for 7–10 days 500 mg tid for 7 days 1000 mg tid for 7 days
Cytomegalovirus infection	Ganciclovir	5 mg/kg bid for 1 day and then 5 mg/kg/day for 7–14 days (transplant patients)
	Valganciclovir	900 mg bid for 21 days and then qd
	Foscarnet	60 mg/kg tid or 90 mg/kg bid for 21–42 days or longer
	Cidofovir	5 mg/kg/week for 2 weeks and then 5 mg/kg/2 weeks (w/ probenecid)

Data from: Balasubramaniam, R., Kuperstein, A. S., & Stoopler, E. T. (2014). Update on oral herpes virus infections. Dent Clin North Am, 58(2), 265–280. https://doi.org/10.1016/j.cden.2013.12.001

HSV herpes simplex virus

6.4.2 Human Papillomavirus (HPV)

Immunosuppressed patients are more susceptible to HPV infections. HPV is a small deoxyribonucleic acid (DNA) virus with at least 25 types that are associated with oral lesions in humans (benign or malignant). The benign lesions induced by HPV include verruca vulgaris (common wart), oral squamous papilloma, and condyloma acuminatum. Oral squamous papilloma presents as a small and cauliflower-like epithelial proliferation of the oral mucosa with a predilection for the soft palate, gingiva, tongue, and lips. It can be keratotic or pink with a pedunculated or sessile base. Oral verruca vulgaris presents as an asymptomatic white lesion with a rough surface. It can be pedunculated or sessile. Lips, gingiva, and hard palate are the most commonly affected sites. Condyloma acuminatum usually occurs on the anogenital mucosa. Oral condylomata may present as sessile, pink, exophytic mass with multiple papillary protrusions, often affecting the labial and palatal mucosa. Management of benign HPV-associated oral lesions is usually with surgical excision. These lesions tend to recur in patients with a compromised immune system.

HPV is responsible for 70% of all oropharyngeal cancers. Most of the HPV-associated oropharyngeal cancers are squamous cell carcinoma associated with HPV 16 persistent infections. When compared to HPV− SCC, these HPV+ SCC primarily present in the lymphoepithelium tissue (tonsils and tongue base) with a predilection of younger population with little to no alcohol or tobacco exposure when compared to HPV− SCC.

Bibliography

1. Balasubramaniam R, Kuperstein AS, Stoopler ET. Update on oral herpes virus infections. Dent Clin N Am. 2014;58(2):265–80. https://doi.org/10.1016/j.cden.2013.12.001.
2. Beech N, Robinson S, Porceddu S, Batstone M. Dental management of patients irradiated for head and neck cancer. Aust Dent J. 2014;59(1):20–8. https://doi.org/10.1111/adj.12134.
3. Bensadoun RJ, Patton LL, Lalla RV, Epstein JB. Oropharyngeal candidiasis in head and neck cancer patients treated with radiation: update 2011. Support Care Cancer. 2011;19(6):737–44. https://doi.org/10.1007/s00520-011-1154-4.
4. Boguslawska-Kapala A, Halaburda K, Rusyan E, Golabek H, Struzycka I. Oral health of adult patients undergoing hematopoietic cell transplantation. Pre-transplant assessment and care. Ann Hematol. 2017;96(7):1135–45. https://doi.org/10.1007/s00277-017-2932-y.
5. Brennan MT, Treister NS, Sollecito TP, Schmidt BL, Patton LL, Mohammadi K, et al. Dental disease before radiotherapy in patients with head and neck cancer: Clinical Registry of Dental Outcomes in Head and Neck Cancer Patients. J Am Dent Assoc. 2017;148(12):868–77. https://doi.org/10.1016/j.adaj.2017.09.011.
6. Clarkson E, Mashkoor F, Abdulateef S. Oral viral infections: diagnosis and management. Dent Clin N Am. 2017;61(2):351–63. https://doi.org/10.1016/j.cden.2016.12.005.
7. Davis BJ. How are odontogenic infections best managed? J Can Dent Assoc. 2010;76:a37.
8. Elad S, Ranna V, Ariyawardana A, Correa ME, Tilly V, Nair RG, et al. A systematic review of oral herpetic viral infections in cancer patients: commonly used outcome measures and interventions. Support Care Cancer. 2017;25(2):687–700. https://doi.org/10.1007/s00520-016-3477-7.
9. Ferguson BL, Barber S, Asher IH, Wood CR. Role of oral microbial infections in oral cancer. Dent Clin N Am. 2017;61(2):425–34. https://doi.org/10.1016/j.cden.2016.12.009.

10. Freifeld AG, Bow EJ, Sepkowitz KA, Boeckh MJ, Ito JI, Mullen CA, et al. Clinical practice guideline for the use of antimicrobial agents in neutropenic patients with cancer: 2010 update by the infectious diseases society of America. Clin Infect Dis. 2011;52(4):e56–93. https://doi.org/10.1093/cid/cir073.
11. Gramolelli S, Schulz TF. The role of Kaposi sarcoma-associated herpesvirus in the pathogenesis of Kaposi sarcoma. J Pathol. 2015;235(2):368–80. https://doi.org/10.1002/path.4441.
12. Kathiravan MK, Salake AB, Chothe AS, Dudhe PB, Watode RP, Mukta MS, Gadhwe S. The biology and chemistry of antifungal agents: a review. Bioorg Med Chem. 2012;20(19):5678–98. https://doi.org/10.1016/j.bmc.2012.04.045.
13. Lalla RV, Latortue MC, Hong CH, Ariyawardana A, D'Amato-Palumbo S, Fischer DJ, et al. A systematic review of oral fungal infections in patients receiving cancer therapy. Support Care Cancer. 2010;18(8):985–92. https://doi.org/10.1007/s00520-010-0892-z.
14. Lalla RV, Patton LL, Dongari-Bagtzoglou A. Oral candidiasis: pathogenesis, clinical presentation, diagnosis and treatment strategies. J Calif Dent Assoc. 2013;41(4):263–8.
15. Lalla RV, Treister N, Sollecito T, Schmidt B, Patton LL, Mohammadi K, et al. Oral complications at 6 months after radiation therapy for head and neck cancer. Oral Dis. 2017;23(8):1134–43. https://doi.org/10.1111/odi.12710.
16. Lerman MA, Laudenbach J, Marty FM, Baden LR, Treister NS. Management of oral infections in cancer patients. Dent Clin N Am. 2008;52(1):129–153, ix. https://doi.org/10.1016/j.cden.2007.10.006.
17. Levi LE, Lalla RV. Dental treatment planning for the patient with oral cancer. Dent Clin N Am. 2018;62(1):121–30. https://doi.org/10.1016/j.cden.2017.08.009.
18. Martins JR, Chagas OL Jr, Velasques BD, Bobrowski AN, Correa MB, Torriani MA. The use of antibiotics in odontogenic infections: what is the best choice? A systematic review. J Oral Maxillofac Surg. 2017;75(12):2606.e2601–11. https://doi.org/10.1016/j.joms.2017.08.017.
19. Millsop JW, Fazel N. Oral candidiasis. Clin Dermatol. 2016;34(4):487–94. https://doi.org/10.1016/j.clindermatol.2016.02.022.
20. Mosel DD, Bauer RL, Lynch DP, Hwang ST. Oral complications in the treatment of cancer patients. Oral Dis. 2011;17(6):550–9. https://doi.org/10.1111/j.1601-0825.2011.01788.x.
21. Mousset S, Buchheidt D, Heinz W, Ruhnke M, Cornely OA, Egerer G, et al. Treatment of invasive fungal infections in cancer patients-updated recommendations of the Infectious Diseases Working Party (AGIHO) of the German Society of Hematology and Oncology (DGHO). Ann Hematol. 2014;93(1):13–32. https://doi.org/10.1007/s00277-013-1867-1.
22. Muzyka BC, Epifanio RN. Update on oral fungal infections. Dent Clin N Am. 2013;57(4):561–81. https://doi.org/10.1016/j.cden.2013.07.002.
23. Nair RG, Salajegheh A, Itthagarun A, Pakneshan S, Brennan MT, Samaranayake LP. Orofacial viral infections—an update for clinicians. Dent Update. 2014;41(6):518–20, 522–4. https://doi.org/10.12968/denu.2014.41.6.518.
24. Ogle OE. Odontogenic infections. Dent Clin N Am. 2017;61(2):235–52. https://doi.org/10.1016/j.cden.2016.11.004.
25. Palmason S, Marty FM, Treister NS. How do we manage oral infections in allogeneic stem cell transplantation and other severely immunocompromised patients? Oral Maxillofac Surg Clin North Am. 2011;23(4):579–599, vii. https://doi.org/10.1016/j.coms.2011.07.012.
26. Pappas PG, Kauffman CA, Andes DR, Clancy CJ, Marr KA, Ostrosky-Zeichner L, et al. Clinical practice guideline for the management of candidiasis: 2016 update by the Infectious Diseases Society of America. Clin Infect Dis. 2016;62(4):e1–50. https://doi.org/10.1093/cid/civ933.
27. Peedikayil FC. Antibiotics in odontogenic infections-an update. J Antimicrol. 2016;2(117):2472–1212.
28. Rajendra Santosh AB, Ogle OE, Williams D, Woodbine EF. Epidemiology of oral and maxillofacial infections. Dent Clin N Am. 2017;61(2):217–33. https://doi.org/10.1016/j.cden.2016.11.003.
29. Rodrigues ME, Henriques M, Silva S. Disinfectants to fight oral candida biofilms. Adv Exp Med Biol. 2016;931:83–93. https://doi.org/10.1007/5584_2016_10.

30. Santosh AB, Reddy BV. Oral mucosal infections: insights into specimen collection and medication management. Dent Clin N Am. 2017;61(2):283–304. https://doi.org/10.1016/j.cden.2016.12.002.
31. Scully C, Samaranayake LP. Emerging and changing viral diseases in the new millennium. Oral Dis. 2016;22(3):171–9. https://doi.org/10.1111/odi.12356.
32. Sroussi HY, Epstein JB, Bensadoun RJ, Saunders DP, Lalla RV, Migliorati CA, et al. Common oral complications of head and neck cancer radiation therapy: mucositis, infections, saliva change, fibrosis, sensory dysfunctions, dental caries, periodontal disease, and osteoradionecrosis. Cancer Med. 2017;6(12):2918–31. https://doi.org/10.1002/cam4.1221.
33. Skiada A, Lanternier F, Groll AH, Pagano L, Zimmerli S, Herbrecht R, et al. Diagnosis and treatment of mucormycosis in patients with hematological malignancies: guidelines from the 3rd European Conference on Infections in Leukemia (ECIL 3). Haematologica. 2013;98(4):492–504. https://doi.org/10.3324/haematol.2012.065110.
34. Stojanov IJ, Woo SB. Human papillomavirus and Epstein-Barr virus associated conditions of the oral mucosa. Semin Diagn Pathol. 2015;32(1):3–11. https://doi.org/10.1053/j.semdp.2014.12.003.
35. Stoopler ET, Sollecito TP. Oral mucosal diseases: evaluation and management. Med Clin North Am. 2014;98(6):1323–52. https://doi.org/10.1016/j.mcna.2014.08.006.
36. Swidergall M, Filler SG. Oropharyngeal candidiasis: fungal invasion and epithelial cell responses. PLoS Pathog. 2017;13(1):e1006056. https://doi.org/10.1371/journal.ppat.1006056.
37. Telles DR, Karki N, Marshall MW. Oral fungal infections: diagnosis and management. Dent Clin N Am. 2017;61(2):319–49. https://doi.org/10.1016/j.cden.2016.12.004.
38. Ullmann AJ, Schmidt-Hieber M, Bertz H, Heinz WJ, Kiehl M, Kruger W, et al. Infectious diseases in allogeneic haematopoietic stem cell transplantation: prevention and prophylaxis strategy guidelines 2016. Ann Hematol. 2016;95(9):1435–55. https://doi.org/10.1007/s00277-016-2711-1.
39. Villa A, Akintoye SO. Dental management of patients who have undergone oral cancer therapy. Dent Clin N Am. 2018;62(1):131–42. https://doi.org/10.1016/j.cden.2017.08.010.
40. Villa A, Hanna GJ. Human papillomavirus and oropharyngeal cancer. Curr Probl Cancer. 2018; https://doi.org/10.1016/j.currproblcancer.2018.06.005.

Salivary Gland Diseases, Hyposalivation, and Xerostomia in Head and Neck Cancer Patients

7

Jillian Rigert and Michael T. Brennan

7.1 Introduction

Due to the superficial location of the salivary glands in the head and neck, salivary glands are often damaged when in the radiation treatment field for head and neck cancer. Radiation doses as low as 10 Gy have been shown to cause partial damage to the glands. The lower limit dose for total and permanent damage varies by study, but general consensus agrees that doses 60 Gy and above typically cause permanent damage to the glands. The amount of damage to the salivary glands is impacted by the cumulative amount of radiation to the area. When salivary glands are damaged, a cascade of side effects may occur in the mouth secondary to hyposalivation and resultant xerostomia. Xerostomia is a common complaint from head and neck cancer patients with a reported 93% prevalence in patients currently undergoing radiation therapy and 74–85% following radiation therapy. Other side effects of hyposalivation secondary to radiation treatment include increased bacteriogenic flora, reduced buffering capacity, increased dental caries and periodontal disease rate, and increased risk for oral infections and ulcerative lesions. Additionally, patients may experience pain, difficulty eating or speaking, and reduced quality of life. Management strategies for hyposalivation and xerostomia have been aimed at salivary gland protection, residual salivary gland stimulation, and symptomatic relief with the use of salivary substitutes and mucosal lubrication. Current management strategies are often limited by low effectiveness, high risk/benefit ratios, and/or high cost burden to patients.

J. Rigert · M. T. Brennan (✉)
Department of Oral Medicine, Atrium Health's Carolinas Medical Center, Charlotte, NC, USA
e-mail: mike.brennan@atriumhealth.org

R. Nair (ed.), *Orofacial Supportive Care in Cancer*,
https://doi.org/10.1007/978-3-030-86510-8_7

7.2 Normal Salivary Gland Function and Role of Saliva

Saliva has several functions in the mouth including lubrication of the mucosal surfaces, mobilization of food debris, formation of food bolus, neutralization of oral environment acidity, remineralization of teeth, and assistance with swallowing and speech. The three major salivary glands (submandibular, parotid, and sublingual) are responsible for 90% of saliva production, while the minor salivary glands contribute the remaining 10%. The submandibular gland contains both mucous and serous glands which generate a mixed mucin-rich and protein-rich saliva, respectively. In contrast, the sublingual gland is composed mainly of mucous cells and contributes mucous-rich saliva, while the parotid gland is composed of mainly serous glands and contributes serous, protein-rich saliva. In normal conditions, the submandibular glands contribute 66% of the saliva at rest which is often referred to as the unstimulated saliva. During stimulated conditions (i.e., during mastication), the parotid gland contributes about 50% of the total saliva production. While the minor salivary glands contribute much less volume of saliva, their proper functioning is important for lubrication of the mucosal surfaces. Damage to the salivary glands leads to hyposalivation and xerostomia which often leads to detrimental consequences for the patients' oral environment and quality of life.

7.2.1 Hyposalivation and Xerostomia

Hyposalivation represents a pathologically low state of salivary secretion and is often defined as an unstimulated flow rate of less than or equal to 0.1 mL saliva/min and/or a stimulated saliva flow rate of less than or equal to 0.7 mL/min. Hyposalivation often leads to xerostomia, the subjective feeling of oral dryness, which may occur when a patient experiences a 45–50% reduction in resting salivary production. Hyposalivation puts patients at risk for increased infections, tooth decay, periodontal disease, mucosal trauma, oral pain/discomfort, difficulty swallowing and speaking, and reduced quality of life. Notably, patients may express feelings of oral dryness without observed oral dryness or measurable hyposalivation which may reflect changes in saliva composition.

7.3 Impact of Cancer Therapy on Salivary Gland Function

7.3.1 Radiation Therapy

The majority of patients receiving radiation for head and neck cancer will experience hyposalivation and resultant xerostomia of at least a mild-moderate severity during and following radiation therapy, with a small percentage of patients reporting severe xerostomia late following radiation treatment. The extent of salivary gland damage and xerostomia is related to the cumulative dose of radiation received by the salivary gland tissue and the volume of salivary gland tissue included in the radiation field. The highest prevalence of salivary hypofunction and xerostomia may be anticipated when all salivary glands are included in the radiation field (i.e., for treatment of nasopharyngeal carcinoma) with low chance of salivary gland recovery if doses reach 60 Gy. The long-term prevalence and severity of hyposalivation and xerostomia may be reduced in patients treated unilaterally, at reduced radiation doses, and/or by sparing normal tissue from radiation fields through the use of 3D conformal radiation therapy or intensity-modulated radiation therapy (IMRT).

A systematic review by Jensen SB et al. found the prevalence of xerostomia from a pooled data of patients undergoing conventional radiotherapy, 3D conformational radiotherapy, and/or intensity-modulated therapy of the head and neck to be 93% during radiation with a slight reduction (73.6–85.3%) 1 month to over 2 years post-treatment. The severity of xerostomia as measured by a visual analog scale (VAS) and grades 1–4 (4 being most severe) revealed highest prevalence of grade 2 xerostomia during radiation treatment to 6 months postradiation, grade 1 xerostomia 6 months to 1 year posttreatment, and a small number of patients experiencing grade 3 and 4 xerostomia late after radiation therapy. Correlating with the timing and severity of xerostomia reported, assessment of salivary flows revealed significant decline in both unstimulated and stimulated flows during radiation treatment, declining further 1–3 months postradiation treatment and slightly improving after 6 months to 2 years after completion of radiation (Fig. 7.1). Studies revealed that stimulated flow rates were consistently higher than unstimulated flow rates,

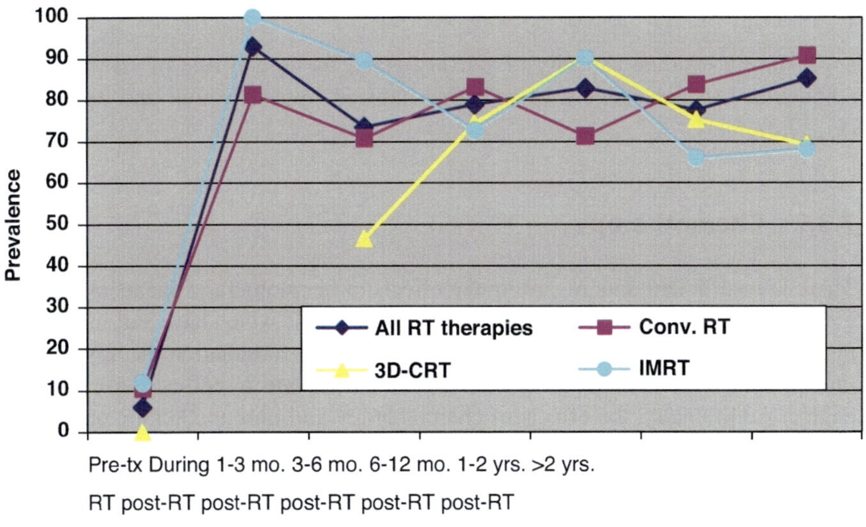

Fig. 7.1 Pooled and weighted prevalences of xerostomia induced by head and neck radiotherapy. *RT* radiotherapy, *Conv.* conventional, *3D-CRT* three-dimensional conformal RT, *IMRT* intensity-modulated RT, *Tx* treatment, *Mo.* months, *Yrs.* years . (*Reprinted by permission from Springer Nature: Jensen SB, Pedersen AM, Vissink A, Andersen E, Brown CG, Davies AN et al. A systematic review of salivary gland hypofunction and xerostomia induced by cancer therapies: prevalence, severity and impact on quality of life. Support Care Cancer. 2010;18(8):1039–60*)

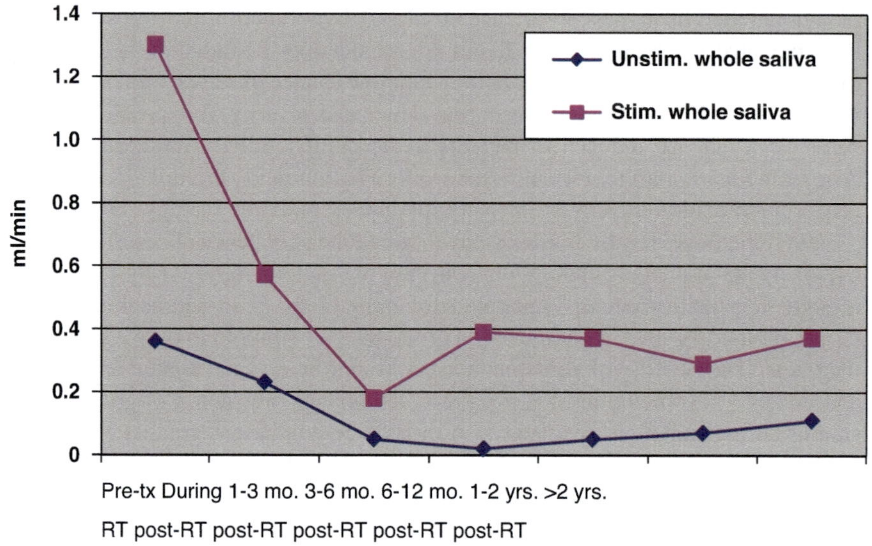

Fig. 7.2 Pooled and weighted data of unstimulated and stimulated whole saliva flow changes during and after head and neck radiotherapy. *Tx* treatment, *RT* radiotherapy, *Mo.* months, *Yrs.* years, *Unstim.* unstimulated, *Stim.* stimulated. (*Reprinted by permission from Springer Nature: Jensen SB, Pedersen AM, Vissink A, Andersen E, Brown CG, Davies AN et al. A systematic review of salivary gland hypofunction and xerostomia induced by cancer therapies: prevalence, severity and impact on quality of life. Support Care Cancer. 2010;18(8):1039–60*)

suggesting a residual capacity of salivary gland tissue and role of salivary gland stimulants for management of radiation-induced hyposalivation and xerostomia (Fig. 7.2).

7.3.2 Chemotherapy

There is insufficient data regarding the effects of chemotherapy agents on salivary gland tissue. Several chemotherapy agents are available which have varying mechanisms of action and impacts on tissue. In comparison to radiation therapy, chemotherapy and immunotherapy may induce salivary gland hypofunction to a lesser degree. Additionally, the effects of chemotherapy and immunotherapy on salivary gland tissue are more likely to be temporary and reversible.

7.3.3 Radioactive Iodine Treatment

Patients with thyroid cancer treated with radioactive iodine may experience hyposalivation and xerostomia due to the accumulation of radioactive iodine in salivary gland tissue with approximately 30–35% prevalence of dry mouth and a 33% reduction of salivary flow after therapy.

7.3.4 Conditioning Total Body Irradiation/Chemotherapy and Hematopoietic Stem Cell Transplantation

A prospective study by Laaksonen M et al. assessed xerostomia and salivary function pre- and post-hematopoietic stem cell transplantation (HSCT). Defining hyposalivation as stimulated whole salivary flow <0.7 mL/min, the prevalence of patients with hyposalivation was highest 6 months post-HSCT (53%) and dropped off to 26% by 24 months post-HSCT. A prospective study of 44 long-term survivors and their donors (median survival = 17.5 years; range = 11–26 years) post-HSCT demonstrated that 53% of patients compared to only 7% of donors reported dry mouth.

7.4 Management of Hyposalivation and Xerostomia

7.4.1 Prevention Strategies

7.4.1.1 Limiting Radiation Doses

While there is variation in the proposed minimum threshold amount of radiation that results in permanent damage to salivary gland tissue, there is general agreement in the literature that radiation doses >60 Gy result in permanent damage. Studies suggest that mean doses ranging from <26 to <40 Gy may result in preservation of some parotid gland function, while mean doses <39 Gy may result in potential preservation of submandibular gland function. Treatments aimed at selective targeting of cancerous cells, such as with IMRT, may assist in limiting cumulative radiation dose to normal tissue by better isolation of target tissue.

7.4.1.2 Intensity-Modulated Radiation Therapy (IMRT)

When available, IMRT is a currently recommended standard treatment for head and neck cancer patients aimed at treatment of disease while preventing xerostomia and salivary gland hypofunction. IMRT uses multiple beams with varying intensity profiles geared at targeting cancer cells while minimizing radiation to normal tissue, such as the salivary glands. As a result, salivary gland tissue may receive less cumulative dose of radiation, and function may be spared. Studies reveal that parotid-sparing IMRT may serve to reduce the prevalence and severity of parotid hyposalivation with resultant reduction in patient experience of xerostomia when patients were followed for more than 1 year. In contrast to patients treated with conventional radiation therapy, patients treated with IMRT showed better improvement of salivary flows over time postradiation indicating that these patients have higher levels of active residual gland remaining posttreatment. Additionally, patients with early-stage disease and unilateral involvement may have sparing of the contralateral submandibular gland with the use of IMRT, though practices are limited to select cases that do not require bilateral radiation. For patients that have advanced disease requiring bilateral radiation and/or radiation to critical lymphatics, IMRT may not be able to spare the function of submandibular gland tissue which results in reduction in unstimulated flow and altered saliva composition. In a recent study by Lalla et al., preliminary results for a larger prospective study of 577 head and neck cancer patients indicated stimulated whole salivary flow declined significantly from 1.09 mL/min pre-RT to 0.47 mL/min 6 months post-RT in head and neck cancer patients treated with IMRT or newer RT modalities. The mean stimulated whole salivary flow at 6 months post-RT for the different RT treatments included 3D conformal RT = 0.38 mL/min, IMRT with or without image guidance = 0.54–0.56 mL/min, and proton therapy = 0.80 mL/min.

7.4.1.3 Amifostine

Amifostine is a radical scavenger that has been shown in rat models to preferably accumulate in salivary gland tissue and have a radioprotective effect. A recent Cochrane Review concluded that there is low-quality evidence to support the use of amifostine to reduce xerostomia at the end of RT and up to 3 months post-RT. Limitations with the use of amifostine, clinically, include possible coincident radioprotection on tumor cells and severe adverse effects including hypotension, nausea, vomiting, and allergy particularly when administered intravenously.

7.4.2 Secretory Stimulants: Muscarinic Agonists

Both pilocarpine and cevimeline are parasympathomimetics that can improve salivary flow and decrease xerostomia. Pilocarpine has been approved for the treatment of radiation-induced xerostomia in several countries. The use of parasympathomimetics is dependent on residual capacity of salivary gland tissue function as the medication works by stimulating the tissue to secrete saliva via targeting agonism of muscarinic receptors on the cell surface. Pilocarpine is commonly prescribed in dosage of 5 mg four times per day with maximum recommended dose being 10 mg per dose and up to 30 mg daily. Cevimeline (30 mg tabs) can be prescribed up to three times per day. Literature data suggests that 50% of patients will benefit from oral pilocarpine postradiation with optimum benefits occurring after 8–12 weeks of use. Topical use of pilocarpine in the forms of pastilles, lozenges, and mouthwashes has also shown promise for treatment of postradiation xerostomia. Benefits of parasympathomimetics are use-dependent and observed improvements in hyposalivation and xerostomia decline with cessation of the medication. Side effects of parasympathomimetics include sweating, headache, increased urinary frequency, vasodilatation, dizziness, dyspepsia, lacrimation, and nausea, and the medications are contraindicated for use in patients with narrow-angle glaucoma, uncontrolled asthma, and gastric ulcers. Close monitoring is required for patients with cardiovascular disease and pulmonary disease. Potential medication interactions should be reviewed prior to use.

7.4.3 Gustatory and Masticatory Salivary Stimulants

For patients that maintain residual function of salivary gland tissue, the use of sugar-free candies and lozenges may increase whole saliva and improve oral dryness post-radiation; however, acidic lozenges increase risk of hard tissue damage (i.e., teeth), and care should be taken with use. Masticatory stimulation with the use of gum is another approach to manage dry mouth, but poses an increased risk for development of myalgia and temporomandibular disorder. Use of gum may be limited if such symptoms develop. Residual salivary gland function is required in order for gustatory and masticatory approaches to be successful.

7.4.4 Saliva Substitutes/Mucosal Lubricants

Saliva substitutes and mucosal lubricants are often used for symptomatic relief of salivary hypostimulation and xerostomia. Products are available in various forms such a mouthwashes, sprays, and gels. These substitutes are composed of various constituents that serve to resemble the glycoprotein and antimicrobial components of saliva such as carboxymethylcellulose and mucin. Saliva substitutes are most beneficial when used in patients with severe xerostomia compared to mild-moderate xerostomia. Higher viscosity products such as gels may provide better, longer lasting nighttime relief, while less viscous substitutes may be preferred during the day. Due to the substitutes' limitations including short duration of relief and cumulative cost burden over time, patients may prefer frequent use of water. A Cochrane Review from 2011 reported that there is insufficient evidence that saliva substitutes are better or worse than placebos. Thus, recommendations for use may be made according to individual patient preference and perceived benefit.

7.4.5 Alternative Management Options

7.4.5.1 Surgical Transfer of Submandibular Gland/ Seikaly-Jha Procedure

Surgical transfer of a submandibular gland into the submental space may be considered for patients treated with radiation that does not include the submental space. A recent phase II study of 40 patients receiving submandibular gland transfer demonstrated good results in the rate of dry mouth and loss of salivary flow from baseline. The technique has been shown to preserve some submandibular function and reduce radiation-induced xerostomia. Preliminary data is promising, though careful considerations for case selection, cost, and surgical risks must be considered.

7.4.5.2 Acupuncture

In patients that have some residual salivary gland function, preliminary research reveals that acupuncture may have a role in improving salivary flow rates, reducing xerostomia, and improving patient quality of life. A systematic review of three randomized controlled trials indicated an improvement of xerostomia compared to control groups and some improvement in salivary flow. Additional studies have reported improvements in xerostomia (55% decrease in patients undergoing IMRT) with sustained effects lasting up to 3 years. The use of acupuncture may be beneficial with low risks of side effects, though more information is needed to substantiate the preliminary research findings.

7.4.5.3 Hyperbaric Oxygen (HBO) Treatment

A cohort of 80 head and neck cancer patients treated with HBO therapy post-radiotherapy demonstrated improvement in dry mouth complaints and a slight increase in unstimulated and stimulated salivary flows. These patients were treated for the prevention or treatment of osteoradionecrosis or soft tissue radiation injury. Two earlier reports reviewed revealed possible decrease in xerostomia when patients were being treated with HBO perioperatively for prevention of osteoradionecrosis of the jaw. Logistics, cost, and side effects will need to be considered before recommending HBO therapy solely for the management of xerostomia and salivary hypofunction.

7.5 Discussion and Conclusion

Salivary gland hypofunction and hyposalivation are common problems for patients being treated for head and neck cancer and lead to deleterious impacts on patients' oral health and quality of life. Prevention and treatment strategies for hyposalivation and xerostomia are limited by low and temporary efficacy, potentially high risk/benefit ratios, and high cumulative cost burdens. To date, the most commonly recommended treatment strategies are prevention of salivary damage via radiation dose-reduction methods such as IMRT with a combination of patient behavioral modifications including increased hydration and use of salivary substitutes. More research needs to be done in order to improve prevention and treatment of hyposalivation and xerostomia in a more effective, lower cost manner.

Bibliography

1. Deasy JO, Moiseenko V, Marks L, Chao KS, Nam J, Eisbruch A. Radiotherapy dose-volume effects on salivary gland function. Int J Radiat Oncol Biol Phys. 2010;76(3 Suppl):S58–63. https://doi.org/10.1016/j.ijrobp.2009.06.090.
2. Jensen SB, Pedersen AM, Vissink A, Andersen E, Brown CG, Davies AN, et al. A systematic review of salivary gland hypofunction and xerostomia induced by cancer therapies: prevalence, severity and impact on quality of life. Support Care Cancer. 2010;18(8):1039–60.
3. Pedersen AM, Bardow A, Jensen SB, Nauntofte B. Saliva and gastrointestinal functions of taste, mastication, swallowing and digestion. Oral Dis. 2002;8(3):117–29.

4. Dawes C, Ong BY. Circadian rhythms in the flow rate and proportional contribution of parotid to whole saliva volume in man. Arch Oral Biol. 1973;18(9):1145–53.
5. Dawes C, Wood CM. The contribution of oral minor mucous gland secretions to the volume of whole saliva in man. Arch Oral Biol. 1973;18(3):337–42.
6. Sreebny LM. Saliva in health and disease: an appraisal and update. Int Dent J. 2000;50(3):140–61.
7. Dawes C. Physiological factors affecting salivary flow rate, oral sugar clearance, and the sensation of dry mouth in man. J Dent Res. 1987;66(Special Issue):648–53.
8. Yeh SA, Huang YJ. Dose escalation for patients with locally advanced nasopharyngeal carcinoma treated with radiotherapy alone. Am J Clin Oncol. 2007;30(4):401–5. https://doi.org/10.1097/COC.0b013e31803377b3.
9. Franzen L, Funegard U, Ericson T, Henriksson R. Parotid gland function during and following radiotherapy of malignancies in the head and neck. A consecutive study of salivary flow and patient discomfort. Eur J Cancer. 1992;28(2–3):457–62.
10. Jensen SB, Pedersen AM, Vissink A, Andersen E, Brown CG, Davies AN, et al. A systematic review of salivary gland hypofunction and xerostomia induced by cancer therapies: management strategies and economic impact. Support Care Cancer. 2010;18(8):1061–79.
11. Jeong SY, Kim HW, Lee SW, Ahn BC, Lee J. Salivary gland function 5 years after radioactive iodine ablation in patients with differentiated thyroid cancer: direct comparison of pre- and postablation scintigraphies and their relation to xerostomia symptoms. Thyroid. 2013;23(5):609–16. https://doi.org/10.1089/thy.2012.0106.
12. Soo Roh S, Wook Kim D, Jin Baek H. Association of xerostomia and ultrasonographic features of the major salivary glands after radioactive iodine ablation for papillary thyroid carcinoma. AJR Am J Roentgenol. 2016;207(5):1077–81. https://doi.org/10.2214/AJR.15.15776.
13. Laaksonen M, Ramseier AM, Rovo A, Jensen SB, Raber-Durlacher JE, Zitzmann NU, et al. Longitudinal assessment of hematopoietic stem cell transplantation and hyposalivation. J Dent Res. 2011;90(10):1177–82. https://doi.org/10.1177/0022034511414156.
14. Daikeler T, Mauramo M, Rovo A, Stern M, Halter J, Buser A, et al. Sicca symptoms and their impact on quality of life among very long-term survivors after hematopoietic SCT. Bone Marrow Transplant. 2013;48(7):988–93. https://doi.org/10.1038/bmt.2012.260.
15. Chao KS, Deasy JO, Markman J, Haynie J, Perez CA, Purdy JA, et al. A prospective study of salivary function sparing in patients with head-and-neck cancers receiving intensity-modulated or three-dimensional radiation therapy: initial results. Int J Radiat Oncol Biol Phys. 2001;49(4):907–16. S0360-3016(00)01441-3 [pii].
16. Eisbruch A, Ten Haken RK, Kim HM, Marsh LH, Ship JA. Dose, volume, and function relationships in parotid salivary glands following conformal and intensity-modulated irradiation of head and neck cancer. Int J Radiat Oncol Biol Phys. 1999;45(3):577–87.
17. Blanco AI, Chao KS, El Naqa I, Franklin GE, Zakarian K, Vicic M, et al. Dose-volume modeling of salivary function in patients with head-and-neck cancer receiving radiotherapy. Int J Radiat Oncol Biol Phys. 2005;62(4):1055–69. https://doi.org/10.1016/j.ijrobp.2004.12.076.
18. Saarilahti K, Kouri M, Collan J, Hamalainen T, Atula T, Joensuu H, et al. Intensity modulated radiotherapy for head and neck cancer: evidence for preserved salivary gland function. Radiother Oncol. 2005;74(3):251–8. https://doi.org/10.1016/j.radonc.2004.11.004.
19. Li Y, Taylor JM, Ten Haken RK, Eisbruch A. The impact of dose on parotid salivary recovery in head and neck cancer patients treated with radiation therapy. Int J Radiat Oncol Biol Phys. 2007;67(3):660–9. S0360-3016(06)02988-9 [pii]. https://doi.org/10.1016/j.ijrobp.2006.09.021.
20. Munter MW, Karger CP, Hoffner SG, Hof H, Thilmann C, Rudat V, et al. Evaluation of salivary gland function after treatment of head-and-neck tumors with intensity-modulated radiotherapy by quantitative pertechnetate scintigraphy. Int J Radiat Oncol Biol Phys. 2004;58(1):175–84.
21. Liu WS, Lee SP, Lee JK, Su MC, Chen GD, Lee HS, et al. Factors influencing the parotid function in nasopharyngeal carcinoma treated with parotid-sparing radiotherapy. Jpn J Clin Oncol. 2006;36(10):626–31. https://doi.org/10.1093/jjco/hyl098.
22. Roesink JM, Moerland MA, Battermann JJ, Hordijk GJ, Terhaard CH. Quantitative dose-volume response analysis of changes in parotid gland function after radiotherapy in the head-and-neck region. Int J Radiat Oncol Biol Phys. 2001;51(4):938–46.

23. Scrimger R. Salivary gland sparing in the treatment of head and neck cancer. Expert Rev Anticancer Ther. 2011;11(9):1437–48. https://doi.org/10.1586/era.11.101.
24. Chao KS, Majhail N, Huang CJ, Simpson JR, Perez CA, Haughey B, et al. Intensity-modulated radiation therapy reduces late salivary toxicity without compromising tumor control in patients with oropharyngeal carcinoma: a comparison with conventional techniques. Radiother Oncol. 2001;61(3):275–80.
25. Wang ZH, Yan C, Zhang ZY, Zhang CP, Hu HS, Tu WY, et al. Impact of salivary gland dosimetry on post-IMRT recovery of saliva output and xerostomia grade for head-and-neck cancer patients treated with or without contralateral submandibular gland sparing: a longitudinal study. Int J Radiat Oncol Biol Phys. 2011;81(5):1479–87. https://doi.org/10.1016/j.ijrobp.2010.07.1990.
26. Saarilahti K, Kouri M, Collan J, Kangasmaki A, Atula T, Joensuu H, et al. Sparing of the submandibular glands by intensity modulated radiotherapy in the treatment of head and neck cancer. Radiother Oncol. 2006;78(3):270–5. https://doi.org/10.1016/j.radonc.2006.02.017.
27. Lalla RV, Treister N, Sollecito T, Schmidt B, Patton LL, Mohammadi K, et al. Oral complications at 6 months after radiation therapy for head and neck cancer. Oral Dis. 2017; https://doi.org/10.1111/odi.12710.
28. Brizel DM, Wasserman TH, Henke M, Strnad V, Rudat V, Monnier A, et al. Phase III randomized trial of amifostine as a radioprotector in head and neck cancer. J Clin Oncol. 2000;18(19):3339–45.
29. Wasserman TH, Brizel DM, Henke M, Monnier A, Eschwege F, Sauer R, et al. Influence of intravenous amifostine on xerostomia, tumor control, and survival after radiotherapy for head-and-neck cancer: 2-year follow-up of a prospective, randomized, phase III trial. Int J Radiat Oncol Biol Phys. 2005;63(4):985–90. https://doi.org/10.1016/j.ijrobp.2005.07.966.
30. Hensley ML, Hagerty KL, Kewalramani T, Green DM, Meropol NJ, Wasserman TH, et al. American Society of Clinical Oncology 2008 clinical practice guideline update: use of chemotherapy and radiation therapy protectants. J Clin Oncol. 2009;27(1):127–45. https://doi.org/10.1200/JCO.2008.17.2627.
31. Brizel DM, Overgaard J. Does amifostine have a role in chemoradiation treatment? Lancet Oncol. 2003;4(6):378–81.
32. Riley P, Glenny AM, Hua F, Worthington HV. Pharmacological interventions for preventing dry mouth and salivary gland dysfunction following radiotherapy. Cochrane Database Syst Rev. 2017;7:CD012744. https://doi.org/10.1002/14651858.CD012744.
33. Takahashi I, Nagai T, Miyaishi K, Maehara Y, Niibe H. Clinical study of the radioprotective effects of Amifostine (YM-08310, WR-2721) on chronic radiation injury. Int J Radiat Oncol Biol Phys. 1986;12(6):935–8.
34. Ozsahin M, Betz M, Matzinger O, Bron L, Luthi F, Pasche P, et al. Feasibility and efficacy of subcutaneous amifostine therapy in patients with head and neck cancer treated with curative accelerated concomitant-boost radiation therapy. Arch Otolaryngol Head Neck Surg. 2006;132(2):141–5. https://doi.org/10.1001/archotol.132.2.141.
35. Law A, Kennedy T, Pellitteri P, Wood C, Christie D, Yumen O. Efficacy and safety of subcutaneous amifostine in minimizing radiation-induced toxicities in patients receiving combined-modality treatment for squamous cell carcinoma of the head and neck. Int J Radiat Oncol Biol Phys. 2007;69(5):1361–8. https://doi.org/10.1016/j.ijrobp.2007.05.052.
36. Chambers MS, Posner M, Jones CU, Biel MA, Hodge KM, Vitti R, et al. Cevimeline for the treatment of postirradiation xerostomia in patients with head and neck cancer. Int J Radiat Oncol Biol Phys. 2007;68(4):1102–9. S0360-3016(07)00149-6 [pii]. https://doi.org/10.1016/j.ijrobp.2007.01.019.
37. Chambers MS, Jones CU, Biel MA, Weber RS, Hodge KM, Chen Y, et al. Open-label, long-term safety study of cevimeline in the treatment of postirradiation xerostomia. Int J Radiat Oncol Biol Phys. 2007;69(5):1369–76. https://doi.org/10.1016/j.ijrobp.2007.05.024.
38. Jham BC, Teixeira IV, Aboud CG, Carvalho AL, Coelho Mde M, Freire AR. A randomized phase III prospective trial of bethanechol to prevent radiotherapy-induced salivary gland damage in patients with head and neck cancer. Oral Oncol. 2007;43(2):137–42. https://doi.org/10.1016/j.oraloncology.2006.01.013.

39. Mercadante V, Al Hamad A, Lodi G, Porter S, Fedele S. Interventions for the management of radiotherapy-induced xerostomia and hyposalivation: a systematic review and meta-analysis. Oral Oncol. 2017;66:64–74. https://doi.org/10.1016/j.oraloncology.2016.12.031.
40. Wiseman LR, Faulds D. Oral pilocarpine: a review of its pharmacological properties and clinical potential in xerostomia. Drugs. 1995;49(1):143–56.
41. Fox PC, Atkinson JC, Macynski AA, Wolff A, Kung DS, Valdez IH, et al. Pilocarpine treatment of salivary gland hypofunction and dry mouth (xerostomia). Arch Intern Med. 1991;151(6):1149–52.
42. Johnson JT, Ferretti GA, Nethery WJ, Valdez IH, Fox PC, Ng D, et al. Oral pilocarpine for post-irradiation xerostomia in patients with head and neck cancer. N Engl J Med. 1993;329(6):390–5.
43. LeVeque FG, Montgomery M, Potter D, Zimmer MB, Rieke JW, Steiger BW, et al. A multicenter, randomized, double-blind, placebo-controlled, dose-titration study of oral pilocarpine for treatment of radiation-induced xerostomia in head and neck cancer patients. J Clin Oncol. 1993;11(6):1124–31.
44. Davies AN, Singer J. A comparison of artificial saliva and pilocarpine in radiation-induced xerostomia. J Laryngol Otol. 1994;108(8):663–5.
45. Hamlar DD, Schuller DE, Gahbauer RA, Buerki RA, Staubus AE, Hall J, et al. Determination of the efficacy of topical oral pilocarpine for postirradiation xerostomia in patients with head and neck carcinoma. Laryngoscope. 1996;106(8):972–6.
46. Taweechaisupapong S, Pesee M, Aromdee C, Laopaiboon M, Khunkitti W. Efficacy of pilocarpine lozenge for post-radiation xerostomia in patients with head and neck cancer. Aust Dent J. 2006;51(4):333–7.
47. Bernardi R, Perin C, Becker FL, Ramos GZ, Gheno GZ, Lopes LR, et al. Effect of pilocarpine mouthwash on salivary flow. Braz J Med Biol Res. 2002;35(1):105–10.
48. Daniels TE, Wu AJ. Xerostomia—clinical evaluation and treatment in general practice. J Calif Dent Assoc. 2000;28(12):933–41.
49. Senahayake F, Piggott K, Hamilton-Miller JM. A pilot study of Salix SST (saliva-stimulating lozenges) in post-irradiation xerostomia. Curr Med Res Opin. 1998;14(3):155–9. https://doi.org/10.1185/03007999809113355.
50. Jensdottir T, Nauntofte B, Buchwald C, Hansen HS, Bardow A. Effects of sucking acidic candies on saliva in unilaterally irradiated pharyngeal cancer patients. Oral Oncol. 2006;42(3):317–22. https://doi.org/10.1016/j.oraloncology.2005.08.009.
51. S-Gravenmade EJ, Roukema PA, Panders AK. The effect of mucin-containing artificial saliva on severe xerostomia. Int J Oral Surg. 1974;3(6):435–9.
52. Regelink G, Vissink A, Reintsema H, Nauta JM. Efficacy of a synthetic polymer saliva substitute in reducing oral complaints of patients suffering from irradiation-induced xerostomia. Quintessence Int. 1998;29(6):383–8.
53. Epstein JB, Stevenson-Moore P. A clinical comparative trial of saliva substitutes in radiation-induced salivary gland hypofunction. Spec Care Dentist. 1992;12(1):21–3.
54. Furness S, Worthington HV, Bryan G, Birchenough S, McMillan R. Interventions for the management of dry mouth: topical therapies. Cochrane Database Syst Rev. 2011;12:CD008934. https://doi.org/10.1002/14651858.CD008934.pub2.
55. Scrimger RA, Seikaly H, Vos LJ, Harris J, O'Connell D, Ghosh S, et al. Combination of submandibular salivary gland transfer and intensity-modulated radiotherapy to reduce dryness of mouth (xerostomia) in patients with head and neck cancer. Head Neck. 2018; https://doi.org/10.1002/hed.25339.
56. Jha N, Seikaly H, Harris J, Williams D, Liu R, McGaw T, et al. Prevention of radiation induced xerostomia by surgical transfer of submandibular salivary gland into the submental space. Radiother Oncol. 2003;66(3):283–9.
57. Pathak KA, Bhalavat RL, Mistry RC, Deshpande MS, Bhalla V, Desai SB, et al. Upfront submandibular salivary gland transfer in pharyngeal cancers. Oral Oncol. 2004;40(9):960–3. https://doi.org/10.1016/j.oraloncology.2004.04.016.

58. Seikaly H, Jha N, Harris JR, Barnaby P, Liu R, Williams D, et al. Long-term outcomes of submandibular gland transfer for prevention of postradiation xerostomia. Arch Otolaryngol Head Neck Surg. 2004;130(8):956–61. https://doi.org/10.1001/archotol.130.8.956.
59. Al-Qahtani K, Hier MP, Sultanum K, Black MJ. The role of submandibular salivary gland transfer in preventing xerostomia in the chemoradiotherapy patient. Oral Surg Oral Med Oral Pathol Oral Radiol Endod. 2006;101(6):753–6. https://doi.org/10.1016/j.tripleo.2005.12.017.
60. Johnstone PA, Peng YP, May BC, Inouye WS, Niemtzow RC. Acupuncture for pilocarpine-resistant xerostomia following radiotherapy for head and neck malignancies. Int J Radiat Oncol Biol Phys. 2001;50(2):353–7.
61. Blom M, Dawidson I, Fernberg JO, Johnson G, Angmar-Mansson B. Acupuncture treatment of patients with radiation-induced xerostomia. Eur J Cancer B Oral Oncol. 1996;32B(3):182–90.
62. Blom M, Lundeberg T. Long-term follow-up of patients treated with acupuncture for xerostomia and the influence of additional treatment. Oral Dis. 2000;6(1):15–24.
63. Cho JH, Chung WK, Kang W, Choi SM, Cho CK, Son CG. Manual acupuncture improved quality of life in cancer patients with radiation-induced xerostomia. J Altern Complement Med. 2008;14(5):523–6. https://doi.org/10.1089/acm.2007.0793.
64. Zhuang L, Yang Z, Zeng X, Zhua X, Chen Z, Liu L, et al. The preventive and therapeutic effect of acupuncture for radiation-induced xerostomia in patients with head and neck cancer: a systematic review. Integr Cancer Ther. 2013;12(3):197–205. https://doi.org/10.1177/1534735412451321.
65. Forner L, Hyldegaard O, von Brockdorff AS, Specht L, Andersen E, Jansen EC, et al. Does hyperbaric oxygen treatment have the potential to increase salivary flow rate and reduce xerostomia in previously irradiated head and neck cancer patients? A pilot study. Oral Oncol. 2011;47(6):546–51. https://doi.org/10.1016/j.oraloncology.2011.03.021.
66. Gerlach NL, Barkhuysen R, Kaanders JH, Janssens GO, Sterk W, Merkx MA. The effect of hyperbaric oxygen therapy on quality of life in oral and oropharyngeal cancer patients treated with radiotherapy. Int J Oral Maxillofac Surg. 2008;37(3):255–9. https://doi.org/10.1016/j.ijom.2007.11.013.
67. Harding SA, Hodder SC, Courtney DJ, Bryson PJ. Impact of perioperative hyperbaric oxygen therapy on the quality of life of maxillofacial patients who undergo surgery in irradiated fields. Int J Oral Maxillofac Surg. 2008;37(7):617–24. https://doi.org/10.1016/j.ijom.2008.04.004.
68. Sasportas LS, Hosford DN, Sodini MA, Waters DJ, Zambricki EA, Barral JK, et al. Cost-effectiveness landscape analysis of treatments addressing xerostomia in patients receiving head and neck radiation therapy. Oral Surg Oral Med Oral Pathol Oral Radiol. 2013;116(1):e37–51. https://doi.org/10.1016/j.oooo.2013.02.017.

Soft Tissue and Hard Tissue Necrosis

8

Mel Mupparapu and Sunday O. Akintoye

8.1 Introduction

Notable among the conditions that cause both soft tissue damage and bone damage during cancer therapy are osteoradionecrosis (ORN) and medication-related osteonecrosis of the jaw (MRONJ). ORN is a condition that occurs as a complication of radiation therapy (RT) in patients undergoing cancer therapy. If not prevented, ORN leads to significant morbidity due to progressive loss of vascularity to the affected region leading to necrosis of the bone and pathologic fracture. After RT, bone undergoes changes that are histologically noted as obliteration of the lumen of vessels and sclerotic changes in their walls. Bone trabeculation is reduced in both width and numbers, and hence there is increase in the size of marrow spaces containing necrotic material. The bony changes are not apparent for a while and, even if they do, are not pathognomonic of radiation injury. Radiographs are of little or no value in the early stages of the disease. ORN ranges from asymptomatic bone exposures that may remain stable for months or years to severe necrosis leading to pathologic fractures. Severe intractable pain is sometimes the only symptom in the absence of any radiographically detectable bony changes of ORN. MRONJ is a clinical condition resulting from the use of medication that would alter the normal physiology of bone turnover. MRONJ can be precipitated by any individual medication that causes direct toxicity to soft and hard tissues or suppression of bone turnover or leads to a change in the acquired immunity leading eventually to delayed wound healing or promoting infection. Some examples of medications that would affect the bone turnover are antiresorptive medications like bisphosphonates and RANK ligand inhibitors (denosumab). Both are primarily antiresorptive in nature. Bisphosphonates are administered both orally and intravenously, but denosumab is administered

M. Mupparapu (✉) · S. O. Akintoye
Department of Oral Medicine, School of Dental Medicine, University of Pennsylvania, Philadelphia, PA, USA
e-mail: mmd@upenn.edu

R. Nair (ed.), *Orofacial Supportive Care in Cancer*,
https://doi.org/10.1007/978-3-030-86510-8_8

subcutaneously. The antiresorptive preparations commonly in use are alendronate (Fosamax®), risedronate (Actonel®), ibandronate (Boniva®), pamidronate (Aredia®), zoledronate (Zometa®, Reclast®), and denosumab (Xgeva®, Prolia®). Denosumab is a humanized monoclonal antibody administered SQ 120 mg every 4 weeks. The other groups of drugs that are implicated in the predisposition for MRONJ are the antiangiogenic medications. Their mechanism of action varies from being tyrosine kinase inhibitors or humanized monoclonal antibodies or being mammalian targets of rapamycin pathway. Commonly used medications are sunitinib, sorafenib, bevacizumab, and sirolimus among others. However, the current understanding of the pathophysiology points to participation of drug interactions and genetic polymorphisms.

8.2 Definitions

ORN can be defined as a condition where the irradiated bone becomes exposed through a break in the overlying mucosa or skin and persists without healing for period of 3–6 months.

MRONJ can be defined as an exposure of the bone that can be probed through and intraoral or extraoral fistula in the oral and maxillofacial region that has persisted for over 8 weeks. A previous history of antiresorptive or antiangiogenic drug use should be present, but there should be no history of RT.

8.3 Current Knowledge

The widespread use of radiotherapy for head and neck cancer as well as bone antiresorptives and antiangiogenic agents have increased the incidence of soft and hard tissue necrosis in oral cancer patients. External and internal insults from radiation, chemotherapeutic regimens, and other chemical agents can induce pathological processes that damage the orofacial soft and hard tissue structures.

Radiation-induced soft tissue necrosis is one of the first complications of head and neck cancer radiotherapy. Soft tissue necrosis is an ulceration or necrosis of the irradiated field and surgical bed or a persistently unhealed high-grade acute oral mucositis. Disruption of the vasculature and connective tissue and reduced repopulation of proliferative stem cells in the irradiated region will delay healing. Hence, severe oral mucositis, tissue fibrosis, or obliteration of minor blood vessels of the oral tissue can promote soft tissue necrosis. Additionally, a subset of patients managed with transoral robotic surgery (TORS) and postoperative RT also often develop soft tissue necrosis. In these patients, several risk factors that increase susceptibility to soft tissue necrosis include the position of the tonsils, resection depth, radiation dose, and severity of mucositis. Patients on antiresorptive therapies to control abnormal bone turnover caused by skeletal cancer metastasis are highly prone to MRONJ. While the exact pathophysiological process of hard tissue necrosis such as ORN and MRONJ is still unclear, the incidence of MRONJ continues to rise relative to other types of osteonecrosis. Notwithstanding, ORN is still a major challenge in spite of careful head and neck cancer treatment planning.

Several pathophysiologic theories regarding oral soft and hard tissue necrosis have been used to support the cellular and molecular processes that occur to the oral tissues during oral cancer therapies. Radiation-induced fibroatrophic process is a theory attributed to the damaging effects of reactive oxygen species on fibroblasts, endothelium, and bone cells that eventually results in soft tissue and bone necrosis. Several other theories have been used to support the hard tissue changes that occur in head and neck cancer patients. The processes leading to ORN were first described as a triad of radiation, trauma, and infection. But this has since been replaced by the theory that radiation induces a hypoxic-hypocellular-hypovascular environment within the bone tissue. This theory combined with the fibroatrophic process supports the sequential damages to oral soft and hard tissues that occur progressively from the skin or mucosa to periosteum, bone, and finally the endothelium within the bone marrow compartment. A combination of local tissue injury, infection, and radiation-induced osteoblast and osteoclast depletion allows ORN to progress unabated. Habitual smoking, alcoholism, and poor oral health are strong risk factors for ORN. Additionally, tooth extraction or any form of surgical probing of the irradiated bone can set off ORN.

At the cellular level, radiation causes the release of free radicals like superoxide (O^-) and hydroxyl (OH^-) that cause radiation-induced cell death and loss of osteoprogenitor cells needed to repair the bone damage. Histologically, the early stages of ORN begin with erythema and vascular hyperemia. This then progresses to vascular damage leading to thrombosis and cell death (Fig. 8.1). Transdifferentiation of bone marrow cells leads to adipocytic infiltration, and deposition of extracellular collagen leads to fibrosis.

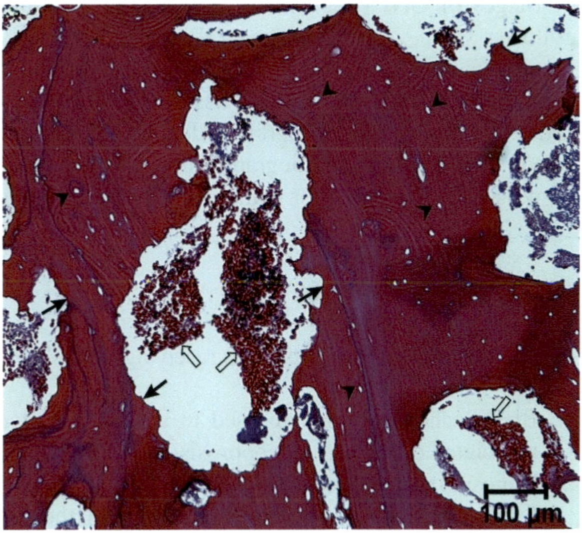

Fig. 8.1 A typical histologic presentation of jaw necrosis in oral cancer patient. There are regions of thrombosis (transparent arrows), empty osteocyte lacunae (black arrowheads), and irregular bone margins characteristic of abnormal bone resorption (black arrows)

8.4 Clinical Presentation

ORN is associated with pain, swelling, and fever depending on the severity of the inflammatory process. The irradiated oral soft tissue becomes thinner and fibrotic and can be readily traumatized. The breakdown of soft and hard tissues can be associated with paresthesia/anesthesia, and it exposes the irradiated bone to further insults that can lead to osteomyelitis. The relatively tenuous blood supply and higher compact bone of the mandible make it more susceptible to ORN than the maxilla. Extensive ORN particularly in the mandible can result in pathologic fracture. For patients with MRONJ, the clinical presentation is often variable ranging from non-exposed bone to severe bone loss and pathologic fracture.

8.5 Classification

8.5.1 ORN Staging

ORN is bone death after irradiation. This is secondary to either reduced vascularity or complete lack of vascularity based on the severity of the radiation injury. The diagnosis of ORN is primarily based on clinical evaluation of signs and symptoms. Although mandible is commonly affected, ORN can affect the maxilla as well. It was noted that the incidence of ORN in conventional RT is about 7.4%, about 5.2% in intensity-modulated RT (IMRT), about 6.8% in chemoradiotherapy, and about 5.3% in brachytherapy. In this evidence-based review, Peterson and associates found no clear guidelines for either prevention or treatment of ORN. There is no universally accepted classification of ORN. Schwartz and Kagan classified ORN based on the clinical presentation and associated complications. The Canadian Cancer Society's clinical classification of ORN is a simple, yet efficient, one.

Stages of ONJ (Fig. 8.1) as defined by the Canadian Cancer Society are as follows:

Grade I (clinical diagnosis): soft tissue necrosis with exposure of bone underneath.
Grade II (clinical and radiographic diagnosis): ORN that is refractory to treatment.
Grade III (clinical and radiographic diagnosis): ORN that affected the entire thickness of the bone with or without a pathologic fracture.

8.5.2 MRONJ Stages

MRONJ has been noted in patients receiving the following categories of medications:

1. Bisphosphonates that are used to treat hypercalcemia of malignancy, tumor-associated osteolysis, osteoporosis, and Paget's disease.
2. Denosumab, a monoclonal antibody that inactivates receptor activator of nuclear factor-kappa B ligand (RANKL), used in the treatment of osteoporosis and tumor-associated osteolysis (TAO).

3. Bevacizumab, another monoclonal antibody that inactivates vascular endothelial growth factor (VEGF), used in cancers like glioblastoma and metastatic breast, renal, lung, and colorectal cancers.
4. Sunitinib, sorafenib, and cabozantinib—tyrosine kinase inhibitors that block VEGF receptor and are used in the treatment of metastatic breast, lung, renal, and colorectal cancers.
5. Everolimus and temsirolimus® that are mTor inhibitors used in the treatment of metastatic renal cell carcinoma.
6. Tocilizumab or atlizumab, a humanized monoclonal antibody that acts against the interleukin-6 receptor (IL-6R). This is an immunosuppressive drug used for the treatment of rheumatoid arthritis (RA) and systemic juvenile idiopathic arthritis (SJIA). In a presented case by Bindakhil and Mupparapu, the patient did not have a history of bisphosphonate therapy but only took tocilizumab 162 mg/day for RA with clinical and radiographic evidence of osteonecrosis status post-extractions in the area. Although this association has not been consistent, it is yet another class of drug that has shown the potential for osteonecrosis.
7. Raloxifene, a second-generation selective estrogen receptor modulator (SERM). This has an estrogen-agonistic effect on the bone and hence increases bone mineral density and mass by decreasing bone resorption. This drug also has estrogen-antagonistic effect in the breast and uterus.

MRONJ was categorized by the American Academy of oral and maxillofacial surgeons (AAOMS) into four clinically distinguishable categories.

Stage 0: No clinical evidence of necrotic bone with nonspecific clinical and radiographic findings. If the periodontal bone loss cannot be attributed to chronic periodontal disease and changes in trabecular pattern are potential clues (Figs. 8.2, 8.3, and 8.4).

Stage 1: Clinically exposed bone that appears necrotic but clinical symptoms are not noted (Figs. 8.5 and 8.6).

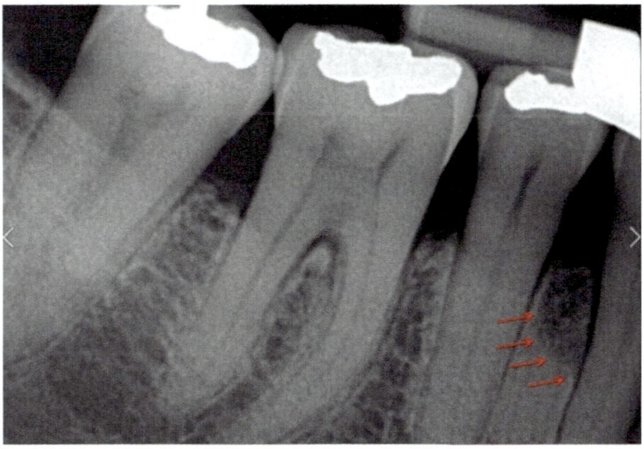

Fig. 8.2 MRONJ stage 0. Cropped intraoral periapical radiograph of right premolar region showing the interdental area between the two premolars. Arrows point to the developing bony pocket

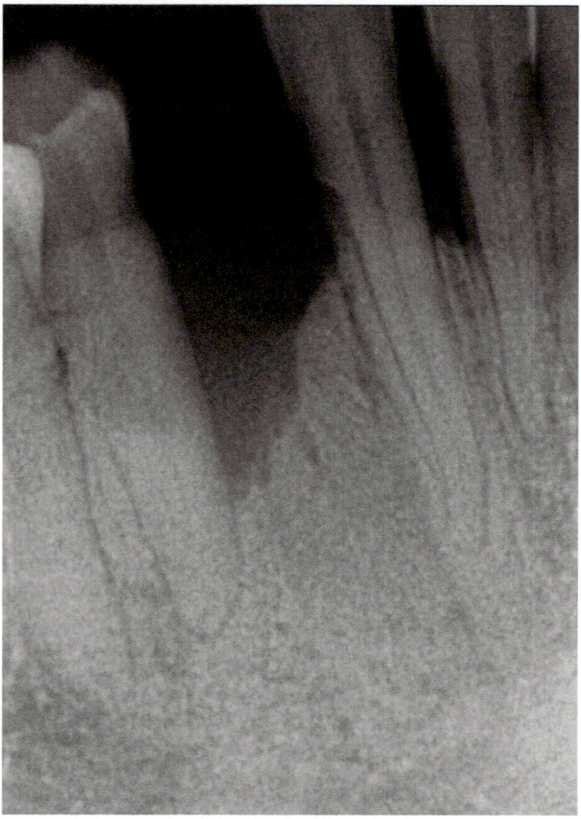

Fig. 8.3 MRONJ stage 0. Intraoral mandibular right lateral-canine periapical radiograph showing the angular bone loss mesial to the first premolar. Note the canine is missing due to a prior extraction. This is a 55-year-old female patient who was on 35 mg weekly dose of alendronate for over 3 years after surgical removal of melanoma left chest. Note the increased sclerosis of bone in the region of the canine and the premolar suggestive of changes consistent with stage 0 MRONJ

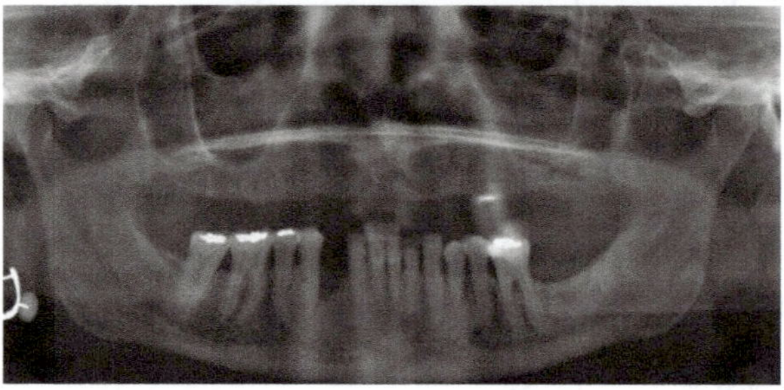

Fig. 8.4 MRONJ stage 0. CBCT axial view. Panoramic radiograph of the same patient in Figs. 8.2 and 8.3. Note the extensive sclerosis of the region between mandibular right lateral incisor and second premolar. Patient was discharged after clear follow-up instructions and good oral hygiene home care. The intervention will be considered successful if the patient's condition does not progress to stage 1 MRONJ

Stage 2: Exposed and necrotic bone with fistulae that probe to the bone and are associated with pain, erythema, and drainage suggestive of infection (Fig. 8.7).

Stage 3: All the clinical signs and symptoms noted in stages 1 and 2, and, in addition, the necrotic bone would be noted extending beyond the region of alveolus.

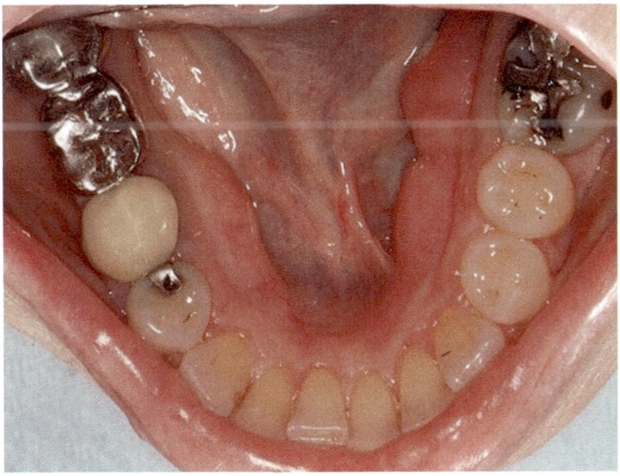

Fig. 8.5 MRONJ stage 1. Intraoral photograph of a patient who was on yearly infusion of 5 mg of zoledronic acid. The soft tissue ulceration was noted on the lingual mucosa over left mandibular torus in relation to mandibular first molar. (Case courtesy of Dr. Takako I. Tanaka, DMD, Hospital of the University of Pennsylvania, Philadelphia, USA)

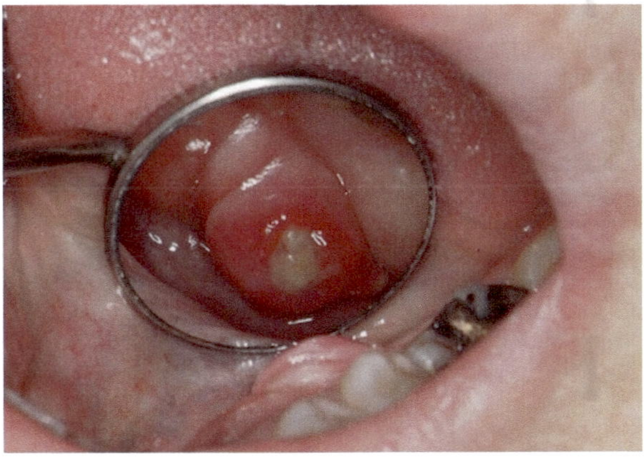

Fig. 8.6 MRONJ stage 1. Close-up view of the mucosal ulceration shown in Fig. 8.5 using a mouth mirror. The denuded and necrotic bone is noted in the center of the ulcer. (Case courtesy of Takako I. Tanaka, DMD, Hospital of the University of Pennsylvania, Philadelphia, USA)

There may be a pathologic fracture, intra- or extraoral fistula, or an osteolysis extending to the inferior border of the mandible or sinus floor (Fig. 8.8).

The potential mechanisms of MRONJ induction can be broadly classified into the following:

1. Compromised bone function due to disturbances in bone turnover and repair.
2. Angiogenesis inhibition leading to delay in wound healing or affecting microinfarctions in soft tissues and bone.
3. Infection promoting cell death in both soft tissues and bone.
4. Soft tissue toxicity due to leaching of the chemicals leading to direct epithelial toxicity.
5. Immune-related effects like interactions between osteoprotegerin ligand and RANKL leading to osteoclastogenesis and resultant bone loss.

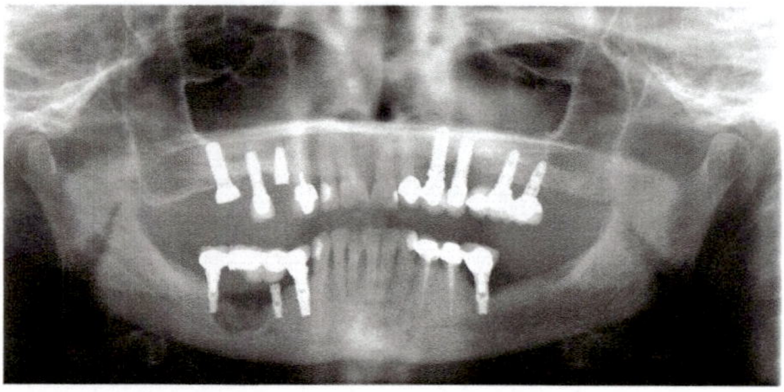

Fig. 8.7 MRONJ stage 2. Necrotic bone in the region of mandibular right premolar region status post-extractions, bone grafting, and implant placement. Patient had a history of oral bisphosphonate use. The necrosis is limited to the alveolus above the inferior alveolar nerve canal

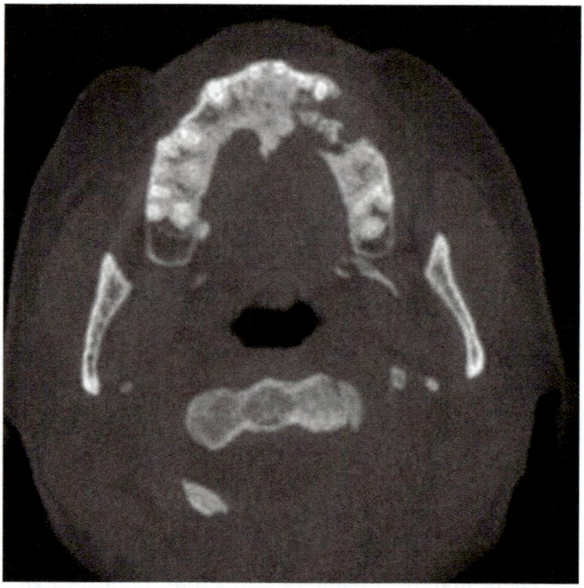

Fig. 8.8 MRONJ stage 3. Note the extensive spread of the osteomyelitis-like appearance of the maxillary bone secondary to oral bisphosphonate use in a middle-aged male patient who reported for dental care. Note the pathologic fracture in the region of maxillary left canine-premolar region. (Case courtesy Steven R. Singer, DDS, Rutgers School of Dental Medicine, Newark, NJ, USA)

8.6 Guidelines for Soft Tissue and Hard Tissue Management

8.6.1 Management of ORN

Prevention of MRONJ is the most important goal in treatment planning patients who are about to receive antiresorptive or antiangiogenic medication. Patients should receive a thorough examination of the oral cavity including radiographic assessment when indicated. It is important to consider patient education during dental care once they are on the above groups of medications. This includes patient motivation, fluoride applications, chlorhexidine mouth rinses, gingival and periodontal care, and elimination of dental caries among other dental care procedures.

Since ORN is a condition that can be easily prevented than treated, all extractions of teeth in the *line of fire or field of irradiation* should be completed at least 3–6 weeks prior to the initiation of the RT. Alveoloplasty should be performed to eliminate any sharp bony fragments, and primary closure should be completed without stretching the oral mucosa. If the extractions were done due to an infection related to the tooth, adequate antibiotic coverage might be necessary before the extractions depending on the severity of the infection. Cessation of at-risk medication prior to tooth extraction or other dentoalveolar procedures has been recommended (drug holiday). After ORN sets in, surgical debridement of the sharp bony edges and conservative bone sequestrectomy may be required. Typically, the patients are referred to an oral and maxillofacial surgeon. Treatment options for ORN include antimicrobial therapy, local resection, sequestrectomy, and hyperbaric oxygen therapy.

The use of hyperbaric oxygen has been debated for its potential effectiveness or lack thereof. A study from the Division of Head and Neck Oncology of the Dana-Farber/Brigham and Women's Cancer Center did not recommend the routine use of HBO for the prevention or management of ORN. They recommend that HBO can be considered for use on a case-by-case for those who failed conservative therapy and had subsequent surgical resection.

8.6.2 Management of MRONJ

Management of MRONJ is mostly symptomatic in stages 1 and 2 along with the use of oral mouth rinse (Chlorhexidine 0.12%), pain control medication, and debridement to relieve soft tissue irritation and infection control. Stage 3 requires antibiotic therapy, pain control, and surgical debridement for long-term palliation of infection and pain. The Royal Australian College of General Practitioners' (RACGP) recommendation for osteoporosis risk assessment, diagnosis, and management looked at the evidence supporting the use of medication for treatment of osteoporosis and the risk for the development of MRONJ. The recommendation is that the benefits of osteoporosis treatment for those at high risk of fractures far outweigh the risk of MRONJ (less than 1–10 cases per 100,000 cases). The recommendation also assures that there is insufficient evidence to interrupt therapy for minor oral surgery or to measure the bone turnover markers to predict onset of MRONJ.

8.6.3 Specific Management Including Follow-Up and Referral

While HBO is a being considered as a helpful adjunct in the management of ORN, several newer treatments have been developed recently to treat MRONJ including:

1. Hyperbaric oxygen: HBO has been found to be a useful adjunct especially in severe cases.
2. Medical ozone therapy (MOT): MOT acts by preserving endogenous antioxidant system and by blocking xanthine or xanthine oxidase system, but this is not considered a substitute for other recommended therapies.

3. Teriparatide: This is recombinant human parathyroid hormone that stimulates osteoclasts and osteoblasts leading to an increase in bone turnover and acts as an osteoanabolic agent.
4. Platelet concentrates: Platelet-rich concentrates enriched with growth factors including VEGF and platelet-derived growth factor (PDGF).
5. Low-level laser therapy with Nd:YAG laser.
6. Platelet-derived growth factor-BB: This is a new key factor involved in angiogenesis and osteoformation. Treatment with PDGF-BB was successful in ovariectomy-induced osteoporotic mouse models where vasculogenesis and bone formation were noted.

Bibliography

1. Worth HM. Principles and practice of oral radiographic interpretation. Chicago: Year Book Medical Publishers; 1963. p. 330–4.
2. O'Dell K, Sinha U. Osteoradionecrosis. Oral Maxillofac Surg Clin North Am. 2011;23:455–64.
3. Mupparapu M, Bindakhil MA. Osteomyelitis of the mandible exhibiting features of medication-related osteonecrosis in a patient with history of tocilizumab treatment. J Orofac Sci. 2018;10:53–5.
4. American Association of Oral and Maxillofacial Surgeons (AAOMS). Medication-related osteonecrosis of the jaw—2014 update. Position paper of the American association of oral and maxillofacial surgeons. Available at: https://www.aaoms.org/docs/govt_affairs/advocacy_white_papers/mronj_position_paper.pdf. Accessed 31 Jul 2020.
5. Mupparapu M. Medication-related osteonecrosis of the jaw (MRONJ): bisphosphonates, antiresorptives, and antiangiogenic agents. What next? Quintessence Int. 2016;47:7–8.
6. Nifosi AF, Zuccarello M, Nifosi L, Saus VH, Nifosi G. Osteonecrosis of the jaw in the era of targeted therapy and immunotherapy in oncology. J Korean Assoc Oral Maxillofac Surg. 2019;45:3–8.
7. Villa A, Akintoye SO. Dental management of patients who have undergone oral cancer therapy. Dent Clin N Am. 2018;62(1):131–42.
8. Omolehinwa TT, Akintoye SO. Chemical and radiation-associated jaw lesions. Dent Clin N Am. 2016;60(1):265–77.
9. Lee YH, Kim YS, Chung MJ, Yu M, Jung SL, Yoo Ie R, Lee YS, Kim MS, Sun DI, Kang JH. Soft tissue necrosis in head and neck cancer patients after transoral robotic surgery or wide excision with primary closure followed by radiation therapy. Medicine (Baltimore). 2016;95(9):e2852.
10. Alterio D, Tagliabue M, Muto M, Zorzi S, Volpe S, Gandini S, Sibio D, Bayir O, Marvaso G, Ferrari A, et al. Soft tissue necrosis in patients treated with transoral robotic surgery and postoperative radiotherapy: preliminary results. Tumori. 2020;106(6):471–9.
11. Delanian S, Lefaix JL. The radiation-induced fibroatrophic process: therapeutic perspective via the antioxidant pathway. Radiother Oncol. 2004;73(2):119–31.
12. Marx RE. Osteoradionecrosis; a new concept of its pathophysiology. J Oral Maxillofac Surg. 1983;41:283–8.
13. McCaul JA. Pharmacologic modalities in the treatment of osteoradionecrosis of the jaw. Oral Maxillofac Surg Clin North Am. 2014;26(2):247–52.
14. Damek-Poprawa M, Both S, Wright AC, Maity A, Akintoye SO. Onset of mandible and tibia osteoradionecrosis: a comparative pilot study in the rat. Oral Surg Oral Med Oral Pathol Oral Radiol. 2013;115(2):201–11.

15. National Cancer Institute. Oral complications of chemotherapy and head/neck radiation (PDQ®)-health professional version. Available at: https://www.cancer.gov/about-cancer/treatment/side-effects/mouth-throat/oral-complications-hp-pdq#cit/section_1.8. Accessed 31 Jul 2020.
16. Peterson DE, Doerr W, Hovan A, et al. Osteoradionecrosis in cancer patients: the evidence base for treatment-dependent frequency, current management strategies, and future studies. Support Care Cancer. 2010;18:1089–98.
17. Schwartz HC, Kagan AR. Osteonecrosis of the mandible: scientific basis for clinical staging. Am J Clin Oncol. 2002;25:168–71.
18. Canadian Cancer Society. Osteoradionecrosis. Available at: https://www.cancer.ca/en/cancer-information/diagnosis-and-treatment/managing-side-effects/osteoradionecrosis/?region=on. Accessed 31 Jul 2020.
19. Lombard T, Neirinckx V, Rogister B, Gilon Y, Wislet S. Medication-related osteonecrosis of the jaw: new insights into molecular mechanisms and cellular therapeutic approaches. Stem Cells Int. 2016;2016:8768162.
20. Baur DA, Altay MA, Teich S, Oswald MS, Quereshy FA. Osteonecrosis of the jaw in a patient on raloxifene: a case report. Quintessence Int. 2015;46:423–8.
21. Pontes HAR, de Souza LL, Uchoa DCC, Cequeira JMM. Mandibular osteonecrosis associated with Raloxifene. J Craniofac Surg. 2018;29:e257–9.
22. Auluck A. How do I manage a patient with osteoradionecrosis? J Can Dent Assoc. 2016;82:g18.
23. Sultan A, Hanna GJ, Margalit DN, Chau N, Goguen LA, et al. The use of hyperbaric oxygen for the prevention and management of osteoradionecrosis of the jaw: a Dana-Farber/Brigham and Women's cancer center multidisciplinary guideline. Oncologist. 2017;22:343–50.
24. Royal Australian College of General Practitioners. Osteoporosis risk assessment, diagnosis and management. Available at: https://www.racgp.org.au/getattachment/5704b636-43c6-4926-8752-402b1641c6f5/Osteoporosis-flowchart.pdf.aspx. Accessed 1 Aug 2020.

Temporomandibular Joint Disorders and Trismus in Head and Neck Cancer Patients

9

Waseem Abboud, George Dimitroulis, and Noam Yarom

9.1 Introduction

The word trismus, from the Greek "trismós," was initially used to describe the grinding and clenching of jaws associated with tetany patients closing their mouths rigidly. Nowadays, it is used to describe restricted jaw movement in general, regardless of etiology, and independent of whether muscle spasm or pain is present or absent. Currently, in the literature, hypomobility and trismus are often used interchangeably. Many conditions can cause restricted mouth opening, and these are usually classified into intra-articular disorders (from the temporomandibular joint) or extra-articular disorders (outside the temporomandibular joint). The underlying etiology may be traumatic, inflammatory, congenital, psychogenic, neoplastic, or iatrogenic. Table 9.1 lists common causes of trismus.

Normal range of motion of the mandible is defined as a mouth opening in the range of 40–50 mm measured between upper and lower incisor teeth and bilateral and protrusive excursions in the range of 8–10 mm. Dijkstra et al. proposed a 35 mm cutoff point where less than this value is considered a restricted mouth opening, thus

W. Abboud
Department of Oral and Maxillofacial Surgery, Sheba Medical Center, Tel-Hashomer, Israel

Institute of Movement Disorders, Department of Neurology, Sheba Medical Center, Tel-Hashomer, Israel
e-mail: waseem.abboud@mail.huji.ac.il

G. Dimitroulis
Maxillofacial Surgery Unit, Department of Surgery, St. Vincent's Hospital—University of Melbourne, Melbourne, VIC, Australia

N. Yarom (✉)
Oral Medicine Unit, Sheba Medical Center, Tel-Hashomer, Israel

School of Dental Medicine, Tel-Aviv University, Tel-Aviv, Israel
e-mail: noamyar@post.tau.ac.il; noam.yarom@sheba.health.gov.il

R. Nair (ed.), *Orofacial Supportive Care in Cancer*,
https://doi.org/10.1007/978-3-030-86510-8_9

Table 9.1 Common causes of restricted mouth opening

Intra-articular pathologies
Internal derangement
Degenerative arthritis (osteoarthritis, osteoarthrosis)
Inflammatory arthritis (rheumatoid, psoriatic, etc.)
Metabolic arthritis (gout, pseudogout)
Septic arthritis (usually from contiguous spread of infection)
Ankylosis
Trauma: Joint effusion, hemarthrosis, condylar fracture, temporal bone fracture, and incorporation of foreign body
Tumor or pseudotumor of temporomandibular joint structures
Postoperative complication of head and neck surgery
Prolonged immobilization
Extra-articular pathologies
Myofascial pain
Myospasm (idiopathic, iatrogenic, neurogenic, reflectory)
Myositis (postsurgical, infectious, traumatic)
Myofibrotic contracture (idiopathic, postradiation, postsurgical)
Myositis ossificans
Coronoid hyperplasia
Jacob's disease
Eagle syndrome (elongation of styloid process)
Facial and jaw bone fractures
Oral submucous fibrosis
Neoplasia adjacent to masticatory muscles, temporomandibular joint, or their innervation
Drugs: phenothiazine, TCAs, metoclopramide, succinylcholine, halothane
Psychogenic trismus (hysteria, conversion syndrome)
Systemic conditions (scleroderma, juvenile idiopathic arthritis, etc.)
Electrolyte imbalances
Postoperative complication of head and neck surgery
Prolonged immobilization

trismus, and many authors have adopted this value. There are jaw-opening and jaw-closing muscles, and these two muscle groups act as antagonists, as neurogenic stimulation of one muscle group reflexly results in neurogenic inhibition of the other. Table 9.2 lists the primary muscles of mastication, their function, origin, insertion, innervation, and adjacent fascial spaces.

Clinicians dealing with head and neck cancer patients encounter restriction of jaw mobility on a daily basis. Trismus may occur as a presenting sign of malignancy, as a sequela of tumor site or growth, as a side effect of oncologic treatment, or as a first sign of recurrence. The prevalence in the different studies varies depending on tumor site, size, diagnostic criteria used to define trismus, and oncologic treatment.

9.2 Implications of Trismus on Cancer Patients

Restricted mouth opening compromises oral intake, oral hygiene, and speech. In addition, oral cavity inspection, either for dental care or for oncologic follow-up, may become significantly impeded in patients with trismus. The implications of

Table 9.2 Jaw-closing and jaw-*opening* muscles

Muscle	Origin	Insertion	Innervation	Neighboring spaces	Main action
Jaw-closing muscles					
Masseter	Zygomatic bone and arch	Lateral surface of mandibular ramus	CN V3	Submasseteric and buccal spaces	Elevation, protrusion, and retrusion of mandible
Temporalis	Temporal fossa (portions of parietal, temporal, frontal, and sphenoid bones) and temporalis fascia	Coronoid process and anterior border of the ascending ramus down to the occlusal surface of the mandible	CN V3	Superficial and deep temporal spaces	Elevation and retrusion of mandible
Medial pterygoid	Medial surface of lateral pterygoid plate, maxillary tuberosity, and pyramidal process of palatine bone	Medial surface of mandibular angle	CN V3	Pterygomandibular space, lateral pharyngeal space, and infratemporal fossa	Elevation and protrusion of mandible Contralateral excursion of mandible with unilateral contraction
Lateral pterygoid (superior head)	Infratemporal surface of the greater sphenoid wing	Superior aspect of the pterygoid fovea, the articular capsule, and the medial aspect of the articular disk	CN V3	Pterygomandibular space and infratemporal fossa	Elevation and retrusion of mandible Contralateral excursion of mandible with unilateral contraction
Jaw-opening muscles					
Lateral pterygoid (inferior head)	Lateral surface of the lateral pterygoid plate	Inferior aspect of the pterygoid fovea and condylar neck	CN V3	Pterygomandibular space and infratemporal fossa	Depression and protrusion of mandible Contralateral excursion of mandible with unilateral contraction
Mylohyoid	Mylohyoid ridge on the medial surface of the mandible	Opposite mylohyoid at the midline raphe and hyoid bone	CN V3	Submandibular, sublingual, and submental spaces	Elevation of hyoid bone and floor of mouth Depression of mandible when hyoid bone held in place by infrahyoid muscles
Digastric	Mastoid process	Digastric fossa of the mandibular symphysis	Anterior belly: CN V3 Posterior belly: CN VII	Submandibular, submental, and lateral pharyngeal spaces	Elevation of hyoid bone Depression and retrusion of mandible when hyoid bone held in place by infrahyoid muscles
Stylohyoid	Styloid process	Body of hyoid bone	CN VII	Submandibular and lateral pharyngeal spaces	Elevation and retraction of hyoid bone
Geniohyoid	Inferior genial tubercle of the mandibular symphysis	Body of hyoid bone	Ansa cervicalis (ventral rami of C1–2 running along CN XII)	Sublingual space	Anterior and superior movement of hyoid bone and tongue Depression of mandible when hyoid bone fixed in place by infrahyoid muscles

both may be detrimental on the patients' well-being, as clinical surveillance is mandatory in many neoplastic diseases, and untreated dental problems predispose the patient to infection and osteomyelitis.

General anesthesia, performed for therapeutic or diagnostic purposes, may become impossible and necessitate fiber-optic awake nasal intubation or tracheotomy.

In patients using an obturator after maxillectomy, trismus may limit prosthetic options for fabricating a suitable appliance and limit proper postoperative maintenance of the obturator by the patient.

Patients with restricted mouth opening may suffer from weight loss and nutritional deficits, which may complicate the healing period, a time at which the body is recovering from extensive surgery, radiation, and possibly chemotherapy. In addition, inability of the patient to eat "normally" increases the risk of social isolation and decreases the quality of life, both of which have a significant psychologic impact on the patients and caregivers.

Finally, trismus may compromise the ability to safely secure an airway and may increase the risk of aspirations.

Trismus is frequently overlooked by clinicians, assuming the reduction in jaw mobility in head and neck cancer patients to be "trivial" or "normal." Many patients may not realize the gradual development of trismus during the initial healing phase, when they are consuming mainly liquids or fed through a nasogastric tube. Many times when patients attempt to resume intake of normal food or get back to normal daily activities, only then the restriction is noted and becomes a major complaint.

9.3 Etiology of Trismus in Cancer Patients

In patients with cancer, trismus can result from local infiltration of primary or metastatic tumor into or adjacent to the masticatory muscles, their neural innervation, or the temporomandibular joint. Similarly, surgery or radiotherapy affecting these structures can also cause trismus.

9.3.1 Mechanical Impediment

Space-occupying lesions, either primary or metastatic tumors, may mechanically interfere with the free movement of the mandible. Malignant tumors with rapid and infiltrative growth cause trismus more frequently than do benign masses. Lesions of the condyle, coronoid process, zygoma, infratemporal fossa, pterygomandibular, and temporal spaces may compromise mobility of the mandible by limiting anterior movement of the condyle or coronoid process during mouth opening. Tumors adjacent to masticatory muscles may restrict their ability to stretch and therefore reduce mouth opening. In addition, infiltration into masticatory muscles, even minimal micro-invasions not detected on imaging, can cause reflex spasms resulting in sustained contractions and trismus.

9.3.2 Neuromuscular Reflectory Spasm

Tumors growing adjacent to the mandibular or maxillary divisions of the trigeminal nerve may produce afferent sensory impulses leading to the principal sensory trigeminal nucleus in the pons. From the pons, the impulses are directed centrally to the sensory cortex (where they are perceived as pain) and peripherally via the motor nucleus of the trigeminal nerve into efferent output to the muscles of mastication. This reflex arch increases the tonus of jaw-closing muscles and causes trismus. The response is bilateral even though the stimulus is unilateral.

The mandibular division of the trigeminal nerve exits the skull via foramen ovale into the infratemporal fossa, and the maxillary division of the trigeminus exits the skull via foramen rotundum into the pterygopalatine fossa and enters the orbit through the inferior orbital fissure. Thus, lesions in the soft palate, peritonsillar area, sinuses, nasopharynx, temporomandibular joint, pinna, pterygopalatine, and infratemporal fossae may cause restricted mouth opening by this so-called reflectory trismus.

9.3.3 Radiation Therapy

Patients receiving radiotherapy for head and neck cancer, whether as a sole treatment or in combination with surgery and chemotherapy, have an increased risk of developing postradiation trismus. The prevalence of trismus for patients receiving therapeutic doses of radiotherapy has been reported to be as high as 45%. Several studies demonstrated that, in general, mouth opening after radiotherapy decreases in the range of 20–30% compared to mouth opening prior to radiotherapy. Mandibular opening worsens as the dose of radiation delivered to the masticatory muscles increases, which is affected by three main factors: the total therapeutic radiation dose, tumor proximity to masticatory structures, and type of radiation technique.

Total therapeutic radiation dose: A correlation exists between the absorbed dose to the masticatory structures and the decrease in mouth opening. While levels in excess of 60 Gy are more likely to cause trismus, Goldstein et al. reported that doses as low as 15 Gy resulted in functional impairment and diminution in opening.

Tumor proximity to masticatory structures: Tumor sites such as the oral cavity, pharynx, base of tongue, tonsils, salivary glands, nasopharynx, and jaws carry an increased risk of radiation-induced trismus, whereas hypopharyngeal and laryngeal tumors carry a relatively decreased risk of this complication.

Type of radiation technique: The newer technologies of external beam radiation, namely, intensity-modulated radiotherapy (IMRT) and image-guided radiotherapy (IGRT), seem to lower the percentage and severity of radiotherapy-induced trismus. These techniques contribute to better control over the pattern of radiation distribution and diminish the radiation dose to healthy structures in close proximity to the tumor. Proton radiation therapy, a more advanced radiotherapy

> technique, holds even more promise with regard to improving coverage to tumor while minimizing radiation to adjacent normal tissues. This technique however is more expensive and is not readily available in most cancer centers. That said, one must be aware that in patients with tumors sited in or next to the mastication structures, even the most sophisticated isodose shaping and sculpting techniques cannot spare adjacent structures from some degree of radiation.

Radiation-induced trismus may begin toward the end of radiotherapy or at any time during the subsequent 24 months; however, most commonly, diminution of mouth opening ensues within weeks of cessation of radiation and deteriorates relatively rapidly in the following 9 months. After this initial period, a continued deterioration continues however more slowly. Wang et al. reported that in the first 9 months after radiotherapy, mouth opening decreases on average by 2.4% per month. In the second year, mouth opening decreases about 0.2% per month, and in the period from 24 to 48 months, mouth opening decreases by 0.1% per month. All in all, in the first year after RT, about two-thirds of the total reduction in mouth opening occurs.

On the cellular level, radiation penetrates human tissue to cause damage via the production of hydroxyl radicals. Initially, apoptosis or clonogenic cell death via free radical-mediated DNA damage occurs. In addition, microvascular endothelial damage (endarteritis obliterans) causes regional loss of vascular perfusion and ischemia. Fibrosis is generally a late complication of radiation therapy that may not manifest clinically for several months after treatment. It is the result of dysregulation of fibroblast activity, stimulation of fibrotic and sclerotic changes, and ultimately atrophy of tissues, an insidious process named radiation-induced fibroatrophic activity.

On the tissue level, radiation damage to the masticatory muscles can cause focal myopathy, and myopathic muscles are prone to painful spasms. Radiation damage to the innervating motor nerve can cause ectopic neural activity, further worsening the muscle contractions. The latter two are further exacerbated by the radiation-induced fibrosis and sclerosis of tendons and ligaments, causing them to lose elasticity, shorten, and contract. The end result is restriction of motion of the masticatory apparatus.

9.3.4 Ablative Procedures

Unfavorable scarring after surgical resection of tumors is not uncommon in head and neck cancer patients. Although advanced reconstructive techniques enable restoration of tissues and function, some degree of limitation may still occur.

A common side effect of extensive buccal mucosa resection is the formation of a fibrotic band connecting the upper and lower vestibules and limiting mouth opening. Reconstruction of this defect by the buccal fat pad lowers the chances of scarring.

Resection of the contents of the infratemporal fossa including condylectomy will inevitably result in diminished mobility of the ipsilateral mandible. Under normal conditions, contraction of both lateral pterygoid muscles results in protrusion and depression of the mandible without deviation. If one side is resected, then protrusion and opening with deviation to the opposite side occurs, regardless whether the defect was reconstructed or not.

Neurosurgical procedures performed through the temporal bone or through skull base that need dissection of the temporalis muscle may result in restricted mouth opening. Dissection of the temporalis above or below the zygomatic arch may result in hypomobility due to muscle fibrosis and pseudo-ankylosis, respectively.

9.3.5 Prolonged Immobilization

Regardless whether the immediate cause of trismus is the proximity of the neoplasia to masticatory structures, the extent of the ablative procedure, or the radiation therapy, sustained mandibular hypomobility will ultimately result in both muscle and joint degeneration. Bensadoun et al. showed that muscles that fail to move through their range of motion for as little as 3 days begin to show signs of atrophy and joints that are immobilized quickly begin to show degenerative changes in joint surfaces.

If increased tonus of the muscles of mastication is also present, then fibrosis and sclerosis of muscles and tendons is further worsened.

9.3.6 Combined Toxicities

Resection of the primary tumor may be combined with neck dissection, radiotherapy, and chemotherapy. The toxicities of these modalities may be cumulative and difficult to separate clinically.

There are several possible factors that may determine a patient's risk for developing clinical manifestations of trismus, including age, overall health, medical and degenerative disorders, and the concomitant use of neurotoxic medications (usually platinum-based) and other drugs (phenothiazines, tricyclic antidepressants, capecitabine).

Electrolyte imbalances, especially hypocalcemia, hypomagnesemia, and hypokalemia, all of which may develop after extensive surgeries and prolonged hospitalization time, can manifest with tetanic contractions of the jaw muscles causing trismus.

9.3.7 Jaw Fracture and Hardware Failure

Radiation renders jaw bones brittle and prone to fractures and osteoradionecrosis. Cancer patients are predisposed to infections which may lead to osteomyelitis and fractures. The residual mandibular bone after the ablative procedure may be thin and prone to crack. Bone metastases weaken the mechanical resistance of the jaws. The plates and screws inserted during surgery to strengthen the jaw or to fixate the bony reconstruction may fail with time and cause an inflammatory resorptive reaction. The main presenting clinical sign of all the previously mentioned scenarios is usually trismus, which generally manifests early before other signs and symptoms appear.

9.4 Prevention of Trismus

Mouth opening should be measured before and after surgery, before and after radiotherapy, and regularly throughout follow-up. When a patient presents with trismus after therapy, it is important to determine whether the restriction is the result of treatment or the first sign of recurrence.

Treatments aimed at relieving trismus after oncologic therapy are generally not very helpful, especially when trismus was induced by radiation. Therefore, prevention is more desirable than treatment.

Minimizing the radiation effects should be a primary goal of treatment. Fabricating a splint for the patient to wear during radiotherapy can be a simple and effective measure toward achieving this objective. The use of dose-sculpting techniques such as IMRT and IGRT decreases radiation doses to adjacent structures involved in mastication without compromising the necessary therapeutic dose. Thus, compared with conventional radiotherapy, it is safe to conclude that new isodose radiation techniques reduce the incidence and severity of radiation-induced trismus.

Concomitant prophylactic coronoidectomy should be considered in extensive surgeries involving the mandibular ramus, maxillary tuberosity, zygomatic arch, or the infratemporal fossa. Scarring and fibrosis of the temporalis muscle, either after surgery, radiotherapy, or prolonged immobilization, has a detrimental effect on development of movement restriction. Prophylactic coronoidectomy performed simultaneously with the ablative procedure should be considered trivial in this patient population.

Satisfactory reconstruction of the defect, even after small resections, decreases the chances of developing scar tissue and fibrotic bands. Surgeons should aim to perform reconstruction immediately after resection whenever feasible, so that normal appearance and function are restored as soon as possible. Late reconstructions carry the risk of achieving comparably inferior outcomes with proportionally larger efforts.

The aim of postsurgical physical therapy is to prevent secondary immobilization of the patient which carries the risk of cicatricial tissue formation, adhesions, and contracture of healing tissues with further limitation of range of motion. It is generally agreed that physical therapy should start soon after radiation therapy ends, before the development of trismus. A broad scientific basis for this recommendation, however, is lacking.

Patients at risk of developing trismus, such as those with tumors close to the temporomandibular joint or masticatory muscles or those who are due to receive radiotherapy to these structures, should be informed of the risks of trismus and educated that their cooperation with preventive and therapeutic measures is important to the success of treatment. These measures are discussed in the following section.

9.5 Treatment of Trismus

The majority of the available literature on the topic of head and neck cancer complications reported trismus to be a common finding in this patient population but with no focus on its management. Recommendations regarding therapeutic modalities and treatment plans lack scientific evidence and are based on clinical experience and good clinical practice. Furthermore, few authors reported trismus to be independent of treatment efforts, and in many cases symptoms resolve or worsen with time, regardless of the interventional therapeutic modality used or the rehabilitation efforts made.

9.5.1 Physical Therapy

Physical therapy is generally regarded as the first-line and mainstay of prevention and treatment for trismus in head and neck cancer patients. The very limited available literature, however, demonstrated modest effectivity, especially in radiation-induced trismus.

Active jaw movement exercises consist of movements driven by the musculature around the joints, without the assistance of external forces. Patients move their lower jaw in the greatest range of motion possible by their muscles and joints, by performing maximal opening, closing, protrusion, and lateral excursions to both sides. Ruler measurements or even the fingers can be used as a reference to goal set the patients.

Passive jaw motion exercises, on the other hand, imply the application of external forces, so that joint movement and muscle stretching occurs without activity of the muscles of mastication. The simplest way to perform this is by using stacked wooden tongue depressors. This method can also be used for goal setting for the patients by the number of tongue blades inserted between the upper and lower incisors. Cases with teeth mobility or edentulism may be less suitable for this method. Other stretching techniques available include commercial devices such as the TheraBite Jaw Motion Rehabilitation System and the Dynasplint Trismus System. Few authors reported fabricating individualized appliances using springs, coils, bands, acrylic cones, and wedges. Whatever the stretching method is, it should be acceptable by patients as their compliance with the program and cooperation with the physical therapist are of paramount importance to the success of rehabilitation.

The third principle used in physical therapy is the "proprioceptive neuromuscular facilitation principle." It is based on the physiological phenomenon that activation of one muscle group (agonist) reflexly causes relaxation of the muscular antagonist affecting the same joint. After repeated attempts to open the mouth against applied resistance, such as the therapist's hand placed on the patient's chin opposing the opening movement, the jaw-closing muscles are inactivated due to the continued stimulation of the jaw-opening muscles. After several opening attempts against external resistance, the patient is asked to widely open the mouth, and immediately a slightly increased number of tongue depressors are inserted between the upper and lower teeth. This type of exercises is better performed with the guidance of a physical therapist. Appliances other than tongue blades could be similarly used.

The question as to when to start physiotherapy has not been answered in the literature. Some authors advised to start rehabilitation exercises as soon as it is practical. Other authors were more specific and advocated performing exercises during the radiation therapy, while others recommended starting exercise programs soon after finishing radiotherapy. That said, all authors agree that initiating physiotherapy a year or more after finishing oncologic treatment significantly lowers the chances of achieving satisfactory results, since maturation of scar tissue leads to substantial resistance to exercises.

During the exercise period, it is important to measure mouth opening regularly to evaluate the improvement of trismus. The clinician should set a realistic goal for the patient, and after reaching it, home-based self-exercises aimed to maintain this range of motion should continue on a daily basis, once or twice a day, for some years. All in all, in radiation-induced trismus, gains in the range of 3–8 mm have been reported in the majority of clinical trials in the literature.

9.5.2 Pharmacologic Therapy

Analgesics, with or without anti-inflammatory properties, should be prescribed at the initial active phase of physiotherapy. Pain needs to be alleviated before starting trismus treatment. Muscle relaxants can also be prescribed concomitantly to ease on the exercises. Benzodiazepines are effective for this purpose.

Pentoxifylline, a methylxanthine derivative, was reported to show some benefit in radiation-induced trismus. This agent improves tissue oxygenation and influences cytokine-mediated inflammation. The literature on this topic however is mixed, with some authors reporting this drug to hold promise for oncologic patients, while others reporting it to be ineffective.

Botulinum toxin injected into masticatory muscles exposed to radiation was shown to alleviate the local pain, however, with no effect on trismus. The toxin probably reduces the painful spasms of myopathic muscles. It could be considered as an adjuvant therapy for radiation-induced trismus, especially during the active phase of physiotherapy.

Cannabis has the ability to decrease depression and anxiety in cancer patients, and few authors reported it to improve appetite and generalized feelings of well-being. In addition, cannabis has been reported to help alleviate muscle spasms and pain; however, an association between its use and an improvement of trismus has not been reported in the literature.

9.5.3 Release Surgery

It is recommended that a coronoidectomy is performed during tumor resection whenever the ablative procedure is extensive and involves the mandibular ramus, the maxillary tuberosity, the zygomatic arch, and the infratemporal fossa, and radiation is expected as an adjuvant therapy. Patients not responding to conservative measures may be advanced to coronoidectomy or temporal muscle myotomy; however, one must be aware that when performed postoperatively, this procedure carries considerable surgical risks in previously irradiated patients.

Fibrosis of the other masticatory muscles, whether due to radiation, scarring, or immobilization, will not be corrected by coronoidectomy and may require myotomy of the specific muscles involved.

Scar resection may be indicated in cases where the conditions after this secondary release surgery are expected to be better compared to the conditions present after the primary resection, especially in terms of reconstructive measures available and patient cooperation with mobilization exercises.

Patient selection for these "release-surgery" procedures cannot be overemphasized. Patients should be motivated and well cooperative, as postoperative physical therapy is intensive, painful, and mandatory to the success of treatment.

9.5.4 Miscellaneous

Forced opening under general anesthesia has been reported. The rationale is to gain an immediate increase of range of motion which is then maintained by intensive physiotherapeutic exercises combined with pharmacologic measures. This procedure however may be complicated by jaw and alveolar ridge fractures and soft tissue injuries.

Heat therapy, applied to the affected area a couple of times a day, combined with rinsing the mouth with warm water has been reported to help relieve the discomfort of trismus.

Micro-current electrotherapy, either combined or without other physiotherapeutic modalities, has been examined in the literature. It probably has a very limited effect on mouth opening.

Several studies evaluated the effectivity of hyperbaric oxygen therapy (HBO) on radiation-induced trismus. HBO is likely ineffective and does not alleviate the restriction.

Low-level laser therapy, a type of photobiostimulation, has been shown to be an effective prophylactic and therapeutic modality for oral mucositis. It reduces its severity and duration. Recently, reports of its potential efficacy in improving trismus and other radiation-induced toxicities have been proposed; however, future studies are still needed to establish this.

9.6 Summary

In patients with cancer, trismus can result from local invasion of primary or metastatic tumor into or adjacent to the masticatory muscles, their neural innervation, or the temporomandibular joint. Similarly, surgery or radiotherapy affecting these structures can also cause trismus.

Although advances in diagnostic modalities, reconstructive surgeries, and radiation techniques have lowered the prevalence and severity of trismus, restricted mouth opening continues to be a common complaint in head and neck cancer patients. In addition to the profound effect on daily activities and psychosocial status of cancer survivors, trismus can have deleterious effects on the physical, psychosocial, and overall survival of the patients.

Caregivers should monitor mouth opening regularly, and whenever suspicion arises, investigation of the underlying cause is warranted. Clinicians should not consider trismus to be a trivial sequela of cancer or its treatment, and efforts at preventing or at least minimizing it should be made. Nowadays, despite numerous publications, the knowledge about prevention and treatment of trismus remains scarce, and the majority of guidelines published rely solely on personal experience and good clinical practice. Future investigation is needed to clarify the optimal management measures for trismus in cancer patients.

Bibliography

1. Aldington S, Harwood M, Cox B, Weatherall M, Beckert L, Hansell A, et al. Cannabis use and cancer of the head and neck: case-control study. Otolaryngol Head Neck Surg. 2008;138(3):374–80.
2. Chang YM, Deek NFAL, Wei FC. Trismus secondary release surgery and microsurgical free flap reconstruction after surgical treatment of head and neck cancer. Clin Plast Surg. 2016;43(4):747–52. https://doi.org/10.1016/j.cps.2016.06.002.
3. Van Der Laan HP, Van De Water TA, Van Herpt HE, Christianen MEMC, Bijl HP, Korevaar EW, et al. The potential of intensity-modulated proton radiotherapy to reduce swallowing dysfunction in the treatment of head and neck cancer: a planning comparative study. Acta Oncol (Madr). 2013;52(3):561–9.
4. Jakobi A, Bandurska-Luque A, Stützer K, Haase R, Löck S, Wack LJ, et al. Identification of patient benefit from proton therapy for advanced head and neck cancer patients based on individual and subgroup normal tissue complication probability analysis. Int J Radiat Oncol Biol Phys. 2015;92(5):1165–74.
5. Zecha JAEM, Raber-Durlacher JE, Nair RG, Epstein JB, Elad S, Hamblin MR, et al. Low-level laser therapy/photobiomodulation in the management of side effects of chemoradiation therapy in head and neck cancer: Part 2: Proposed applications and treatment protocols. Support Care Cancer. 2016;24(6):2793–805.
6. González-Arriagada WA, Ramos LMA, Andrade MAC, Lopes MA. Efficacy of low-level laser therapy as an auxiliary tool for management of acute side effects of head and neck radiotherapy. J Cosmet Laser Ther. 2018;20(2):117–22. https://doi.org/10.1080/14764172.2017.1376097.

7. Zhang H, Xie M, Archibald SD, Jackson BS, Gupta MK. Association of marijuana use with psychosocial and quality of life outcomes among patients with head and neck cancer. JAMA Otolaryngol Head Neck Surg. 2018;144(11):1017–22.
8. Jakobi A, Lühr A, Stützer K, Bandurska-Luque A, Löck S, Krause M, et al. Increase in tumor control and normal tissue complication probabilities in advanced head-and-neck cancer for dose-escalated intensity-modulated photon and proton therapy. Front Oncol. 2015;5(November):1–9. Available from: http://journal.frontiersin.org/Article/10.3389/fonc.2015.00256/abstract.
9. Scherpenhuizen A, Van Waes AMA, Janssen LM, Van Cann EM, Stegeman I. The effect of exercise therapy in head and neck cancer patients in the treatment of radiotherapy-induced trismus: a systematic review. Oral Oncol. 2015;51(8):745–50. https://doi.org/10.1016/j.oraloncology.2015.05.001.
10. Nieder C, Zimmermann FB, Adam M, Molls M. The role of pentoxifylline as a modifier of radiation therapy. Cancer Treat Rev. 2005;31(6):448–55.
11. Elliott DA, Nabavizadeh N, Romer JL, Chen Y, Holland JM. Medical marijuana use in head and neck squamous cell carcinoma patients treated with radiotherapy. Support Care Cancer. 2016;24(8):3517–24. https://doi.org/10.1007/s00520-016-3180-8.
12. Goldstein M, Maxymiw W, Cummings B, Wood R. The effects of antitumor irradiation on mandibular opening and mobility: a prospective study of 58 patients. Oral Surg Oral Med Oral Pathol Oral Radiol Endod. 1999;88(3):365–73.
13. Bensadoun RJ, Riesenbeck D, Lockhart PB, Elting LS, Spijkervet FKL, Brennan MT. A systematic review of trismus induced by cancer therapies in head and neck cancer patients. Support Care Cancer. 2010;18(8):1033–8.
14. Wang CJ, Huang EY, Hsu HC, Chen HC, Fang FM, Hsiung CY. The degree and time-course assessment of radiation-induced trismus occurring after radiotherapy for nasopharyngeal cancer. Laryngoscope. 2005;115(8):1458–60.
15. Satheeshkumar PS, Mohan MP, Jacob J. Restricted mouth opening and trismus in oral oncology. Oral Surg Oral Med Oral Pathol Oral Radiol. 2014;117(6):709–15. https://doi.org/10.1016/j.oooo.2014.02.031.
16. Stubblefield MD. Radiation fibrosis syndrome: neuromuscular and musculoskeletal complications in cancer survivors. PM R. 2011;3(11):1041–54. https://doi.org/10.1016/j.pmrj.2011.08.535.
17. Rapidis AD, Dijkstra PU, Roodenburg JLN, Rodrigo JP, Rinaldo A, Strojan P, et al. Trismus in patients with head and neck cancer: etiopathogenesis, diagnosis and management. Clin Otolaryngol. 2015;40(6):516–26.
18. Dijkstra PU, Kalk WWI, Roodenburg JLN. Trismus in head and neck oncology: a systematic review. Oral Oncol. 2004;40(9):879–89.
19. Dijkstra PU, Huisman PM, Roodenburg JLN. Criteria for trismus in head and neck oncology. Int J Oral Maxillofac Surg. 2006;35(4):337–42.
20. Loh SY, Mcleod RWJ, Elhassan HA. Trismus following different treatment modalities for head and neck cancer: a systematic review of subjective measures. Eur Arch Oto Rhino Laryngol. 2017;274(7):2695–707.
21. Dhanrajani PJ, Jonadel O. Trismus: aetiology. Differential Dent Update. 2002;29:88–9, 94.
22. Roberts DS, Egerton JR. The aetiology and pathogenesis of ovine foot-rot. J Comp Pathol. 1969;79:217–27. Available from: http://www.sciencedirect.com/science/article/pii/0021997569900085.
23. Abboud W, Yahalom R, Leiba M, Greenberg G, Yarom N. Temporomandibular joint involvement in patients with multiple myeloma—a retrospective study. Int J Oral Maxillofac Surg. 2016;45(12):1545–50. Available from: http://linkinghub.elsevier.com/retrieve/pii/S0901502716301126.
24. Abboud WA, Yarom N, Yahalom R, Joachim M, Reiter S, Koren O, et al. Comparison of two physiotherapy programmes for rehabilitation after temporomandibular joint arthroscopy. Int J Oral Maxillofac Surg. 2018;47(6):755–61. https://doi.org/10.1016/j.ijom.2017.10.019.

10 Drug-Specific Orofacial Complications of Novel Anti-cancer Therapies

Harry M. Gasper and Jasotha Sanmugarajah

10.1 Introduction

In recent years,there has been a revolution in cancer treatment. Research has greatly expanded understanding of the mechanisms through which neoplastic growth occurs, most famously summarized by Hanahan and Weinberg in their landmark paper on hallmarks of cancer [1]. This and the knowledge interaction of neoplastic cells with the stroma surrounding a tumor have identified new potentially druggable targets [2, 3], and biochemical technology has allowed new ways of delivering drugs to these targets [4]. The result of this has been a massive expansion in the number of drugs approved for market, with 51 new drugs approved by the FDA for the treatment of solid organ cancer between 2000 and 2015 [5].

Some medications target specific pathways of cellular function either through antibody-mediated delivery to extracellular receptors, for example, cetuximab (an EGFR antagonist) [6], or through small-molecule-mediated delivery to intracellular targets, for example, erlotinib (a tyrosine kinase inhibitor targeting the intracellular signaling domain of EGFR) [7]. Increasingly drugs are being designed with multiple targets. The number of medications available in the treatment of cancer is increasing rapidly year on year, and there are now targeted agents in regular use for many different cancers including, but not limited to, lung cancer, breast cancer, renal cancer, thyroid cancer, melanoma, and colorectal cancer [8–13]. While these drugs are designed to target specific pathways in cancer cells, it is inevitable that unwanted effects can occur, which both relate to the method of delivery and to the target which they are designed to interact with [14].

H. M. Gasper · J. Sanmugarajah (✉)
Medical Oncology, Gold Coast University Hospital, Gold Coast, QLD, Australia
e-mail: Jasotha.sanmugarajah@health.qld.gov.au

R. Nair (ed.), *Orofacial Supportive Care in Cancer*,
https://doi.org/10.1007/978-3-030-86510-8_10

Another area of growing importance has been the interaction of the immune system with cancer cells. It is known that there is an interaction of the functioning immune system with cancer cells [15], and the ability of cancers to evade immune-mediated cell death is now recognized as a hallmark of cancer [16, 17]. Recent advances have led to the development of drugs designed to target immune evasion and potentiate the response of the immune system to the cancer. Immune-oncology with inhibition of the CTLA-4 and PDL-1 immune checkpoint inhibitors is set to be a growing feature of anti-cancer treatment across a wide range of tumour streams.

For clinicians who come into contact with cancer patients, an awareness of the potential for orofacial adverse events is vital since it may have implications for quality of life and compromise the safety of other treatments or procedures. Complications related to the mouth and face can lead to some patients having to delay or even cease their anti-cancer drug or other drugs, such as analgesia, leading to substandard outcomes. Poor mouth care may also lead to malnutrition which can be a serious cause of morbidity and even death. Despite the potential for harm, the effect of drugs on the mouth and related areas is often underreported or underestimated by patients and physicians alike. Although the evidence base for specific or facial toxicities related to newer agents is currently limited, the body of literature describing overall toxicities is increasing. As more agents are released, some with new mechanisms of action, the adverse effects experienced will change and clinicians will be required to adapt to new potential toxicities. In this chapter we will provide a brief introduction to some of the newer anti-cancer agents in use and a guide to the type and management of the orofacial side effects one might expect to see.

10.2 Targeted Therapy: MABs and TKIs

10.2.1 Introduction

Monoclonal antibody drug conjugates (MABs) and small molecule kinase inhibitors (TKIs) have allowed the introduction of a wave of drugs which target specific pathways in cancer cells. While MABs interact with these pathways via the extracellular domain of their receptors, small molecules are designed to interact with the intracellular tyrosine kinases [18]. Most of the drugs in use currently target either cellular proliferation and growth or vascular formation within the tumor environments. While some adverse effects associated with these molecules will be familiar from conventional cytotoxic medications, there are some nuances in presentation and clinical course that healthcare practitioners should be aware of.

In this part of the chapter, we will explore some of these pathways and drugs targeting them, as well as some of the complications one may expect to encounter with them. An overview summarizing the drugs, targets, and the cancers they are associated with can be found in Table 10.1 at the end of this section.

Table 10.1 Complications associated with common drugs targeting angiogenesis

	Bevacizumab		Sunitinib		Pazopanib		Sorafenib	
	All Grade	G3–4	All Grade	G3–4	All Grade	G3–4	All Grade	G3–4
Hypertension	23.6%	7.9%						
Hemorrhage	30.4%	3.5%						
Thromboembolic events	11.9%	6.3%	1.7%				1.3%	
Stomatitis	4%	0%	16.5–27%	1–4%	14–27%	1%	7–19%	0–3%
Dysgeusia	N/R	N/R	20–49%	0–1%	26–49%	<1%	3–8%	N/R
Xerostomia	N/R	N/R	10–11%	N/R	0–10%	N/R	4–8%	N/R

10.3 Angiogenesis

10.3.1 Introduction

Tumors require the development of new vasculature in order for neoplastic growth to progress beyond the limits of the existing supporting blood vessels, and this is fuelled by hypoxia [19]. Cancer cells demonstrate upregulated activity in many pathways, commonly vascular endothelial growth factor (VEGF) leading to changes in the intra-tumoral environment and multiple effects including the growth of new blood vessels and the release of signaling molecules such as chemokines. Targeting angiogenesis as a method of treating cancer involves several agents in current use [20], which are MABS such as bevacizumab and kinase inhibitors such as sunitinib and pazopanib, as well as others in mainstream use or late stages of development. MABs are primarily used as adjuncts to chemotherapy, where they are suspected to enhance delivery of cytotoxic drug into the tumor through remodeling of the intra-tumoral vasculature. Current FDA indications include renal cell carcinoma, hepatocellular carcinoma, colorectal cancer, glioblastoma multiforme, and others [21–24].

Side effects related to the use of anti-angiogenic agents are mostly vascular related events. The most common and most important reported events include hypertension and thromboembolic complications, including cerebrovascular accident. Although not specifically related to orofacial problems directly, impairment of wound healing has been well described and should be considered before undertaking any procedures [25]. Of equal importance is the potential for ONJ (osteonecrosis of the jaw) which, although relatively rare, is a known side effect of these agents. With the use of the TKIs, oral issues are not infrequently observed and mostly involve mucosal surfaces with stomatitis, dysgeusia, and xerostomia seen in up to a quarter of patients taking Sunitinib [26], but it should be noted that these are largely low-grade events that can be managed with simple measures. Interestingly, the incidence of stomatitis seems to be much less with monoclonal antibody conjugates such as bevacizumab, while dysgeusia and xerostomia are rarely reported.

Rates of the most common adverse events associated with the use of anti-angiogenic agents are summarized in Table 10.1.

While the majority of the oral issues related to the use of angiogenesis agents are low grade, management mostly consists of conservative measures including good dental hygiene and avoidance of exacerbating substances such as alcohol. In some cases, dose adjustment or temporary cessation of the agent may be required. Practitioners should also be aware of the potential for hypertension, hemorrhage, or other vascular events and screen for the risk of bleeding prior to carrying out any procedures. Finally, all clinicians should be aware that bevacizumab is often primarily used as an adjunct to standard therapies, including chemotherapy, and therefore oral health issues that arise may relate to the therapy with which it is being combined.

10.4 The Epidermal Growth Factor Receptor Family

This family of receptors is of great importance in the current understanding of neoplastic growth. There are several members of the family, and they are implicated in many different cancers. Activation of the extracellular domain of EGFR receptors leads to intracellular responses and subsequent activation of multiple cascades including MAPK and PI3K-AKT pathways which are involved in proliferation, cell growth, and anti-apoptotic mechanisms [27]. Targeting the EGFR receptor is a strategy currently employed in lung cancer and colorectal cancer [6, 28], while the HER2neu receptor (a member of the EGFR family) is targeted in breast cancer and gastric cancer [29, 30]. As with most cellular receptors, molecules can be employed to target the extracellular or intracellular domain of the protein, with monoclonal antibodies or tyrosine kinase inhibitors, respectively. Another interesting way in which HER2 has been utilized is via antibody-drug conjugates, whereby an active anti-cancer drug is attached to a HER2 antibody, with the intention of delivering the drug directly to the cell, an example of which is trastuzumab emtansine used in advanced breast cancer [31]. With some of these molecules, mucocutaneous adverse effects are very important, while with others they seem to occur with very low frequency. We will explore each class of drug in turn in the next part of this chapter.

10.5 Monoclonal Antibodies Targeting EGFR

Cetuximab and panitumumab have an established role in the treatment of colorectal cancer for individuals who have wild-type RAS mutations [6, 32]. Published literature indicates that oral problems are rare with these agents, despite the fact that cutaneous problems are seen commonly [33]. Low-grade stomatitis can occur and is usually easily manageable with simple measures; on the other hand, dysgeusia appears to be more common, albeit often low grade, and xerostomia is seen in a minority. Dysgeusia is rarely dose limiting but can be a source of very poor quality of life and in some cases may lead to more severe secondary problems including malnutrition. Although when used in isolation these drugs are relatively well tolerated in terms of mouth care, they are often used in combination with chemotherapy or radiotherapy, and this of course increases the potential for side effects markedly. Mucositis is especially common in those having radiotherapy in combination with cetuximab [34], and this is dealt with in other parts of this book. Specific management related to mucositis, dysgeusia, and xerostomia can be found later in this chapter.

10.6 Tyrosine Kinase Inhibitors Targeting EGFR/HER2

TKIs such as gefitinib, erlotinib, and osimertinib are utilized for their anti-cancer effect in lung cancer and are being explored in other cancers, with newer agents in development [35]. Fortunately for these relatively narrow-spectrum agents, the incidence of issues related to mouth care is limited to low numbers with mucositis predominating [36]. Some of the newer agents have a broader spectrum of EGFR/HER blockade, and mucositis, dysgeusia, and xerostomia are seen more frequently. Lapatinib, used in the treatment of breast cancer, is combined with capecitabine chemotherapy leading to greater stomatitis events [37]. While in study populations it has been seen that rates of high grade complications do not exceed 10%, and dose reductions have rarely been required, it is important to consider that these results may underestimate the true complication rates in the general population.

10.7 Targeting the BRAF Mutation

BRAF mutations are found in multiple cancers and in general can be thought to convey a poor prognosis. BRAF is an important early step in the MAPK/RAS pathway that is involved in cellular proliferation, resistance to cell death, metastasis, and other processes that contribute to malignant growth [38]. In recent years, the advent of drugs which target the BRAF cascade has led to clinical meaningful improvements in survival in melanoma, hoping for similar effects in other cancers [39]. BRAF inhibitors such as dabrafenib or vemurafenib can be given alone, or in combination with MEK inhibitors, for example, trametinib and cobimetinib. When given as a combination, an advantage is seen in the form of fewer cutaneous lesions and longer progression-free survival [40].

Direct mucosal damage appears to be relatively infrequent with the use of BRAF inhibitors, both alone and in combination with MEK inhibitors. Most of the toxicities related to the mouth are concerned with the development of hyperplasia (non-malignant growth) which can manifest orally as simple gingival hyperplasia or hyperkeratotic lesions [41]. More serious is the potential for secondary malignant growth and the development of squamous cell carcinoma, although this risk seems to be much reduced when these drugs are used in combination with MEK inhibitors. When used as a combination, an important side effect is the development of fever [42], which although unrelated to the oral mucosa should still be recognized, as it necessitates temporary withdrawal of the drug and discussion with the oncologist treating patients.

10.8 Immune Checkpoint Inhibitors

The role of the immune system in the treatment of cancer has been investigated intensely, and attempts to employ the immune response in the treatment of cancer using interferon and intravesical Bacille Calmette-Guérin (BCG) have shown some success in the past [43, 44]. However, in recent years there has been a breakthrough in harnessing the immune system with the advent of immune checkpoint inhibitors, which have seen effective and durable responses across a range of cancers. Avoidance of immune destruction is a hallmark of cancer, and ground-breaking research has demonstrated that cancers interact with T lymphocytes leading to inhibitory signals that result in the cytotoxic mechanism becoming downregulated [45]. There are multiple signaling molecules through which this can occur, but currently targets in mainstream use are CTLA4 and PD1/PDL1 due to the creation of drugs which can interact with these targets [46]. The number of indications for these agents is increasing rapidly, and they are set to be used in all settings of cancer treatment, both adjuvant and palliative.

For details regarding the immunology of cancer cells, it is recommended to consult an immunology reference; however the mechanism of action of the CTLA4 and PD1 inhibitors (Fig. 10.1a, b) is to prevent the deactivation of T cells responding to antigens (CTLA4) and to prolong the anti-tumor response (PD1/PD-L1).

For medical practitioners treating patients who are receiving these agents, the important thing to recognize is that, by preventing downregulation of the immune system response and thus having an overall more active immune system, the potential for side effects related to autoimmune phenomenon is raised, and this is where the majority of problems arise [48]. CTLA4-targeting molecules were the first to be tested and are associated with impressive tumor responses in melanoma [49]. However, as they are not antigen specific, they are associated with high levels of adverse events, reaching above 50% grade 3 and 4 event rates [50]. PD1-targeting drugs work at the level of the T-cell interaction with the antigen, in this case being the cancer cell and prevention exhaustion of the T-cell response. As such PD1 and PDL1 inhibitors have been seen to have fewer autoimmune event rates, although they do still occur. Immune checkpoint inhibitors are also used in combination, which has been associated with higher response rates, at the expense of greater toxicity [51]. Responses are also being seen in other cancers and there are an increasing number of indications for these molecules [52].

→

Fig. 10.1 (**a**) CTLA-4 inhibition prevents early deactivation of T cells responding to tumor antigens presented by APCs. Activated T cells can migrate to the tumor site and mount effective antitumor immune responses. Activation of T cells with cross-reactivity to host antigens may cause immunologic AEs. (**b**) PD-1 and PD-L1 checkpoint inhibition. PD-1 checkpoint inhibitors will prevent PD-1:PD-L1- and PD-1:PD-L2-mediated deactivation of T cells. PD-L1 checkpoint inhibitors will prevent PD-1:PD-L1-mediated deactivation of T cells. PD-1 pathway inhibition can restore antitumor immune responses directly at the tumor site and also facilitate T-cell activation in lymph nodes or other sites. Activation of T cells with cross-reactivity to host antigens may cause immunologic AEs. (Taken from Luke, J. J., & Ott, P. A. (2015). PD-1 pathway inhibitors: the next generation of immunotherapy for advanced melanoma. Oncotarget, 6(6), 3479–92 [47])

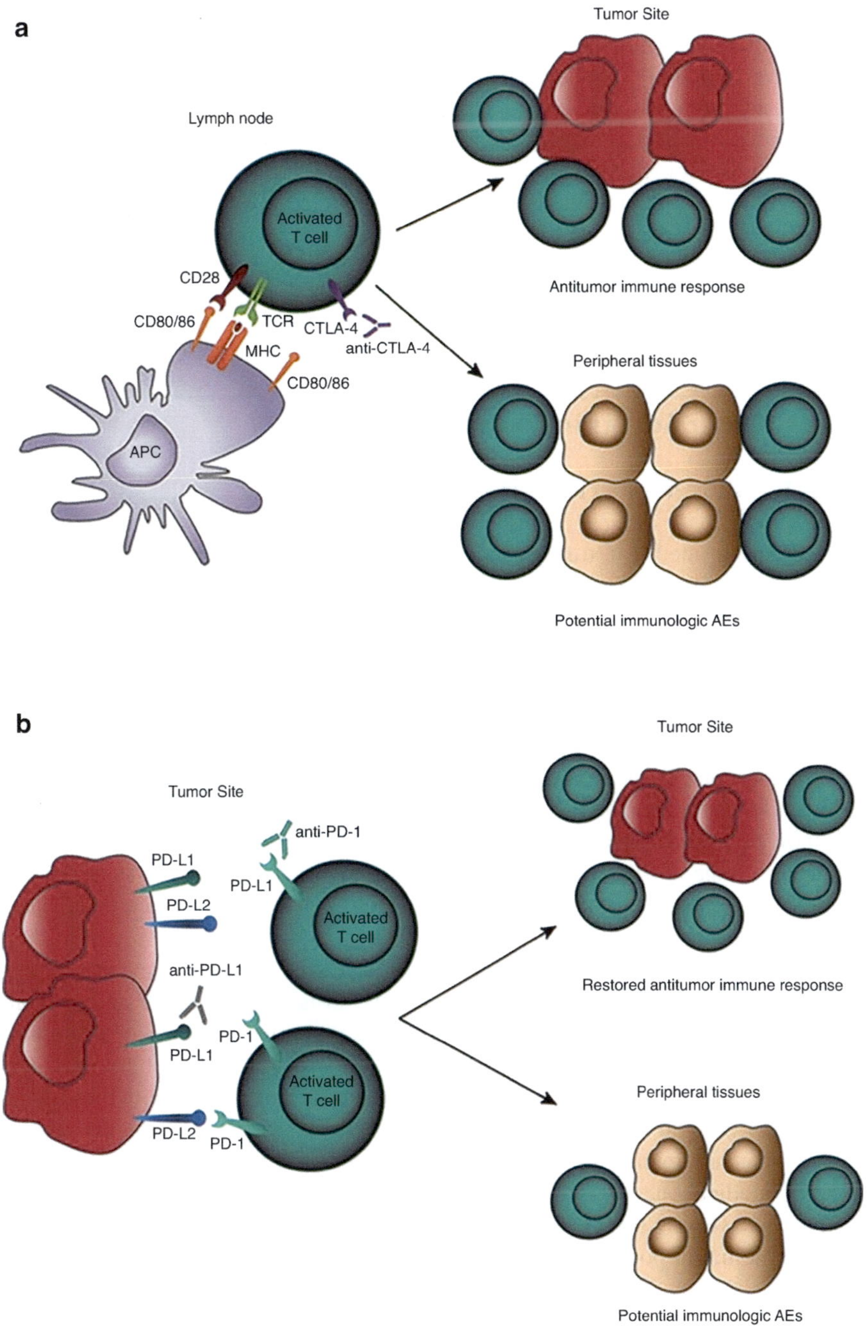
a
Lymph node
Activated T cell
CD28
CD80/86
TCR
CTLA-4
anti-CTLA-4
MHC
CD80/86
APC
Tumor Site
Antitumor immune response
Peripheral tissues
Potential immunologic AEs
b
Tumor Site
PD-L1
PD-L2
anti-PD-1
PD-L1
Activated T cell
anti-PD-L1
PD-1
PD-L1
Activated T cell
PD-L2
PD-1
Tumor Site
Restored antitumor immune response
Peripheral tissues
Potential immunologic AEs

Common adverse events associated with the use of immune therapy are colitis, pneumonitis, nephritis, thyroid disorders, rashes, rheumatic problems, and fatigue [53]. These tend to occur mainly in a predictable time course in the first months of therapy, although they can develop at any time. The development of side effects has been shown to correlate with greater anti-tumor response [54]. Nevertheless, with increasing use, it is becoming clear that any tissue of the body can become a target for the immune system when using these agents. In terms of the specific oral health implications of these drugs, fortunately noted side effects are few and rarely severe and relate mostly to autoimmune inflammation of mucosal and local structures; this includes xerostomia, Sjogren's-like syndrome, lichenoid reactions, pigment dysgeusia, and parotid gland inflammation [55].

10.9 Other Agents in Current Use

10.9.1 Multi-kinase Inhibitors

Of increasing interest in treating cancer are drugs with multiple targets. There are already many drugs in mainstream use that have been designed to act on several pathways. Two such examples are the multi-kinase inhibitors lenvatinib and vandetanib. Lenvatinib targets include VEGF 1–3, FGFR 1–4, PDGFR, RET, and KIT, while vandetanib targets RET, VEGF, and EGFR kinases [13, 56]. Clinical indications for these drugs currently include metastatic thyroid cancer, renal cell cancer, and hepatocellular cancer with the number of indications likely to grow as more evidence becomes available.

Both lenvatinib and vandetanib have been evaluated for efficacy in phase III trials showing impressive anti-tumor activity. Despite the undoubtable efficacy, toxicity was an issue in trials with reported rates of any treatment-related adverse event as high as 97% in the treatment group; nonetheless, it should be noted that discontinuation rates were still low.

Toxicities related to multi-kinase inhibitors consist of vascular events, including hypertension, and thromboembolic events; in addition, fatigue and asthenia are also common [57]. In relation the orofacial toxicities, the rates of dry mouth and stomatitis were 13-20% for Lenvatinib and Vandetinib nasopharyngitis was reported in 11%. In general, oral events seem to be relatively few with these drugs and, when they do occur, are not generally serious. If serious problems were to occur, standard management of mucositis applies. It is recommended that the treating medical oncologist should be consulted before attempting any procedures on patients who are taking these drugs due to the potential risk of serious complications including poor wound healing, venous thrombosis, and osteonecrosis of the jaw.

10.9.2 ALK Inhibitors

Fusions of EML4-ALK genes are found in around 5% of patients with non-small-cell lung cancer and are predominantly seen in female Asian patients. The ALK inhibitors crizotinib, ceritinib, and alectinib are currently used to treat patients with these genetic abnormalities, as well as those with ROS1 mutations. Dysgeusia and stomatitis were noted in up to 26% of patients taking these agents; however high-grade events were very uncommon [58, 59].

10.9.3 Poly (ADP-Ribose) Polymerase Inhibitors

PARP inhibitors are drugs which inhibit a cellular pathway involved in DNA damage repair. They are used primarily in patients who have germline or somatic deficiencies in DNA repair in order to enhance the effect of DNA damaging cytotoxic drugs or to prevent alternative pathways of DNA repair. The result of this is increased DNA mutation leading to apoptosis. This has been a successful strategy in many cancers including breast, ovarian, and prostate cancer. Clinical trials seem to suggest low rates of mucositis, dysgeusia, and nasopharyngitis occur at 10–15% [60].

10.10 Drugs Targeting the Cell Cycle

There are two main classes of drug currently used which target cell cycle kinetics. MTOR inhibitors are used in breast cancer and renal cell cancer, and CDK4/6 inhibitors are used in breast cancer. CDK4/6 inhibitors are relatively new, and currently there are three drugs available for use in advanced breast cancer: abemaciclib, palbociclib, and ribociclib [61]. Side effects that commonly occur include asthenia, diarrhea, and neutropenia and generally can be managed with dose reductions or temporary withdrawal. There is not currently a large body of evidence regarding oral health implications, but care should be taken before attempting procedural work.

In contrast to this, MTOR inhibitors have a range of mucosal side effects which can lead to significant morbidity and treatment adjustment. Examples include everolimus, used in the treatment of renal cell cancer and breast cancer [62, 63]. The adverse effects commonly described with these agents (and oral TKIs) were elegantly summarized by Boers-Doets and colleagues [64]. Stomatitis and mucosal inflammation are common with the use of these drugs, although they are often manageable. MTOR inhibitor-associated stomatitis (MIAS) is a well-described syndrome with clearly defined symptomology, clinical course, and treatment, which is discussed in greater detail further on in this chapter. Management of mucositis, dysgeusia, and other inflammatory problems is the same as with other drugs.

10.11 Examples and Management of Specific Orofacial Complications

10.11.1 Stomatitis

10.11.1.1 Background

Stomatitis has been defined in other sections of this book but briefly is a broad term that relates to breakdown of the oral mucosa manifested as inflammation, ulceration, dryness, and general discomfort. Stomatitis has been reported to occur in up to 29% of patients who are treated with oral tyrosine kinase inhibitors, particularly sunitinib, sorafenib, and cabozantinib. Interestingly, it is rarely seen with MABs such as bevacizumab. High-grade stomatitis can be extremely uncomfortable for the patient and lead to morbidity, both through the local effects and also the secondary problems of reduced oral intake. The development of adverse effects with TKIs used to treat renal cancer has been shown to correlate with increased efficacy of the drug.

The clinical presentation of stomatitis can be varied due to the broad array of symptoms associated with the term. However, in most cases there seems to be the rapid development of a generalized oral discomfort which can be painful and is often burning in nature. Symptoms often develop within weeks of starting the therapy but can be seen up to 2 months later. There may be erythema on visual inspection, and if ulceration is seen, it is often a linear lingual ulceration of the nonkeratinized mucosa. Very often, the symptoms will tend to resolve slowly, even without direct intervention.

10.11.1.2 Management

Management of stomatitis related to oral TKIs is much the same as management of stomatitis from other causes and involves treating the symptoms, aiding oral intake, and in some cases adjustment of the treatment intensity. In refractory or severe cases, a dose reduction may be required and is usually a successful management strategy. In phase III trials, treatment discontinuation due to oral stomatitis appears to be minimal. As with all mucosal issues, good mouth hygiene is recommended along with avoidance of potential precipitants.

10.11.2 mTor Inhibitor-Associated Stomatitis (MIAS)

10.11.2.1 Background

The mTOR inhibitors everolimus, temsirolimus, and deferolimus are generally used as a potentiating agent in combination with other therapies, although anticancer activity is noted with their use as a solo agent. Side effects are common with the use of these drugs with cutaneous and mucosal side effects particularly problematic. Much experience has been gained in this area through the use of

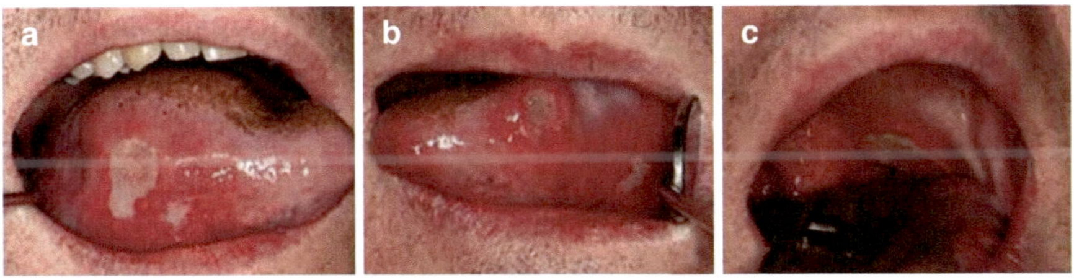

Fig. 10.2 mTOR inhibitor-associated stomatitis (**a**–**c**). Adapted from clinical presentation and management of mTOR inhibitor associted stomatitis. Marcio Augusto de Oliveira et al. Oral Oncology, 2011-10-01, Volume 47, Issue 10, Pages 998–1003, Copyright © 2011 Elsevier Ltd. [67]

mTOR inhibitors in the treatment of cancer; mTOR inhibitor-associated stomatitis (MIAS) is a distinct syndrome that has a specific presentation and management.

MIAS is seen in up to 50% of patients receiving mTOR inhibitors and is described with all the drugs within this class [65]. The highest incidence is seen with everolimus, where documented incidence in the literature of all-grade MIAS has reached greater than 60%. MIAS is unique compared with stomatitis associated with other drugs and follows a predictable clinical course [66].

Typically, the onset is within the first cycle of starting the drug and has a median onset of around 10 days; a phenomenon of a second onset is also seen in a large number of patients. Ulceration is noted with characteristic well-circumscribed, rounded painful ulcers (Fig. 10.2) which may be single or multiple. The ulcers mostly affect the non-keratinized mucosa, measure a few millimeters in their greatest dimension, and have a clearly demarcated gray central area with an erythematous halo surrounding, similar in appearance to aphthous ulcers. In contrast to stomatitis induced by chemotherapy, the gastrointestinal mucosa is usually spared, and the ulcers tend to be less diffuse.

10.11.2.2 Management

Management of MIAS can be divided into two streams: prevention and treatment of established disease [55, 67]. Given the predictability of stomatitis with the use if these agents, and the significant morbidity associated with its development, prophylactic measures should be considered standard of care when prescribing mTOR inhibitors. Initial management includes a thorough dental examination including the teeth and gums, with appropriate treatment of any issues identified. Basic oral hygiene should be promoted in common with all the stomatitis measures described previously and patients should be encouraged to avoid food or drink that may exacerbate inflammation of the oral mucosa. This includes spicy food, very hot food, alcohol, and alcohol-containing products (i.e., mouthwashes) and tobacco products. Zero alcohol mouthwashes, salt water rinses, or sodium bicarbonate are often useful in primary prevention.

Treatment of established mIAS is stratified according to grade [67]; for low grade events simple measures suffice and observation with resolution of the symptoms is often seen. Grade 2 and above events may require topical steroids either with local application of high potency steroid containing creams if the lesions are reasonably isolated, or dexamethasone-based mouthwashes for more diffuse ulceration. In severe cases, oral steroid is indicated along with dose interruption and subsequent reduction, always in consultation with the treating medical oncologist. Suggested doses on the basis of clinical trial evidence are pulses of prednisolone 30–60 mg for 1 week with a slow wean thereafter. Treatment should generally be accompanied by appropriate analgesic agents such as topical local anesthetic solutions, nonsteroidal anti-inflammatories, or other analgesic solutions. Other potential treatment modalities include intra-lesion steroid injections and low-level laser therapy. It should also be noted that, in severe cases, alternative routes of administration for treatments should be considered, as the oral route may be too painful and strong analgesic preparations, including opiates, and local anesthetic preparations may be required.

10.11.3 Dysgeusia and Xerostomia

Dysgeusia refers to changes in taste, while xerostomia refers to the lack of secretions leading to a feeling of dryness. Patients may underreport these symptoms because they attribute them to other things such as their cancer and clinical practitioners underestimating their importance. At the least, these symptoms are uncomfortable, and sometimes for patients, if severe, malnutrition can develop very quickly due to undereating. Specific management includes the use of artificial lubricants, avoidance of certain foods which may worsen dryness, over-seasoning of food, and use of supplements to ensure adequate oral intake. Referral to a dietician may be of use, and in a very unresponsive case a dose reduction or cessation of the agent may be required.

10.11.4 Immune-Related Adverse Events

Guidelines related specifically to oral adverse events from the immune therapies are not available due to the scarcity of data, which represents both the fact that oral issues are relatively rare and that we are yet to gather the evidence required. Nonetheless there are international guidelines from all major oncology societies that can guide general principles [68, 69]. If patients are receiving immune therapy, it is prudent to be vigilant for any unusual symptoms that may develop.

As a general rule, the first step in management is to assess the severity and rule out any potential alternative causes for the issue. Generally, baseline bloods should be sought as well as a thorough history and examination. If rheumatologic problems are suspected, there may an indication to test for autoantibodies if the severity is deemed to be high. The clinician should also be aware of other issues that can arise, including Addisonian syndromes, organ failure, and other rarer toxicities. Guidelines for assessment and management of the common toxicities can be found at all major oncology societies web pages. In very severe cases of toxicity, admission and high dose steroids are used. It goes without saying that, if any immune-related toxicity is suspected, all attempts should be made to contact the oncologist treating patients.

10.12 Conclusion

Medical treatment of cancer is in a new era of expansion and rapid development of therapeutics. Newer anti-cancer agents have different mechanisms of action and therefore different toxicities to traditional cytotoxic treatments. Knowledge of these is vital in those who are involved in caring for such patients, and oral health is an important and often neglected area. Drugs may have implications directly or indirectly on this. While having a background level of understanding regarding new agents is important, it is also key to remember that consultation with treating teams is advised if any doubt exists as to the nature of a drug which your patient is taking.

Key Points

- Newer anti-cancer agents involve different oral health side effects than older cytotoxic agents, and the frequency of high-grade events is generally lower.
- Targeted anti-cancer agents are often associated with mucositis, xerostomia, and dysgeusia. While often self-limiting, they can be severe and lead to significant morbidity.
- Management of oral toxicities consists of good oral hygiene and preventative measures, topical and systemic analgesia in established disease, and topical or systemic corticosteroids if severe or refractory. Antimicrobials should be considered if secondary infection is suspected.
- Immune checkpoint inhibitors are well tolerated but may lead to unusual side effects. Awareness of these agents will aid in the identification of such problems.
- Consultation with treating teams is recommended if any doubt persists regarding the safety and oral health implications of newer anti-cancer agents.

Small-molecule drugs and MABs in routine clinical use (including phase III trials):

Drug class	Examples	Uses
VEGF inhibitors (MAB)	Bevacizumab	Colorectal cancer, GBM, lung cancer
VEGF inhibitors (TKI)	Sunitinib, pazopanib, axitinib	Renal cell carcinoma
ALK inhibitors	Alectinib, crizotinib, ceritinib	ALK-mutated lung cancer
EGFR inhibitors (TKI)	Erlotinib, osimertinib, gefitinib, afatinib	EGFR-mutated lung cancer
EGFR inhibitors (MAB)	Cetuximab, panitumumab	RAS wild-type colorectal cancer, head and neck cancer
Multi-kinase inhibitors	Lenvatinib, vandetanib, cabozantinib, regorafenib, sorafenib	Medullary thyroid cancer, renal cell cancer, colorectal cancer, hepatocellular cancer
Mammalian target of rapamycin inhibitors	Everolimus, temsirolimus	Renal cell carcinoma, breast cancer
HER2 inhibitors (MABs)	Trastuzumab, pertuzumab	Breast cancer, gastric cancer
HER2 inhibitors (TKI)	Lapatinib, neratinib	Breast cancer
PD1 inhibitors	Nivolumab, pembrolizumab	Melanoma, lung cancer, renal cell carcinoma, bladder cancer, head and neck cancer
PDL-1 inhibitors	Atezolizumab, avelumab durvalumab	Lung cancer, Merkel cell cancer
CTLA4 inhibitors	Ipilimumab, tremelimumab	Lung cancer, renal cell carcinoma, bladder cancer
Hedgehog inhibitors	Vismodegib	Basal cell carcinoma
PARP inhibitors	Olaparib, niraparib	Ovarian cancer, BRCA-associated cancer
CDK4/6 inhibitors	Palbociclib, abemaciclib, ribociclib	Advanced breast cancer

Bibliography

1. Hanahan D, Weinberg RA. The hallmarks of cancer. Cell. 2000;110:57–70.
2. Gibbs JB. Mechanism-based target identification and drug discovery in cancer research. Science. 2000;287:1969–73.
3. Kummar S. Drug development in oncology: classical cytotoxics and molecularly targeted agents. Br J Clin Pharmacol. 2006;62:15–26.
4. Perona R. Cell signalling: growth factors and tyrosine kinase receptors. Clin Transl Oncol. 2006;8:77–82.
5. Vivot A. Clinical benefit, price and approval characteristics of FDA-approved new drugs for treating advanced solid cancer, 2000–2015. Ann Oncol. 2017;28:1111–6.
6. Jonker DJ. Cetuximab for the treatment of colorectal cancer. N Engl J Med. 2007;357:2040–8.
7. Shepherd F. Erlotinib in previously treated non-small-cell lung cancer. N Engl J Med. 2005;353:123–32.
8. Ocana A. Preclinical development of molecular targeted agents for cancer. Nat Rev Clin Oncolol. 2007;8:200–9.
9. Tol J. Chemotherapy, bevacizumab, and cetuximab in metastatic colorectal cancer. N Engl J Med. 2009;360:563–72.

10. Leyland-Jones B. Pharmacokinetics, safety, and efficacy of trastuzumab administered every three weeks in combination with paclitaxel. J Clin Oncol. 2003;21:3965–71.
11. Long GV. Dabrafenib and trametinib versus dabrafenib and placebo for Val600 BRAF-mutant melanoma: a multicentre, double-blind, phase 3 randomised controlled trial. Lancet. 2015;386:444–51.
12. Motzer RJ. Sunitinib versus interferon alfa in metastatic renal-cell carcinoma. N Engl J Med. 2007;356:115–24.
13. Schlumberger M. Lenvatinib versus placebo in radioiodine—refractory thyroid cancer. N Engl J Med. 2015;372:621–30.
14. Park SR. Safety and feasibility of targeted agent combinations in solid tumours. Nat Rev Clin Oncol. 2013;10:154–68.
15. Kim R. Cancer immunoediting from immune surveillance to immune escape. Immunology. 2007;121:1–14.
16. Hanahan D, Weinberg R. Hallmarks of cancer: the next generation. Cell. 2011;144:646–74.
17. Sahin U. Human neoplasms elicit multiple specific immune responses in the autologous host. Proc Natl Acad Sci U S A. 1995;92:474–84.
18. Zwick E. Receptor tyrosine kinase signalling as a target for cancer intervention strategies. Endocr Relat Cancer. 2001;8(3):161–73.
19. Folkman J. Tumour angiogenesis: therapeutic implications. N Engl J Med. 1971;285:1182–6.
20. Ferrara N. Vascular endothelial growth factor as a target for anticancer therapy. Oncologist (Suppl). 2004;9:2–10.
21. Motzer R. Pazopanib versus sunitinib in metastatic renal-cell carcinoma. N Engl J Med. 2013;369:1722–31.
22. LLovet JM. Sorafenib in advanced hepatocellular carcinoma. N Engl J Med. 2008;359:378–90.
23. Hurwitz H. Bevacizumab plus irinotecan, fluorouracil, and leucovorin for metastatic colorectal cancer. N Engl J Med. 2004;350:2335–42.
24. Wong ET. Bevacizumab for recurrent glioblastoma multiforme: a meta-analysis. J Natl Compr Cancer Netw. 2011;9:403–7.
25. Bose D. Vascular endothelial growth factor targeted therapy in the perioperative setting: implications for patient care. Lancet Oncol. 2010;11(4):373–82.
26. Cella D. Quality of life in patients with metastatic renal cell carcinoma treated with sunitinib or interferon alfa: results from a phase III randomized trial. J Clin Oncol. 2008;26(22):3763–9.
27. Normanno N. Epidermal growth factor receptor (EGFR) signaling in cancer. Gene. 2006;17(366):2–16.
28. Zhou C. Erlotinib versus chemotherapy as first-line treatment for patients with advanced EGFR mutation-positive non-small-cell lung cancer (OPTIMAL, CTONG-0802): a multicentre, open-label, randomised, phase 3 study. Lancet Oncol. 2011;12(8):735–42.
29. Slamon D. Adjuvant trastuzumab in HER2-positive breast cancer. N Engl J Med. 2011;365(14):1273–83.
30. Bang Y. Trastuzumab in combination with chemotherapy versus chemotherapy alone for treatment of HER2-positive advanced gastric or gastro-oesophageal junction cancer (ToGA): a phase 3, open-label, randomised controlled trial. Lancet. 2010;376(9742):687–97.
31. Krop IE. Trastuzumab emtansine versus treatment of physician's choice for pretreated HER2-positive advanced breast cancer (TH3RESA): a randomised, open-label, phase 3 trial. Lancet Oncol. 2014;15(7):689–99.
32. Peters TJ. Panitumumab versus cetuximab in patients with chemotherapy-refractory wild-type KRAS exon 2 metastatic colorectal cancer (ASPECCT): a randomised, multicentre, open-label, non-inferiority phase 3 study. Lancet Oncol. 2014;15(6):569–79.
33. Fakih M. Adverse events associated with anti-EGFR therapies for the treatment of metastatic colorectal cancer. Curr Oncol. 2010;14(Suppl 1):S18–30.
34. Pryor DI. Enhanced toxicity with concurrent cetuximab and radiotherapy in head and neck cancer. Radiother Oncol. 2009;90(2):172–6.
35. Sequist LV. Second-generation epidermal growth factor receptor tyrosine kinase inhibitors in non-small cell lung cancer. Oncologist. 2007;12(3):325–30.

36. Nan X. EGFR TKI as first-line treatment for patients with advanced EGFR mutation-positive non-small-cell lung cancer. Oncotarget. 2017;8(43):75712–26.
37. Geyer CE. Lapatinib plus capecitabine for HER2-positive advanced breast cancer. N Engl J Med. 2006;355(26):2733–43.
38. Davies H. Mutations of the BRAF gene in human cancer. Nature. 2002;417(6892):949–54.
39. Long VG. Dabrafenib plus trametinib versus dabrafenib monotherapy in patients with metastatic BRAF V600E/K-mutant melanoma: long-term survival and safety analysis of a phase 3 study. Ann Oncol. 2017;27(3):1631–9.
40. Rompoti N. Combination of BRAF inhibitors and brain radiotherapy in patients with metastatic melanoma shows minimal acute toxicity. J Clin Oncol. 2013;31(30):3844–5.
41. Dréno B. Incidence, course, and management of toxicities associated with cobimetinib in combination with vemurafenib in the coBRIM study. Ann Oncol. 2017;28(5):1137–44.
42. Lee C. Features and management of pyrexia with combined dabrafenib and trametinib in metastatic melanoma. Melanoma Res. 2014;24(5):468–74.
43. Catalona WJ. Risks and benefits of repeated courses of intravesical bacillus Calmette-Guerin therapy for superficial bladder cancer. J Urol. 1987;137(2):220–4.
44. Mocellin S. Interferon alpha adjuvant therapy in patients with high-risk melanoma: a systematic review and meta-analysis. J Natl Cancer Inst. 2010;102(7):493–501.
45. Messerschmidt JL. How cancers escape immune destruction and mechanisms of action for the new significantly active immune therapies: helping nonimmunologists decipher recent advances. Oncologist. 2016;21(2):233–43.
46. Torphy R. Newly emerging immune checkpoints: promises for future cancer therapy. Int J Mol Sci. 2017;18(12):2642.
47. Luke J, Ott P. PD-1 pathway inhibitors: the next generation of immunotherapy for advanced melanoma. Oncotarget. 2015;6(6):3479–92.
48. Champiat S. Management of immune checkpoint blockade dysimmune toxicities: a collaborative position paper. Ann Oncol. 2016;27(4):559–74.
49. Hodi FS. Improved survival with ipilimumab in patients with metastatic melanoma. N Engl J Med. 2010;363(8):711–23.
50. Wolchok JD. Ipilimumab efficacy and safety in patients with advanced melanoma: a retrospective analysis of HLA subtype from four trials. Cancer Immun. 2010;10:9.
51. Postow MA. Nivolumab and Ipilimumab versus Ipilimumab in untreated melanoma. N Engl J Med. 2015;372(21):2006–17.
52. Barbee MS. Current status and future directions of the immune checkpoint inhibitors ipilimumab, pembrolizumab, and nivolumab in oncology. Ann Pharmacother. 2015;49(8):907–37.
53. Nishijima TF. Safety and tolerability of PD-1/PD-L1 inhibitors compared with chemotherapy in patients with advanced cancer: a meta-analysis. Oncologist. 2017;22(4):470–9.
54. Downey S. Prognostic factors related to clinical response in patients with metastatic melanoma treated by CTL-associated antigen-4 blockade. Clin Cancer Res. 2007;13(22):6681–8.
55. Vigarios E. Oral mucosal changes induced by anticancer targeted therapies and immune checkpoint inhibitors. Support Care Cancer. 2017;25(5):1713–39.
56. Wells SA. Vandetanib in patients with locally advanced or metastatic medullary thyroid cancer: a randomized, double-blind phase III trial. J Clin Oncol. 2012;30(2):134–41.
57. Grande E. Vandetanib in advanced medullary thyroid cancer: review of adverse event management strategies. Adv Ther. 2013;30(11):945–66.
58. Costa RB. Systematic review and meta-analysis of selected toxicities of approved ALK inhibitors in metastatic non-small cell lung cancer. Oncotarget. 2018;9(31):22137–46.
59. Solange P. Alectinib versus crizotinib in untreated ALK-positive non-small-cell lung cancer. N Engl J Med. 2017;377(9):829–38.
60. Lederman JA. Overall survival in patients with platinum-sensitive recurrent serous ovarian cancer receiving olaparib maintenance monotherapy: an updated analysis from a randomised, placebo-controlled, double-blind phase 2 trial. Lancet Oncol. 2016;17(11):1579–89.
61. Kwapisz D. Cyclin-dependent kinase 4/6 inhibitors in breast cancer: palbociclib, ribociclib, and abemaciclib. Breast Cancer Res Treat. 2017;166(1):41–54.

62. Rugo HS. Incidence and time course of everolimus-related adverse events in postmenopausal women with hormone receptor-positive advanced breast cancer: insights from BOLERO-2. Ann Oncol. 2014;25(4):808–15.
63. Motzer R. Efficacy of everolimus in advanced renal cell carcinoma: a double-blind, randomised, placebo-controlled phase III trial. Lancet. 2008;372(9637):449–56.
64. Boers-Doets C. Oral adverse events associated with tyrosine kinase and mammalian target of rapamycin inhibitors in renal cell carcinoma: a structured literature review. Oncologist. 2012;17:135–44.
65. Martins F. A review of oral toxicity associated with mTOR inhibitor therapy in cancer patients. Oral Oncol. 2013;49(4):293–8.
66. Sonis S. Preliminary characterization of oral lesions associated with inhibitors of mammalian target of rapamycin in cancer patients. Cancer. 2010;116(1):210–5.
67. Oliviera MD. Clinical presentation and management of mTOR inhibitor-associated stomatitis. Oral Oncol. 2011;47(10):998–1003.
68. Haanen JB. Management of toxicities from immunotherapy: ESMO Clinical Practice Guidelines for diagnosis, treatment and follow-up. Ann Oncol. 2017;28(Suppl 4):iv119–42.
69. Brahmer J. Management of immune-related adverse events in patients treated with immune checkpoint inhibitor therapy: American Society of Clinical Oncology Clinical Practice Guideline. J Clin Oncol. 2018;36(17):1714–68.

Dysphagia in Head and Neck Cancer

11

Barbara A. Murphy, Kyle Mannion, and Kenneth Niermann

11.1 Introduction

Dysphagia, the sensation of abnormal swallowing, is a well-recognized and common side effect of head and neck cancer and its therapy. The perception of "difficulty swallowing" incorporates multiple constructs that are integral to the swallow experience, including (1) perception of increased work, attention, or time required for swallowing, (2) adverse impact of secretions (either hyper- or hyposalivation), (3) changes in mucosal sensation, (4) pain (odynophagia) or mucosal sensitivity, (5) difficulty with mastication due to trismus or loss of dentition, (6) altered taste and smell, and (7) anxiety or fear of choking. In clinical practice it is important to ask patients about all factors contributing to "difficulty swallowing" to ensure that the appropriate etiologic factors are being addressed. This chapter will largely address dysphagia as it relates to physiologic loss of function in structures critical for normal oropharyngeal swallowing.

B. A. Murphy
Medical Oncology, Department of Medicine, Vanderbilt University Medical Center, Nashville, TN, USA
e-mail: barbara.murphy@vumc.org

K. Mannion
Department of Otolaryngology, Vanderbilt University Medical Center, Nashville, TN, USA

K. Niermann (✉)
Department of Radiation Oncology, Vanderbilt University Medical Center, Nashville, TN, USA
e-mail: ken.niermann@vumc.org

R. Nair (ed.), *Orofacial Supportive Care in Cancer*,
https://doi.org/10.1007/978-3-030-86510-8_11

11.2 Assessment

Assessment of swallow function is performed by speech and swallow therapists, also known as a speech-language pathologist (SLP). The SLP undertakes a *clinical evaluation* of swallow function. This may be augmented by the use of *instrumental assessments* that include the modified barium swallow (MBS) and flexible endoscopic evaluation of swallow (FEES) [1–3]. Both the MBS and the FEES have unique advantages and disadvantages; thus the choice of which technique to use is dependent on the clinical question and the patient characteristics. Specific advantages to the FEEs include the ability to directly visualize the mucosa, sensory testing, and direct visualization of secretions [4].

A number of *self-report measures* have been developed for the comprehensive assessment of swallow function in the clinical and research setting [5]. Some tools are designed to assess swallow dysfunction in the general population, while others are directed specifically to head and neck cancer patients. Tools vary in length from a few items to several dozens. The items quarry a wide array of topics including swallowing, chewing, choking, aspiration, impact on food intake, pain, and the emotional and social impact of swallow dysfunction. The ultimate choice of a tool to assess dysphagia in the research setting is dependent on the constructs to be tested and the patient burden. In an analysis of the psychometric properties of selected dysphagia-specific tools, the Swallowing Quality of Life (SWAL-QOL) survey and the Dysphagia Handicap Index (DHI) had the highest psychometric ratings [5].

General quality of life tools and symptoms scales directed specifically at the head and neck cancer population incorporate items that capture or screen for dysphagia. The tools usually have no more than a few items directed at swallow function; thus, they may be effective in the clinical setting as screening tools. There is mounting evidence that patient report or dysphagia correlates with anatomical impairment and/or aspiration [6]. Thus, screening for dysphagia using brief patient reported outcomes measures may be useful in identifying patients who merit further evaluation. Studies evaluating the utility and cost-effectiveness of dysphagia screening are needed.

11.3 Pathophysiology

Diverse physiological insults, both tumor and treatment related, may contribute to dysphagia in head and neck cancer patients [7]. Some insults are transient and resolving spontaneously, while others may lead to long-term dysfunction. For any individual patient, it is critical to tease out the potential contributing factors in order to ensure early interventions for treatable causes and to set realistic expectations for function recovery.

11.3.1 Tissue Loss

Invasive tumors destroy structures that are required for normal swallow function including soft tissues, cartilage, bone, nerves, lymphatics, and vasculature. If tissue damage is severe, functional recovery may not be feasible. It may be difficult to predict the degree to which normal tissue will recover until treatment has been undertaken and rehabilitation completed. That being said, poor swallow function at diagnosis is an adverse prognostic indicator for long-term function. Similarly, an oncological surgical resection may require the extirpation of structures that are critical for normal deglutition. The degree of function loss is determined by the site and extent of resection. In general, the more extensive the resection, the greater the adverse effects on swallow function. Reconstructive procedures may compensate for tissue loss and improve functional outcome. Additionally, aggressive rehabilitation efforts may allow patients to use compensatory measures to accommodate tumor-related or surgical deficits.

11.3.2 Tissue Damage

In addition to overt tissue loss, head and neck cancers and cancer therapy may be associated damage to normal residual tissues. Pathological processes that adversely impact residual tissue function include soft tissue edema, lymphedema, and fibrosis [8, 9]. While acute edema caused by inflammation usually subsides once the inflammation has resolved, lymphedema and fibrosis can lead to permanent soft tissue changes that impair tissue compliance, distort anatomy, and inhibit normal movement. This may in turn lead to dysphagia [7, 10].

Lymphedema is characterized by tissue swelling due to the accumulation of fluid in the interstitial spaces as a result of damage to lymphatic structures. Lymphedema may also be seen when the amount of fluid deposited in the intestinal space overwhelms the capacity of lymphatic channels. Early on, lymphedema results in soft, reducible tissue swelling. Over time, adipose hypertrophy and hyperplasia develop. This is accompanied by scar tissue formation which results in firm, non-reducible tissue swelling. At this stage, lymphedema is less amenable to intervention such as manual lymph drainage, therapeutic bandaging, or compression garments. The hallmark of fibrosis is the deposition of pauci-cellular matrix which is firm to touch. Fibrotic tissues are less pliable resulting in decreased range of motion and, when severe, contraction.

Regardless of the underlying pathophysiology, there are specific physiological changes that are characteristically noted in head and neck cancer patients with dysphagia [11]. The most commonly reported physiologic swallow deficits include reduced laryngeal excursion, dysfunction of the base of tongue, decreased pharyngeal contraction, and decreases epiglottic movement [11].

11.4 Impact

The critical adverse outcomes related to dysphagia in the head and neck cancer population include (1) need for enteral or parenteral nutrition either acutely during treatment or long term, (2) nutritional deficiencies, (3) anatomical complications (stricture and aspiration), (4) treatment interruptions, and (5) psychosocial impact.

11.4.1 Weight Loss and Feeding Tube Placement

Weight loss and malnutrition are common in head and neck cancer patients. Weight loss at presentation or during therapy is associated with adverse outcomes, most importantly a decrease in survival [12, 13]. The etiology of weight loss is usually multifactorial and includes cancer and treatment-related cachexia, chemosensory alterations, nausea and vomiting, constipation, psychological issues such as anxiety and depression, and socioeconomic issues such as financial constraints and lack of caregiver support [14]. Although these factors may contribute in varying degrees to weight loss or malnutrition in individual patients, dysphagia and odynophagia remain the dominant cause of weight loss and the primary reason for feeding tube placement [14–16].

The severity of dysphagia and the need for feeding tube placement vary based on a number of factors including primary site, tumor stage, and treatment parameters [17]. Patients with significant weight loss in the setting of moderate to severe dysphagia at the time of diagnosis must be assessed for immediate feeding tube placement. For patients with intact swallow function who are undergoing primary resection, nasogastric feeding tubes may be placed at the time of surgery to allow soft tissue healing and recovery of swallow function. For patients with intact swallow function undergoing either definitive or adjuvant radiation (± chemotherapy), the optimal timing of feeding tube placement has yet to be determined [18, 19]. Clinicians may opt for either prophylactic feeding tube placement (prior to initiation of therapy) or reactive feeding tube placement (at the time of demonstrated weight loss or significant dysphagia). Most reports indicate that prophylactic feeding tube placement results in decrease weight loss [20]; however, ongoing use of intrinsic muscle of swallowing is critical for maintaining muscle function and to promote lymph flow. Patients with a feeding tube in place may have decreased swallow effort leading to muscle atrophy, lymphedema, and fibrosis. This in turn may lead to increased long-term feeding tube dependence [21]. Conversely, patients receiving reactive feeding tubes may lose substantially more weight but may have a lower rate of long-term feeding tube use. Regardless of the approach used, all patients undergoing radiation should be instructed to perform swallow exercises on a daily basis per instructions of their SLP.

11.4.2 Nutritional Deficiency

Patients with mild to moderate dysphagia may achieve adequate caloric intake through diet modifications; however, adequate caloric intake for weight maintenance does not guarantee a replete diet [22]. Dietary modifications may be adaptive or maladaptive. Working together, the SLP and the dietician can advise the patient with dysphagia about dietary adaptations that ensure replete and safe oral intake. Unfortunately, many patients with dysphagia self-restrict food types and constancies resulting in dietary insufficiencies. Patients may or may not be aware of the presence or severity of dietary adaptations [23]. The degree to which patients are aware of dietary restrictions depends on the rapidity and cause of symptom development. Patients are usually aware of dietary changes that develop quickly as a result of rapidly progressing tumors, surgical procedures, or radiation therapy. However, when dysphagia progresses slowly, patients may be unaware of resulting longstanding macro- and micronutrient deficiencies. Periodic dietary assessment should be undertaken in all patients with any degree of dysphagia.

11.4.3 Stricture

Head and neck cancer patients treated with either surgery or radiation may develop stricture or stenosis at the level of the hypopharynx or the upper esophagus. The incidence varies between studies; however in a recent meta-analysis, 10.6% of patients developed stricture. Stricture is most often diagnosed with a modified barium swallow. Treatment with esophageal dilation is effective in over 70% of patients; however, repeat dilatation procedures may be needed [24].

11.4.4 Aspiration

Aspiration is a common and potentially life-threatening acute and chronic complication of dysphagia in head and neck cancer patients. Although patients may have overt symptoms of aspiration such as coughing after drinking or eating, many patients will have subclinical or "silent" aspiration. Aspiration should be considered in any head and neck cancer patient presenting with a pneumonia. Workup includes assessment using either a MBS or FEES. Swallow therapy, use of compensatory measure, and dietary modifications may limit aspiration allowing for oral nutrition. If aspiration persists despite these measures, patient may require either feeding tube placement or toilette laryngectomy to prevent pulmonary complications from chronic aspiration.

11.4.5 Treatment Delays and Interruptions

Nutritional issues related to mucositis, odynophagia, and dysphagia are one of the critical causal factors for radiation treatment interruptions [25]. The delay of initiation of head and neck cancer therapy and treatment interruptions have an adverse impact on disease outcomes [26, 27]. Factors that may contribute to treatment delays or interruptions, including odynophagia and dysphagia, must be aggressively addressed.

11.4.6 Psychosocial Impact

Dysphagia has a profound psychosocial impact on patients and their caregivers. Dysphagia and/or the presence of a feeding tube has been shown to be associated with decreased quality of life, poor body image [28, 29], and mood disorders among patients [30]. Patients with dysphagia or a feeding tube may require assistance of caregivers [31]. Caregivers provide a wide array of services including meal preparation, tube feeding administration, and monitoring of caloric intake and weight [32]. This adds to caregiver burden and psychological distress [33]. Dysphagia may also result in social anxiety and isolation [34].

11.5 Prevalence of Dysphagia

11.5.1 Baseline

A significant percentage of head and neck cancer patients have some degree of swallowing dysfunction at the time of diagnosis [35]. On self-report measures, 59% of patients complain of swallow difficulties [36]. Patients with higher T-stage and either an oral cavity or pharyngeal lesion were more likely to have impaired swallow function [36].

11.5.2 Acute and Early Recovery

The prevalence of dysphagia during and immediately after completion of therapy is highly variable and depends on a large number of disease, treatment, and patient-related factors. That being said, dysphagia is sufficiently ubiquitous in the head and neck cancer population in which routine screening and assessment are recommended for all patients before, during, and immediately after definitive therapy. It is important to pay particular attention to those patients at high risk for swallowing impairment. Disease-related factors that correlate with swallow function include the T-stage, N-stage, presence of baseline dysphagia, and age [37]. For patients undergoing primary surgery, swallow outcome is impacted by the site and volume of tissue removed as well as the use of reconstructive techniques. For patients undergoing primary or adjuvant radiation, the prevalence and severity of dysphagia are dependent on the radiation dose to anatomic structures that are critical for swallowing. Attempts have been made to define radiation treatment parameters that would minimize long-term dysphagia: there is general consensus that limiting the radiation dose to the pharyngeal constrictors is a reasonable precaution but validation of these recommendations is necessary [38]. In general, multimodality therapy, including concurrent chemoradiation, is associated with higher rates of dysphagia when compared to single modality treatment.

11.5.3 Late Post-treatment Dysphagia

The contemporary use of multimodality therapy led to improved survival in head and neck cancer patients, but it was subsequently recognized that treatment was associated with marked incidence and severity of dysphagia in long-term survivors. Data from early trials spanning from 1992 to 1999 reported high rates of long-term dysphagia and its sequela (most prominently aspiration pneumonia and pneumonitis) [39]. This resulted in the investigation of preventive strategies to mitigate the impact of cancer and its therapy on swallow function including (1) the use of tissue protective agents, (2) the use of pre-habilitation/rehabilitation programs, (3) the use of conformal radiation therapy to minimize radiation to structures critical for swallowing, and (4) the development of surgical techniques to spare tissue and function. These techniques, which are described below, continue to develop and evolve rapidly. A SEER database review evaluating data spanning from 2002 to 2011 was recently reported [40]. This review provides a more contemporary picture of the frequency of important outcome measures including dysphagia, stricture, aspiration, and aspiration pneumonia/pneumonitis. Recognizing that late effects beyond 5 years remain an important and poorly studied outcome, the authors chose to confine the study period to 2 years post-treatment. Dysphagia, stricture, and pneumonia were reported in 45%, 10%, and 9% of patients, respectively, supporting the ongoing need to develop both preventive and treatment strategies to minimize the adverse impact of treatment [40]. These results underscore the need for continued aggressive assessment and management of dysphagia and its sequelae in long-term survivors.

11.6 Odynophagia

Pain on swallowing (odynophagia) may lead to significant alteration in swallow function. The etiology of odynophagia may include tumor-related pain, treatment-related pain, infection, dental abnormalities, and bone deficiency. Many patients will have multiple pain generators creating a management challenge for both the clinician and patient. Patients may report tumor-related odynophagia at the time of diagnosis: under these circumstances, successful treatment of the malignancy may alleviate the patient symptoms. It should be noted, however, that patients with pain at presentation are more likely to experience chronic pain. In addition to cancer itself, both surgery and radiation may lead to acute and chronic odynophagia. While spontaneous pain usually subsides to a moderate level by 1 month post-treatment, functional pain remains problematic regardless of treatment type [41].

11.6.1 Mucositis-Associated Odynophagia

Radiation therapy causes an acute, superficial inflammation of the mucosa on the surfaces within the involved radiation field. Mucositis is the dominant etiology of acute radiation-induced odynophagia. A thorough understanding of the clinical manifestations and patterns of mucositis may aid the clinician in managing patient symptoms and expectations.

11.6.1.1 Site-Specific Considerations

Base of tongue cancer requires high doses of radiation to be delivered to the primary tumor site in the oropharynx, and the mid-to-posterior dorsal surface of the tongue and posterior pharyngeal wall are the most affected.

For a *floor of mouth cancer*, the distribution of mucositis is characteristically on the lateral edges of the tongue, and the floor of mouth itself, which does not contain mucosal membranes, is spared from the effects of mucositis.

Well-lateralized *tonsil cancers* require radiation that results in mucositis that appears more severely on the affected side (right vs. left) of the soft palate, tongue base, and posterior pharyngeal wall.

Hypopharyngeal and laryngeal cancers require radiation plans that cause mucositis that is mostly in the region of the lower pharynx, with sparing of the mucosal surfaces of the oral cavity and oropharynx.

11.6.1.2 Technique-Specific Considerations

The technique of radiation delivery impacts the distribution of mucositis-induced dysphagia. The two main types of radiation plans are (1) conventional three-dimensional conformal radiation therapy (3D-CRT) and (2) intensity-modulated radiation therapy (IMRT). Most modern radiation plans for cancers of the head and neck are formulated using IMRT, because this technique employs dynamically shaped beams spread out through multiple beam angles or beam arcs in order to diffuse the entrance and exit radiation dose through multiple tissue plains. The desired target regions receive the desired prescription dose by means of an additive "cross-fire" effect of these multiple radiation beams from multiple angles. This technique results in radiation of a larger volume of tissue to a lower dose. Conventional 3D-CRT consists of simple, static, laterally opposed beams. This results in high dose delivery to all tissue in the path of the beams. With conventional 3D-CRT, mucositis will be localized within the beam path.

11.6.1.3 Time Course of Oral Mucositis

There are characteristic temporal patterns of the appearance and evolution of mucositis injury that occurs in a definitive radiation/chemotherapy treatment plan. The first sign of mucosal pain is noted at approximately 2000 cGy of delivered radiation therapy, or 1.5–2 weeks after the first dose of daily radiation. Typically at this time, there is not any apparent inflammation, and the patient typically is able to continue to eat soft solid foods and drink beverages with relatively little difficulty. On the third week of radiation therapy, erythematous and ulcerative lesions appear. The inflammation becomes more confluent by the fourth to fifth week. At this stage both dysphagia and odynophagia worsen to the point where oral intake is compromised and dietary adaptations or a feeding tube are required for nutritional support. Erythema and ulceration usually resolve within 4–8 weeks after completion of treatment. This corresponds to improvement in both odynophagia and dysphagia.

11.7 Mucosal Sensitivity

Patients may have persistent oropharyngeal pain after resolution of radiation-induced inflammatory lesions. Mucosal sensitivity is a peripheral neuropathic pain syndrome described as burning pain that is worsened by hot, spiced, or acidic food.

It is also worsened by dry air. Persistent pain on swallowing due to mucosal sensitivity may prevent patients from progression of diet or performance of swallow exercises. Use of adjunctive pain medications such as gabapentin; avoidance of hot, spicy, or acidic foods; or use of a humidifier for hydration may help alleviate symptoms.

11.8 Management: The Need for a Systematic Team Approach

Head and neck cancer patients should be treated by a multidisciplinary team of health care providers which should include speech and language pathologists and dieticians. Because of patient heterogeneity as well as differences in available resources and expertise, ideal interventional strategies to ensure optimal swallow outcomes are difficult to define. Nonetheless, there are a number of general recommendations for care that should be considered in all patients [42, 43].

11.8.1 Pharmacological Therapy

Pharmacologic agents can be useful in managing symptoms that adversely impact swallow function. This includes analgesic agents for treating tumor- or treatment-related pain; agents to address excess secretions or xerostomia; anti-inflammatory agents; and antibiotics or antifungals for treating oral infections. Patients undergoing treatment have rapidly evolving symptom control needs; thus frequent assessment by a dedicated physician, nurse practitioner, or nurse with experience in the medical management of head and neck cancer-related symptoms and functional deficits is critical for optimal outcomes.

For patients undergoing definitive or adjuvant radiation for head and neck cancer, dysphagia and odynophagia are frequently caused by mucositis. It may therefore be hypothesized that by preventing the development of mucositis, there may also be a subsequent decrease in swallowing abnormalities both acutely and long term. A number of pharmacological agents have been tested to determine their ability to decrease oral mucositis due to chemoradiation in the head and neck cancer population. These include amifostine and palifermin. Although there is preliminary data indicating improved swallow outcome with these agents, the data is not sufficiently compelling to warrant standard use of these agents.

11.8.2 Surgical Considerations

Surgical techniques that potentially spare tissue or prevent the need for primary or adjuvant radiation therapy may improve swallow outcomes. The location of the cancer and the extent and type of tissues involved are the greatest determinant of surgical impact, as tumor cannot be left behind to spare surgical morbidity. Less invasive approaches that avoid traumatizing normal tissues to access a tumor (such as transoral robotic surgery) have made some impact on lessening the aftermath of surgical extirpation but do not lessen the need to clear the cancer completely. Therefore, reconstruction of the resultant defects has a greater impact on long- and short-term swallowing function. While resection of adynamic structures like the mandible can be easily reconstructed with little to no impact on swallowing, reconstruction of dynamic tissues like the tongue and soft palate has potential for dramatic impact on swallowing. Current reconstructive techniques allow for replacement of mucosal surface area soft tissue volume, but they do not have the ability to restore the native function of the tissues replaced. The goal of reconstruction in the upper aerodigestive tract is to maximize the function of the normal tissues left behind and give them the best potential to compensate for the lost tissues. This may involve replacing more surface area than was removed to maximize mobility, or potentially less surface area and more volume than the resected tissues to guide food away from the abnormal side toward the retained normal tissues. In making these decisions, the experience of the reconstructive surgeon can dramatically impact swallow outcomes. In addition, baseline swallow dysfunction and protracted duration of postoperative feeding tube placement adversely correlate with swallow function [44].

11.8.3 The Role of the Radiation Oncology Team, Including Radiation Dosimetrists and Medical Physicist

The goal of every radiation therapy plan is to maximize the delivered dose to the intended target while minimizing radiation exposure to adjacent critical structures and normal tissues. In developing a treatment plan, the radiation oncologist uses the series of CT slices (with any applicable overlaid MRI and/or PET scans) to contour the target(s) to be treated as well as all of the regional critical anatomical structures.

The defined radiation targets may be prescribed to receive various levels of radiation dose, as outlined here:

70 Gy to gross unresected tumor
60 Gy to a postoperative bed
50–55 Gy prophylactic dose to clinically uninvolved lymph nodes at risk for microscopic spread of cancer

Multiple organs must also be contoured to calculate radiation exposure. This includes the pharyngeal constrictors which are critical for swallow function. Radiation treatment plans are carefully prepared by the radiation dosimetrist and the medical physicist, with quantification of radiation exposure to specific organs than may be adjacent to the targets, including the following

Optic chiasm, optic nerves	50 Gy maximum dose
Optic lens	10 Gy maximum dose
Brain	60 Gy maximum dose
Eyes	45 Gy maximum dose
Cochlea	36 Gy maximum dose
Brainstem	50 Gy maximum dose
Spinal cord	40 Gy maximum dose
Oral cavity	40 Gy mean dose
Parotid glands	26 Gy mean dose
Submandibular glands	26 Gy mean dose
Pharyngeal constrictors	45 Gy mean dose
Brachial plexus	66 Gy maximum dose
Trachea	60 Gy maximum dose
Esophagus	55 Gy maximum dose

It is not always possible to meet both the prescribed target dose(s) and desired dose constraints to critical structures, especially if the target is large or if it is especially close to a critical structure. In these cases, priorities must be set, weighing all clinical considerations for the patient. For instance, it may be acceptable to exceed the tolerance dose for a single parotid gland on the side of a tonsil or base of tongue tumor; in a case such as this, there would be high priority to spare the contralateral parotid gland to preserve as much salivary function as possible. It is helpful if the entire multidisciplinary team taking care of the patient is informed of the dose level of the radiation plan and the expected side acute and chronic toxicities. A dose-volume histogram (DVH) report is part of the radiation planning documents that catalogue the varying levels of radiation doses to the respective critical structures. This report may be shared by the radiation oncologist with the rest of the care team to help anticipate adverse effects and treat them proactively. For example, if a patient is planned for definitive radiation therapy to the base of tongue, the speech and language pathologist may be consulted for swallow education and a prescription of preventive swallowing exercises.

11.8.4 The Role of the Speech and Language Pathologist

11.8.4.1 Education

As our understanding of the frequency, severity, and long-term impact of swallow dysfunction in head and neck cancer patients evolves, so too does the role of the speech and language pathologist (SLP). Patients must be educated about the potential impact of head and neck cancer and its treatment on swallow function: increasingly, the SLP will serve this role as a part of a multidisciplinary supportive care team. It is critical to set realistic expectations in order to prepare patients emotionally for the profound impact on diet and the potential need for placement of a feeding tube. In addition, education can also motivate patients to adhere to self-care programs designed to minimize long-term functional deficits. The SLP will also educate patient about the signs and symptoms of aspiration [42]. Treating clinicians as well as members of the multidisciplinary supportive care team should be versed in the educational content provided by their local SLP so that they can provide reinforcement, monitor compliance, and identify knowledge gaps that need further education.

11.8.4.2 Assessment of Swallow Function

Head and neck cancer patients with locally advanced disease or those with any indication of dysphagia, odynophagia, or aspiration should undergo immediate swallow evaluation. Assessment will usually begin with a clinical swallow evaluation. During the evaluation, the SLP will determine whether there is evidence of swallow dysfunction or if there is an indication for further evaluation with instrumental assessment with a MBS or FEES.

11.8.4.3 Rehabilitation: Compensatory Measures and Swallow Exercises

If swallow dysfunction is noted during swallow evaluation, compensatory measures will be assessed for efficacy and recommended if indicated. Increasing data would support the initiation of swallow exercises with radiation to maximize swallow function. The effectiveness of rehabilitation programs may be adversely impacted by poor compliance. Incorporation of methods to optimize compliance may also improve swallow outcome [45]. The treatment team should be aware of and support the recommendations of the SLP by underscoring the importance of routine daily practice and encouragement of adherence to their self-care regimen.

11.8.4.4 Dietary Recommendations

One of the critical roles of the SLP is to ensure a safe diet. The SLP may therefore make recommendations for dietary restrictions. Under these circumstances, it is critical for the SLP to work with the dietician to ensure dietary intake that is nutritionally replete. If a patient is unsafe to swallow, the SLP will notify the treating team that alternative methods for nutritional support will be needed. This usually takes the form of a nasogastric or gastric feeding tube. On occasion, patients may require either a jejunostomy tube or parenteral nutrition.

11.8.4.5 Barriers to Care

There are a number of barriers to effective and timely provision of swallow therapy. First and foremost, swallow therapy is a costly service. Care is usually provided one-on-one by a certified speech and language pathologist. Because dysphagia secondary to head and neck cancer poses unique clinical challenges, the treating SLP should ideally have experience in the management of this challenging cohort of patients. Unfortunately, there are insufficient certified SLPs with experience in the management of head and neck cancer patients to meet this clinical challenge. Obtaining appropriate care is most challenging in rural communities. Alternative models of care need to be explored and tested.

Second, head and neck cancer patients experience a wide array of symptom control problems. This creates two distinct challenges: time and capacity. Treatment itself is time-intensive, limiting the patients' available time for therapy appointments or self-care programs that involve patient-directed practice. More importantly, symptoms themselves may limit the patient's capacity to follow through with complex self-care programs. For example, fatigue, which is ubiquitous in the head and neck cancer population, may interfere with the ability to complete daily exercise. Unfortunately, fatigue is most severe during and in the early post-treatment period when rehabilitation efforts are most critical. Odynophagia, which affects the vast majority of head and neck cancer patients treated with combined modality therapy, may also limit the ability to comply with prescribed swallow exercises. Patients develop soft tissue swelling and radiation dermatitis: this results in marked decrease movement of the jaw, neck, and shoulders. Due to physical constrains, patients may be unable to perform range of motion and swallow exercises.

In addition to physical and symptom constraints, patients develop marked cognitive and neuropsychiatric symptoms that make it difficult for them to manage pre-habilitation and rehabilitation efforts. Data would indicate that 9% of head and neck cancer patients have documented delirium during radiation-based combined modality therapy, and between 40% and 50% self-report symptoms of delirium at some point during their treatment course. Similar to the breast cancer population, neurocognitive dysfunction is present at baseline in 40% of head and neck cancer patients. While these abnormalities may improve post-treatment, a cohort of patients will have symptoms that last long term. Anxiety and depression, which are frequent in the head and neck population, may both impact swallow therapy efforts. Patients may avoid swallowing due to fear of choking. Depression may be associated with lack of motivation and apathy leading to noncompliance with recommended exercises. Caregivers can assist in this effort; however, they too are challenged. In developing a caregiver burden task inventory, we identified a wide array tasks required of HNC caregivers. Dysphagia and the requirement for feeding placement and management create substantial caregiver burden in patients already experiencing significant care needs [46]. In addition to neurocognitive limitations, patients also experience physical limitations.

11.8.4.6 Telemedicine: Cost-Effectiveness and Alternative Models of Care Delivery

The use of technology to provide care has been made possible by the rapid dissemination of technology that supports HIPPA-compliant medical services to patients through computers, smart phones, and smart pads. By facilitating real-time video conferencing, these technologies allow patients to receive face-to-face services at a distance and at times that are convenient for both the patient and provider. Issues such as transportation and caregiver time are therefore addressed; however, telemedicine does not address the issue of lack of SLPs experienced in the management of head and neck cancer patients.

The concept of telemedicine can be taken further by the development of web-based videos that provide patients with programs of care that take the place of face-to-face swallow therapy. The advantage of this type of program is that it can be developed by experts and disseminated widely to patients in need. This clearly addresses the issue of cost and staffing; however, it relies on the patient to be motivated and capable of a home-based practice. One randomized pilot study compared three delivery systems for a prophylactic swallow therapy program during radiation treatment: patient-direct (n = 27), clinician-directed (n = 26), and SwallowIT, an IT-based swallow therapy program (n = 26). During the patient-directed care model, patients were given a 1-h education session and instruction in swallow exercises. Patients then practiced independently twice a day. In the clinician-directed program, patients received the same education, but they also received face-to-face instruction 5 days per week. In the SwallowIT program, they received baseline education and then conducted twice a day exercises using an electronic therapy session. As expected, the cost of administering the patient-directed swallow program was the least costly ($1062.98 Australian) followed by the SwallowIT Program ($1613.08 Australian). The clinician-directed program was the most costly ($3514.18 Australian). Both the clinician-directed and the SwallowIT program had improved QOL at the end of treatment when compared to the patient-directed swallow therapy [47].

11.9 Summary

Dysphagia is a common and highly impactful acute and late toxicity of head and neck cancer therapy. At baseline, patients should be assessed for swallow dysfunction by an experienced SLP. Compensatory measures and a program of exercise should be provided if indicated. Because of the high rate of acute and long-term swallow dysfunction, head and neck cancer patients should undergo repeated assessment of swallow function during and after cancer treatment is completed. Patients with dysphagia should be set up with a program of self-care (to include exercises and compensatory measures) and monitored for adverse sequelae including aspiration and dietary insufficiencies.

Bibliography

1. Simental AA, Carrau RL. Assessment of swallowing function in patients with head and neck cancer. Curr Oncol Rep. 2004;6:162–5.
2. Baijens LW, Speyer R, Pilz W, Roodenburg N. FEES protocol derived estimates of sensitivity: aspiration in dysphagic patients. Dysphagia. 2014;29:583–90.
3. Brady S, Donzelli J. The modified barium swallow and the functional endoscopic evaluation of swallowing. Otolaryngol Clin N Am. 2013;46:1009–22.
4. Hiss SG, Postma GN. Fiberoptic endoscopic evaluation of swallowing. Laryngoscope. 2003;113:1386–93.
5. Timmerman AA, Speyer R, Heijnen BJ, Klijn-Zwijnenberg IR. Psychometric characteristics of health-related quality-of-life questionnaires in oropharyngeal dysphagia. Dysphagia. 2014;29:183–98.
6. Hedstrom J, Tuomi L, Finizia C, Olsson C. Correlations between patient-reported dysphagia screening and penetration-aspiration scores in head and neck cancer patients post-oncological treatment. Dysphagia. 2018;33:206–15.
7. King SN, Dunlap NE, Tennant PA, Pitts T. Pathophysiology of radiation-induced dysphagia in head and neck cancer. Dysphagia. 2016;31:339–51.

8. Ridner SH, Dietrich MS, Sonis ST, Murphy B. Biomarkers associated with lymphedema and fibrosis in patients with cancer of the head and neck. Lymphat Res Biol. 2018;16(6):516–24.
9. Deng J, Ridner S, Rothman R, et al. Perceived symptom experience in head and neck cancer patients with lymphedema. J Palliat Med. 2016;19:1267–74.
10. Jackson LK, Ridner SH, Deng J, et al. Internal lymphedema correlates with subjective and objective measures of dysphagia in head and neck cancer patients. J Palliat Med. 2016;19:949–56.
11. Wall LR, Ward EC, Cartmill B, Hill AJ. Physiological changes to the swallowing mechanism following (chemo)radiotherapy for head and neck cancer: a systematic review. Dysphagia. 2013;28:481–93.
12. van Bokhorst-de van der S, van Leeuwen PA, Kuik DJ, et al. The impact of nutritional status on the prognoses of patients with advanced head and neck cancer. Cancer. 1999;86:519–27.
13. Orell-Kotikangas H, Osterlund P, Makitie O, et al. Cachexia at diagnosis is associated with poor survival in head and neck cancer patients. Acta Otolaryngol. 2017;137:778–85.
14. Bressan V, Stevanin S, Bianchi M, Aleo G, Bagnasco A, Sasso L. The effects of swallowing disorders, dysgeusia, oral mucositis and xerostomia on nutritional status, oral intake and weight loss in head and neck cancer patients: a systematic review. Cancer Treat Rev. 2016;45:105–19.
15. Zhao JZ, Zheng H, Li LY, Zhang LY, Zhao Y, Jiang N. Predictors for weight loss in head and neck cancer patients undergoing radiotherapy: a systematic review. Cancer Nurs. 2015;38:E37–45.
16. Kubrak C, Olson K, Jha N, et al. Clinical determinants of weight loss in patients receiving radiation and chemoirradiation for head and neck cancer: a prospective longitudinal view. Head Neck. 2013;35:695–703.
17. Wopken K, Bijl HP, Langendijk JA. Prognostic factors for tube feeding dependence after curative (chemo-) radiation in head and neck cancer: a systematic review of literature. Radiotherapy Oncol. 2018;126:56–67.
18. Locher JL, Bonner JA, Carroll WR, et al. Prophylactic percutaneous endoscopic gastrostomy tube placement in treatment of head and neck cancer: a comprehensive review and call for evidence-based medicine. JPEN J Parenter Enteral Nutr. 2011;35:365–74.
19. Shaw SM, Flowers H, O'Sullivan B, Hope A, Liu LW, Martino R. The effect of prophylactic percutaneous endoscopic gastrostomy (PEG) tube placement on swallowing and swallow-related outcomes in patients undergoing radiotherapy for head and neck cancer: a systematic review. Dysphagia. 2015;30:152–75.
20. Rutter CE, Yovino S, Taylor R, et al. Impact of early percutaneous endoscopic gastrostomy tube placement on nutritional status and hospitalization in patients with head and neck cancer receiving definitive chemoradiation therapy. Head Neck. 2011;33:1441–7.
21. Chen AM, Li BQ, Lau DH, et al. Evaluating the role of prophylactic gastrostomy tube placement prior to definitive chemoradiotherapy for head and neck cancer. Int J Radiat Oncol Biol Phys. 2010;78:1026–32.
22. Ganzer H, Touger-Decker R, Byham-Gray L, Murphy BA, Epstein JB. The eating experience after treatment for head and neck cancer: a review of the literature. Oral Oncol. 2015;51:634–42.
23. Ganzer H, Rothpletz-Puglia P, Byham-Gray L, Murphy BA, Touger-Decker R. The eating experience in long-term survivors of head and neck cancer: a mixed-methods study. Support Care Cancer. 2015;23:3257–68.
24. Moss WJ, Pang J, Orosco RK, et al. Esophageal dilation in head and neck cancer patients: a systematic review and meta-analysis. Laryngoscope. 2018;128:111–7.
25. Bese NS, Hendry J, Jeremic B. Effects of prolongation of overall treatment time due to unplanned interruptions during radiotherapy of different tumor sites and practical methods for compensation. Int J Radiat Oncol Biol Phys. 2007;68:654–61.
26. Thomas K, Martin T, Gao A, Ahn C, Wilhelm H, Schwartz DL. Interruptions of head and neck radiotherapy across insured and indigent patient populations. J Oncol Pract. 2017;13:e319–e28.
27. Coca-Pelaz A, Takes RP, Hutcheson K, et al. Head and neck cancer: a review of the impact of treatment delay on outcome. Adv Ther. 2018;35:153–60.

28. Rhoten BA, Deng J, Dietrich MS, Murphy B, Ridner SH. Body image and depressive symptoms in patients with head and neck cancer: an important relationship. Support Care Cancer. 2014;22:3053–60.
29. Rhoten BA, Murphy B, Ridner SH. Body image in patients with head and neck cancer: a review of the literature. Oral Oncol. 2013;49:753–60.
30. Molassiotis A, Rogers M. Symptom experience and regaining normality in the first year following a diagnosis of head and neck cancer: a qualitative longitudinal study. Palliat Support Care. 2012;10:197–204.
31. Bond SM, Schumacher K, Sherrod A, et al. Development of the head and neck cancer caregiving task inventory. Eur J Oncol Nurs. 2016;24:29–38.
32. Patterson JM, Rapley T, Carding PN, Wilson JA, McColl E. Head and neck cancer and dysphagia; caring for carers. Psychooncology. 2013;22:1815–20.
33. Castellanos EH, Dietrich MS, Bond SM, et al. Impact of patient symptoms and caregiving tasks on psychological distress in caregivers for head and neck cancer (HNC). Psychooncology. 2019;28(3):511–7.
34. Breenan MT, Spijkervet FKL, Elting LS. Systemic reviews and guidelines for oral complications of cancer therapies: current challenges and future opportunities. Support Care Cancer. 2010;18:977–8.
35. Lango MN, Egleston B, Fang C, et al. Baseline health perceptions, dysphagia, and survival in patients with head and neck cancer. Cancer. 2014;120:840–7.
36. Pauloski BR, Rademaker AW, Logemann JA, et al. Pretreatment swallowing function in patients with head and neck cancer. Head Neck. 2000;22:474–82.
37. Mortensen HR, Overgaard J, Jensen K, et al. Factors associated with acute and late dysphagia in the DAHANCA 6 & 7 randomized trial with accelerated radiotherapy for head and neck cancer. Acta Oncol. 2013;52:1535–42.
38. Batth SS, Caudell JJ, Chen AM. Practical considerations in reducing swallowing dysfunction following concurrent chemoradiotherapy with intensity-modulated radiotherapy for head and neck cancer. Head Neck. 2014;36:291–8.
39. Francis DO, Weymuller EA Jr, Parvathaneni U, Merati AL, Yueh B. Dysphagia, stricture, and pneumonia in head and neck cancer patients: does treatment modality matter? Ann Otol Rhinol Laryngol. 2010;119:391–7.
40. Hutcheson KA, Nurgalieva Z, Zhao H, et al. Two-year prevalence of dysphagia and related outcomes in head and neck cancer survivors: an updated SEER-Medicare analysis. Head Neck. 2019;41(2):479–87.
41. Chen SC, Liao CT, Chang JT. Orofacial pain and predictors in oral squamous cell carcinoma patients receiving treatment. Oral Oncol. 2011;47:131–5.
42. Schindler A, Denaro N, Russi EG, et al. Dysphagia in head and neck cancer patients treated with radiotherapy and systemic therapies: literature review and consensus. Crit Rev Oncol Hematol. 2015;96:372–84.
43. Clarke P, Radford K, Coffey M, Stewart M. Speech and swallow rehabilitation in head and neck cancer: United Kingdom National Multidisciplinary Guidelines. J Laryngol Otol. 2016;130:S176–s80.
44. Owen S, Puvanendran M, Meikle D, et al. Baseline swallowing measures predict recovery at 6 weeks after transoral robotic surgery for head and neck cancer. Clin Otolaryngol. 2017;42:366–72.
45. Govender R, Smith CH, Taylor SA, Barratt H, Gardner B. Swallowing interventions for the treatment of dysphagia after head and neck cancer: a systematic review of behavioural strategies used to promote patient adherence to swallowing exercises. BMC Cancer. 2017;17:43.
46. Bond SM, Schumacher K, Sherrod A, Dietrich MS, Wells N, Lindau RH 3rd, Murphy BA. Development of the Head and Neck Cancer Caregiving Task Inventory. Eur J Oncol Nurs. 2016;24:29–38. https://doi.org/10.1016/j.ejon.2016.08.004. Epub 2016 Aug 27. PMID: 27697275.
47. Wall LR, Kularatna S, Ward EC, et al. Economic analysis of a three-arm RCT exploring the delivery of intensive, prophylactic swallowing therapy to patients with head and neck cancer during (chemo)radiotherapy. Dysphagia. 2019;34(5):627–39.

Chemosensory Dysfunction in Head and Neck Cancer Patients

12

Kenneth Niermann and Barbara A. Murphy

12.1 Introduction

Discerning smells, tastes, and flavors is an essential part of the human experience. For patients who are afflicted with cancers of the head and neck, chemosensory disorders are common yet marginalized adverse effects of cancer and its therapy [1]. To complicate the picture, distortion of the sense of smell (dysosmia) and taste (dysgeusia) may result from not only the underlying cancer but also cancer treatment. Chemotherapy, radiation therapy, surgery, and pharmacologic agents may cause or contribute to symptom severity. For some patients, chemosensory dysfunction is temporary; for others it may be permanent [2]. The impact of chemosensory dysfunction in the oncology setting is significant: it affects not only gastronomic satisfaction but also leads to diminished appetite, malnourishment, and an overall decrease in quality of life [3, 4].

Effectively managing patients with HNC experiencing chemosensory dysfunction requires an understanding of the physiology of chemosensory function, knowledge pertaining to the mechanisms of injury, and an appreciation of how chemosensory dysfunction impacts overall health. More importantly, it is critical for clinicians to understand the expected time course of symptom development and recovery. This allows clinicians to set realistic expectations for patients regarding the extent and time course of functional recovery. Complete and accurate

K. Niermann (✉)
Department of Radiation Oncology, Vanderbilt University Medical Center, Nashville, TN, USA
e-mail: ken.niermann@vumc.org

B. A. Murphy
Medical Oncology, Department of Medicine, Vanderbilt University Medical Center, Nashville, TN, USA
e-mail: barbara.murphy@vumc.org

R. Nair (ed.), *Orofacial Supportive Care in Cancer*,
https://doi.org/10.1007/978-3-030-86510-8_12

information can help patients anticipate and cope with dysosmia and dysgeusia during the course of definitive therapy and subsequent recovery. Furthermore it allows health practitioners to implement appropriate interventions in a timely manner.

12.2 Anatomy of Smell and Taste

The sensory system allows communication with the external world through visual, auditory, tactile, and chemosensory input. Chemosensory input is facilitated through olfaction and taste apparatus. Small molecules or chemicals bind to and activate chemical receptors in taste buds and olfactory epithelium which in turn activate neural networks allowing the processing of sensory input. In effect, when we detect a smell or taste, we are responding to external molecular triggers. Input from the olfactory, gustatory, and trigeminal afferent nerves coalesce within the orbitofrontal cortex [5]. Thus, the detection of external molecular triggers is able to elicit both physiological and behavioral response.

The olfactory neuroepithelium is located in the superior portion of the nasal cavity. Olfactory neurons arise from the olfactory nerve (crania nerve I) and the ophthalmic and maxillary branches of the trigeminal nerve (cranial nerve V). A complex array of olfactory receptors are activated by odorants, resulting in an action potential and signal transduction to primary and secondary olfactory regions within the brain. A wide array of anatomical and functional regions are activated by olfactory neurons. This explains the broad and complex behavioral and physiological impact of odorants.

Gustatory receptor cells are the essential neuroepithelial receptor cells in taste function. They are present on various papillae on the dorsal surface and lateral edges of the tongue and also on the posterior oropharyngeal wall and upper esophagus. Multiple gustatory receptor cells are grouped together in a single taste bud, which has hairlike extensions projecting into a pore on the tongue's overlying epithelium. When food is dissolved in saliva, it comes into contact with gustatory hairs within the pores. Each of the gustatory receptor cells is individually differentiated for one of the five sensations of taste: sweet, salty, sour, bitter, and umami. Distinct taste sensations serve important roles in maintaining nutrition balance and preventing ingestion of toxins: sweet taste identifies carbohydrates which are sources of energy, salt taste may be critical in regulating electrolytes, umami detects high-protein food sources that are rich in amino acids, and sour or bitter tastes identify potential toxins [6].

Classically, the "tongue map" has been used to define separate and discrete regions of the tongue that are each responsible for separate tastes. A more thorough understanding of the organization of gustatory nerves reveals that all taste buds contain receptors for each of the five sensations of taste, but the proportion varies. Gustatory receptor cells transmit sensory information via the seventh, ninth, and tenth cranial nerves to the gustatory centers of the brain as outlined in Table 12.1 [7].

Table 12.1 Neuroanatomy of taste sensation

Cranial nerve 7 "facial nerve"	Taste sensation for the anterior two-thirds of the tongue is carried by the chorda tympani branch of CN7 Taste sensation for the palate is carried by the superficial petrosal nerve branch of CN7
Cranial nerve 9 "glossopharyngeal nerve"	Taste sensation for posterior one-third of the tongue
Cranial nerve 10 "vagus nerve"	Taste sensation for the uvula, epiglottis, pharynx, and larynx
Cranial nerve 5 "trigeminal nerve"	Burning sensation of hot pepper in the mouth and nasal cavity
Central processing of taste	CN7, CN9, and CN10 converge at the medulla portion of the brainstem Nerve fibers from the medulla connect to the thalamus Nerve fibers from the thalamus connect to the frontal lobe of the brain, where taste is processed

12.3 Impact of Chemosensory Dysfunction

Chemosensation has a profound impact on multiple dimensions. First and foremost, taste and smell impact food choice and associated enjoyment. Patients with significant chemosensory dysfunction may experience a decrease in caloric intake with associated weight loss or changes in diet with associated nutrient deficiencies. Chemosensory activation is important for initiation of the cephalic phase of digestion. It plays a critical role in safety by assisting in the identification and avoidance of dangerous toxins. It is also integral in normal human behaviors and interaction including mating, reproduction, and infant bonding [8].

12.4 Measurement of Taste and Smell

Smell and taste dysfunction can range from mild degrees of loss (hyposmia and hypogeusia) to total loss of function (anosmia and ageusia). In addition, patients may report altered sensory input (dysosmia and dysgeusia). Alterations in smell and taste can be assessed using self-report or objective measures. Self-report measures vary in content and complexity. There are a number of tools that have been developed specifically to measure self-reported olfactory and gustatory function, including the Questionnaire on Odor, Taste, and Appetite and the Taste and Smell Complaint survey. In addition, several general symptoms and quality-of-life measures developed for head and neck cancer patients include items directed at taste and smell. Self-reported changes in smell and taste may not reflect chemosensory receptor function; however they do reflect patient experience, and [9] as such they may predict behavior more accurately.

Olfactory and gustatory testing is a complex and time-consuming process. Objective measures of olfaction assess three specific functional abilities: odor discrimination, odor detection threshold, and odor identification. Objective measures

Table 12.2 Substances used for physiologic taste testing

Sweet	Sucrose
Salty	Sodium chloride
Sour	Citric acid HCl
Bitter	Quinine sulfate Urea Caffeine
Umami (savory)	Glutamate

of taste include taste sensitivity (detection threshold and recognition threshold for the five taste qualities) and taste intensity (Table 12.2).

In addition to taste and olfaction, other outcome measures should be evaluated, including constructs such flavor and the pleasure derived from food [10]. Flavor is a complex concept that incorporates multiple factors including taste, smell, and sensory input such as texture and temperature. Similarly, pleasure (liking) related to chemosensation and its antithesis are influenced by a host of biopsychosocial factors. These include conditioned responses associated with positive or negative experiences. In the oncologic population, chemotherapy may act as a conditioning event resulting in food aversions.

12.5 Causes of Chemosensory Dysfunction

Chemosensory dysfunction is often multifactorial; thus it is important to consider each potential contributing factor. This is particularly true of HNC patients who are exposed to numerous pharmacological and non-pharmacological interventions that are associated with high rates of chemosensory dysfunction as noted below. A few commonly cited causes of olfactory and gustatory dysfunction include but not limited to the following:

Genetic conditions that contribute to chemosensory dysfunction.
Familial dysautonomia.
Hereditary ataxia.
Machado-Joseph disease.
Guillain-Barre syndrome.
Cancer: Taste abnormalities have been documented in patients prior to the initiation of therapy.
Age: Diminished chemosensory function has been associated with the normal aging process [11]. Dysfunction is more prominent in men than women.
Drugs: Drugs usually cause chemosensory abnormalities by occupying taste or odorant receptors. Discontinuation of drug therapy usually results in return of function [12].
Cigarette use: Use of cigarettes is strongly associated with a decline in chemosensory function [13].

Altered salivary composition or flow.
Environmental conditions and exposures.
Allergic rhinitis and chronic rhinosinusitis.
Viral infections [14].
Altitude sickness.
Oral hygiene and dental health: The microbiota of the oral cavity and associated tongue coating may alter taste function [15, 16].
Head trauma, seizures, or neurodegenerative disorders.

12.6 Head and Neck Cancer-Specific Causes of Chemosensory Dysfunction

12.6.1 Tumor-Induced Nerve Damage

When tumors are locally invasive, they may interrupt taste by compression or erosion of the aforementioned cranial nerves. When this occurs, the patient may experience a chemosensory dysfunction that is unilateral in nature. In the case of dysgeusia, abnormalities may be confined to a specific distribution, depending on the nerve(s) affected. Each cranial nerve is susceptible at any point along its path. When a tumor compresses any large-caliber cranial nerve, taste may be partially or completely disrupted in that nerve's sensory distribution. Because cranial nerves carry other important stimuli and function, the exact location of nerve compression or damage may be pin-pointed based on other accompanying neurologic sequelae. Sites of tumors known to cause gustatory dysfunction include parotid tumors causing CN VII palsy ("Bell palsy"), tumors in the cerebellopontine angle, meningiomas, neurinomas, tumors in the submandibular region, and tumors of the skull base. In addition to alterations in cranial nerve function, tumors may cause alterations in airflow or mucociliary function resulting in decreased delivery of molecular triggers to receptors. Bacterial infection or changes in microbiota may also result in altered chemosensory function.

Nerve-induced chemosensory dysfunction typically gets worse over time as a tumor's local effects become more severe. However, it is common to see reversal of nerve-induced dysfunction days to weeks after the initiation of various cancer therapies, including steroids, chemotherapy, and radiation therapy.

12.6.2 Surgery-Induced Chemosensory Dysfunction

Surgery may cause dysfunction through direct and indirect damage to the chemosensory apparatus. Surgical procedures (including biopsy, excision, debulking, or gross resection of tumor and/or involved regional lymph nodes) that result in extirpation, transection, or trauma to cranial nerves at any level along pathway may cause altered chemosensory function. Dysfunction due to nerve damage may be permanent. Cranial nerves can also be compressed in the setting of post-surgical swelling and inflammation. In this setting, dysfunction generally resolves over a period of weeks. Surgical procedures may also affect taste and smell through other mechanisms. In a study of patients undergoing total laryngectomy, 100% of patients noted hyposmia and 54% noted hypogeusia [17]. Hyposmia was felt to be due to loss of nasal airflow and damage to olfactory mucosa. Hypogeusia was felt to be due to altered functionality within the central nervous system [5].

12.6.3 Radiation-Induced Injury

Radiation therapy when directed to or through the oral cavity directly damages the DNA of any cells in its path, including the chemosensory cells and the adjacent epithelial cells. Most cells of the human body have a significant, but finite, capacity to repair DNA damage that results from the insult of ionizing radiation. With repeated daily radiation treatments, these DNA repair processes cannot keep up with damage caused by radiation, and a portion of the cells may die. Damage to chemosensory cells manifests as dysgeusia and dysosmia.

The development of taste dysfunction during radiation therapy has a characteristic time course [18]. Adverse effect of radiation on chemosensory cells occurs after approximately 20 Gy; thus, there are usually no alterations in taste during the first 2 weeks of therapy. Starting week 3, patients develop mild taste changes which progresses to a moderate level of severity by week 4. Bitter sensation is most sensitive to damage and slowest to recover. Salty sensation is the most resilient, followed by sweet. Thus, patients may complain that food has become overly salty tasting. At this point, patients may begin to alter food choices and decrease caloric intake due to the loss of pleasure with eating. By week 5, patients may complain of complete loss of taste or dramatically altered taste sensation. Some patients will complain that food tastes “bad”; this may result in food aversion and dramatic decrease in oral intake. Patients also complain of loss of desire for food. While this may be in part related to treatment associated anorexia, diminished taste clearly plays a role [19]. Taste alterations, when severe, may result in gagging or retching with food intake. Under these circumstances, feeding tube placement is needed to maintain nutritional status.

Depending on the overall dose of radiation received, restoration of chemosensory function from radiation-induced DNA damage may occur gradually over 3–12 months. Patients who have relatively lower doses of radiation therapy to the oral cavity, including patients with primary tumors in the larynx (as opposed to the oropharynx), tend to demonstrate faster recovery. Patients receiving high doses of radiation therapy may develop permanent and severe function loss. In one study of HNC survivors greater than 6 months out from completion of therapy, 82.6% of patients noted some degree of altered taste and 39.1% indicated that taste alterations were moderate to severe; 28.3%, 34.8%, and 28.3% indicated that taste changes have a moderate to severe impact on the desire to eat, caused alterations in food choice, and led to a decrease in food intake, respectively [20]. That being said, data would indicate that patients are able to adapt to these changes long term and that the impact on overall quality of life is minimal for most patients [21].

Data on altered olfactory function with radiation is more limited. The trajectory of smell dysfunction has not been well established. The degree and duration of symptoms are related to the site of the tumor. Patients who have tumor volumes in or near the nasal passage, nasopharynx, and/or paranasal cavities are more susceptible to dysosmia due to the high therapeutic dosage of radiation required in these regions. In patients greater than 6 months post treatment, 40.4% of patients note an alteration in smell with 27.7% of patients rating symptoms as moderate to severe. Dysosmia results in altered food choices in 37% of patients with 17.4% describing alterations as moderate to severe [20].

12.7 Chemotherapy-Induced Chemosensory Dysfunction

It is widely recognized that chemotherapy as a single modality alters both taste and smell. Although patients endorse altered taste and smell on self-report measures, objective data measuring alterations in taste sensitivity after chemotherapy administration is variable and inconclusive. Data regarding pleasure derived from food (liking) does show a trend toward a decrease following chemotherapy [10]. Thus, the question remains: is the perception of taste change associated with chemotherapy due to an effect on chemosensory receptor function or is this a higher order effect impacting constructs such as flavor and pleasure? Uniform protocols and procedures for testing chemosensory function, pleasure (liking), and flavor are needed to answer this question.

12.8 Intervention Strategies for Chemosensory Dysfunction

Management for chemosensory dysfunction centers largely on supportive measures. Since there is little literature supporting these measures, recommendations are based on clinical experience and expert opinion [22]. Patients should be informed prior to initiation of therapy about the risks of chemosensory dysfunction, the chance for recovery, and the impact on function. Patients should be instructed to maintain good oral hygiene and routine evaluation by oral health providers before, during, and after the course of therapy. Education should be provided about the potential impact on nutritional status. While nutrition deficiencies are not universally noted in non-malignant chemosensory dysfunction, in the oncology population, significant dietary impact may be noted. Thus, patients with clinical significant levels of dysfunction may merit nutritional counseling. Dietary intake and weight should be monitored. Flavor enhancement may be attempted to increase the appeal and pleasure of food.

A number of studies have evaluated the use of nutraceuticals and pharmaceuticals for the prevention and treatment of chemosensory disorders. The most commonly investigated nutraceutical, zinc supplements, was evaluated in a randomized phase III trial in head and neck cancer patients undergoing therapy. Furthermore, in recent meta-analyses, zinc supplementation failed to improve taste acuity in both idiopathic and zinc-deficient patients [23, 24].

12.9 Prevention of Taste Dysfunction

12.9.1 Cytoprotection

Amifostine, a cytoprotective agent, has been investigated in patients undergoing chemotherapy and/or radiation therapy to the head and neck. Preclinical data in mice receiving chemotherapy with cyclophosphamide support the potential for amifostine to protect the taste apparatus [25]. A prospective study conducted between 1995 and 2000 demonstrated a decrease in taste alterations and xerostomia [26].

12.9.2 Radiation Dosimetry and Xerostomia-Related Dysgeusia

Proper gustatory function is heavily dependent on the function of the saliva glands. Saliva performs an important function of the transmission of taste by dissolving food particles and allowing them to be presented to through the openings of the papillae to the hair fibers of the taste buds. Without normal saliva, the oropharyngeal surfaces are dry, and liquid and solid food particles pass through the oropharynx with limited opportunity to interface with the taste buds. Saliva is produced by multiple salivary glands located in the oropharyngeal region. The most important salivary glands are the left and right parotid glands which supply 70% of the volume of saliva. However, the submandibular and accessary salivary glands contribute 25% and 5% to the overall salivary volume, respectively. Surgical removal of any of the above glands permanently affects overall availability of saliva. All of the saliva glands are also sensitive to radiation therapy. Radiation has a direct and partially damaging effect on salivary glands.

For a patient who is undergoing radiation therapy to the head and neck region, it is standard to perform an analysis of the amount of radiation that may be delivered to the parotid and submandibular glands. There are a number of important principles in radiation planning that impact salivary function. One common analysis that is done prior to the initiation of a radiation treatment plan is a calculation of the mean parotid dose being delivered to each of the bilateral parotid glands. If tumor is located on right side of tongue base, the parotid on that side may need to be "sacrificed," and the parotid gland on the contralateral side will be spared. For a patient that undergoes parotid resection on one side, radiation planning techniques may be employed to keep the dose as low as possible to the contralateral intact parotid gland. When cancer is located bilaterally near both parotid glands, it may be impossible to spare either parotid gland. For patients that have parotid glands treated above threshold tolerance (goal is to maintain a mean dose of <26 Gy), salivary function will be more severe. For patients with bilaterally radiated (or surgically excised) parotid glands, the main remaining salivary function is the submandibular gland function. For these patients, who rely mostly on submandibular gland function for saliva flow, saliva function has a daily pattern of good saliva function in the morning, resulting from the patient lying supine at night while sleeping and the submandibular gland lubricating the mouth and oropharynx with the help of gravity and subsequent more severe dryness of the mouth during the course of the day.

12.10 Conclusions

Chemosensory dysfunction is a common acute and late effect of head and neck cancer therapy. Because HNC patients experience a myriad of clinical significant symptoms and functional deficits, chemosensory dysfunction is often overlooked or undiagnosed. As patients recover from the acute effects of therapy, the long-term impact and implications of chemosensory dysfunction becomes relevant. Whether recognized or not, patients' overall health, safety, and quality of life may be adversely impacted. Strategies to cope with chemosensory dysfunction may be maladaptive and harmful in the long run. As the number of HNC survivors increases, addressing chemosensory dysfunction becomes more critical.

Bibliography

1. Wong HM. Oral complications and management strategies for patients undergoing cancer therapy. ScientificWorldJournal. 2014;2014:581795.
2. Lalla RV, et al. Oral complications at 6 months after radiation therapy for head and neck cancer. Oral Dis. 2017;23(8):1134–43.
3. Baharvand M, et al. Taste alteration and impact on quality of life after head and neck radiotherapy. J Oral Pathol Med. 2013;42(1):106–12.
4. Hutton JL, Baracos VE, Wismer WV. Chemosensory dysfunction is a primary factor in the evolution of declining nutritional status and quality of life in patients with advanced cancer. J Pain Symptom Manag. 2007;33(2):156–65.
5. Landis BN, et al. Chemosensory interaction: acquired olfactory impairment is associated with decreased taste function. J Neurol. 2010;257(8):1303–8.
6. Chandrashekar J, et al. The receptors and cells for mammalian taste. Nature. 2006;444(7117):288–94.
7. Heckmann JG, et al. Neurological aspects of taste disorders. Arch Neurol. 2003;60(5):667–71.
8. Patel RM, Pinto JM. Olfaction: anatomy, physiology, and disease. Clin Anat. 2014;27(1):54–60.
9. Spotten LE, et al. Subjective and objective taste and smell changes in cancer. Ann Oncol. 2017;28(5):969–84.
10. Boltong A, Keast R. The influence of chemotherapy on taste perception and food hedonics: a systematic review. Cancer Treat Rev. 2012;38(2):152–63.
11. Schiffman SS. Taste and smell losses in normal aging and disease. JAMA. 1997;278(16):1357–62.
12. Henkin RI. Drug-induced taste and smell disorders. Incidence, mechanisms and management related primarily to treatment of sensory receptor dysfunction. Drug Saf. 1994;11(5):318–77.
13. Doty RL, Shaman P, Dann M. Development of the University of Pennsylvania Smell Identification Test: a standardized microencapsulated test of olfactory function. Physiol Behav. 1984;32:489–502.
14. Cavazzana A, et al. Postinfectious olfactory loss: a retrospective study on 791 patients. Laryngoscope. 2018;128(1):10–5.
15. Asakawa M, et al. Tongue microbiota and oral health status in community-dwelling elderly adults. mSphere. 2018;3(4):e00332–18.
16. Seerangaiyan K, et al. Tongue cleaning increases the perceived intensity of salty taste. J Nutr Health Aging. 2018;22(7):802–4.
17. Riva G, et al. Smell and taste impairment after total laryngectomy. Ann Otol Rhinol Laryngol. 2017;126(7):548–54.
18. Negi P, et al. Pattern of gustatory impairment and its recovery after head and neck irradiation. Iran J Otorhinolaryngol. 2017;29(95):319–27.
19. Ganzer H, et al. The eating experience after treatment for head and neck cancer: a review of the literature. Oral Oncol. 2015;51(7):634–42.

20. Cooperstein E, Gibert J, Epstein JB, Dietrich MS, Bond SM, Ridner SH, Wells N, Cmelak A, Murphy BA. Vanderbilt head and neck symptom survey version 2.0: report of the development and initial testing of a subscale for assessment of oral health. Head Neck. 2012;34(6):797–804.
21. Ganzer H, et al. The eating experience in long-term survivors of head and neck cancer: a mixed-methods study. Support Care Cancer. 2015;23(11):3257–68.
22. McLaughlin L. Taste dysfunction and eating behaviors in survivors of head and neck cancer treatment. Medsurg Nurs. 2014;23(3):165–70, 184.
23. Michelson M, Veitz-Keenan A. Taste disturbances – are there any effective treatments? Evidence Based Dentistry. 2018;19:60.
24. Kumbargere Nagraj S, et al. Interventions for managing taste disturbances. Cochrane Database Syst Rev. 2017;12:Cd010470.
25. Mukherjee N, et al. Pre-treatment with amifostine protects against cyclophosphamide-induced disruption of taste in mice. PLoS One. 2013;8(4):e61607.
26. Buntzel J, et al. Influence of amifostine on late radiation-toxicity in head and neck cancer—a follow-up study. Anticancer Res. 2007;27(4a):1953–6.

13 Orofacial Supportive Care in Paediatric Cancer

Alessandra Majorana and Elena Bardellini

13.1 Introduction

For the past 30 years, the major effort of paediatric oncologists has been to enhance the survival curve of children affected by cancer. Considering all the affected children and all the tumour kinds regardless of the stage of disease, the chance to be cured from a paediatric neoplastic disease is 70%.

Childhood cancers are a small proportion of the total number of cancer cases worldwide accounting for about 2% of the total number registered. Cancers occurring before the age of 15 are considered paediatric, but recently most centres treat children until they are 18 years old. The most common cause of the death from disease in childhood is cancer, with an incidence of a new case every 150,000 inhabitants.

13.2 Paediatric Cancer

The distribution and the types of cancers that occur in the paediatric population are very different from those that occur in adult populations.

A. Majorana (✉) · E. Bardellini
Department of Medical and Surgical Specialities, Radiological Sciences and Public Health, Dental School, University of Brescia, Brescia, Italy
e-mail: alessandra.majorana@unibs.it; elena.bardellini@unibs.it

R. Nair (ed.), *Orofacial Supportive Care in Cancer*,
https://doi.org/10.1007/978-3-030-86510-8_13

The most frequent neoplasms are acute leukaemia, lymphocytic and non-lymphocytic leukaemia, Hodgkin's diseases, non-Hodgkin's lymphoma, CNS tumours, neuroblastoma, retinoblastoma, Wilm's tumour and bone sarcomas.

13.2.1 Acute Leukaemias

The acute leukaemias are the result of accumulation of early myeloid or lymphoid precursors in the bone marrow, blood and other tissues. Acute leukaemia may arise de novo or as the terminal event in a number of pre-existing blood disorders. Clinical features at presentation are infections, haemorrhage and anaemia together with coexisting organ symptoms. Infections are frequent, and there are often bacterial infections affecting the skin, pharynx, perianal and perineal regions and mucosae. The disease is divided in acute myeloid leukaemia (AML) and acute lymphoblastic leukaemia (ALL), subdivided in various categories depending on surface immunological features and molecular patterns.

The treatment plan differs between the two forms of leukaemia. As for AML, the therapy consists of a high-dose regimen utilizing chemotherapeutical drugs in blocks. Once remission is achieved, consolidation consists in intensive combination chemotherapy. If an HLA-matching sibling is available, allogeneic bone marrow transplantation may be carried out, while autologous transplant or further consolidation therapy is considered for those without a familial compatible donor.

The overall survival of children affected by acute leukaemias ranges from 60% (AML) to 75% (ALL).

13.2.2 Hodgkin's Disease

Hodgkin's disease, typical of the adolescents (70% incidence), usually presents with painless supraclavicular or cervical lymphadenopathy. The majority of patients have a mediastinal involvement. Often the affected children show systemic symptoms such as anorexia, fever, unexplained weight loss and night sweats. Histologic subtypes define four groups: lymphocytic predominance, mixed cellularity, lymphocytic depletion and nodular sclerosis.

Once histologic diagnosis of the disease through node biopsy has been performed, the role of staging is critical to address therapy.

Currently the survival rate of patients affected by Hodgkin's disease is between 70% and 90%.

13.2.3 Non-Hodgkin's Lymphoma

Non-Hodgkin's lymphomas are a heterogeneous group of neoplasms that origin from the lymphatic tissue and characterized by different immunologic, cytogenetic, histological and clinical patterns. They constitute the 60% of all lymphomas affecting children and represent 10% of all neoplastic diseases present in children, being the third more frequent. The incidence is of seven cases on a million children less than 15 years of age.

The treatment of NHL in children is based on a multidrug chemotherapeutical approach, and recently with the BFM-oriented protocols the survival rate exceeds 80%.

13.2.4 Ewing Sarcoma

Ewing sarcoma is generally an undifferentiated bone tumour, but it can generate also from soft tissues. The clinical presentation is characterized by pain and swelling of the soft tissues corresponding to the long bones and of the trunk. The high incidence of metastasis (80%) reported in the pre-chemotherapeutic era suggested the hypothesis that most children at diagnosis present micro-metastasis.

13.2.5 Rhabdomyosarcoma

Rhabdomyosarcoma is thought to arise from primitive mesenchymal cells committed to develop into striated muscle. Nearly 20–30% of the cases present metastasis at diagnosis.

It is the commonest form of soft tissue sarcoma in children and young adults and accounts approximately 4–5% of all children malignancy with an annual incidence of 5.3 per million children and a mean age of about 5 years.

A multimodality approach involving surgery, chemotherapy and radiotherapy is necessary.

13.2.6 Neuroblastoma

Neuroblastoma is a relatively frequent tumour of childhood with an incidence raging between 8% and 10% of tumours. Eight cases per million are expected every year. Neuroblastoma comes from the sympathetic nervous system chain. Primary localization of the tumour varies and depends on age. The diagnosis is often posed at the age of 5 years. The disease can present as primary (19%), regional (13%) or metastatic (68%).

Surgery can be curative at stage one, but in all cases chemotherapy is needed. In high-risk disease, the overall survival does not exceed 15%.

13.3 Current Knowledge

As concerns antitumor chemotherapy, a requisite could be the specificity for the target, to eliminate the neoplastic cells not affecting the others. This ideal prerequisite is uneven since the vast majority of molecules are not capable to act against exclusively cancer cells. Since the chemotherapeutical agents inhibit in most cases the cellular proliferation, as a side effect they inhibit the growth of hair, the replication of the cells constituting the mucosae, and decrease the number of blood cells.

The major treatment schedules differ since the biology of childhood tumours is different.

In very high-risk patients, there is indication to proceed to stem cell transplantation that allows to bypass the haematological toxicity of a certain drug by reinfusion stem cells or harvested from the same patient or harvested from an HLA-matched donor. In this case stem cells reduce the infectious risks but cannot prevent totally the risk of presenting severe mucositis.

13.4 Clinical Presentation

While early diagnosis and advances in the cancer therapy for children continue to improve resulting in higher survival rate, oral complications remain a significant cause of morbidity and potential mortality.

Cancer therapy-related oral complications are common consequences in paediatric patients undergoing cancer treatment, who present acute and long-term oral side effects more than adults with an incidence of about 30–100%.

Oral complications can occur at all stages of cancer therapy, and they can interfere significantly with good prognosis.

Mucositis, oral infections, taste dysfunction, xerostomia and bleeding are recognized as common acute sequelae with risks for severe pain, malnutrition and potential source of systemic infections resulting in increased hospitalization and higher costs of care.

Several dental and skeletal developmental abnormalities are well documented in long-term paediatric cancer survivors, and in allogenic transplant children, healing can take longer specially in instances where oral acute or chronic GvHD occurs.

13.5 Complications

13.5.1 Early Complications

13.5.1.1 Oral Mucositis

Oral mucositis is one of the most debilitating complications in children receiving cancer therapy, occurring in 40–80% of cases, and it is higher in patients undergoing myeloablative chemotherapy prior to HSCT and/or simultaneous radiotherapy.

In children and adolescents, the risk of mucositis is higher compared with adults probably due to the high incidence of haematological malignancies, more intensive and aggressive cancer protocols and higher mitotic index of epithelial basal cells. Despite this, the mucositis in paediatric patients tends to resolve more quickly.

Pathogenesis of mucositis results from a physiopathologic process involving rapidly dividing epithelial basal cells, starting from chemoradiation therapy-induced damage.

Several risk factors related to host status can influence the development and severity of mucositis such as age, female gender, poor nutritional status, type of malignancy, drug-induced xerostomia, previous mouth damage, poor oral hygiene and genetic predisposition.

Drug-induced mucositis is related to particularly stomatotoxic chemotherapeutic agents and their dosage and schedule.

Finally, radiotherapy-related risk factors depend on dose, fractioning and site of radiotherapy, radiation combined with chemotherapy and conditioning regimens in HSCT recipients.

Oral mucositis becomes clinically evident at 4–5 days following chemotherapy infusion and generally peaks at 7–14 days after. Uncomplicated mucositis resolves spontaneously within 3 weeks after chemotherapy is ended.

Often mucositis is not limited to that period, but it may develop into a longer lasting pathology with devastating effects on the patient's recovery and hampering complete well- being for years.

Radiation-induced mucositis develops later; it starts at a cumulative dose of 10 Gy, peaks at 30 Gy of radiations dose and requires 3–6 weeks after the completion of radiotherapy for healing of oral tissues. Chronic mucositis occurs rarely after radiotherapy.

Children undergoing cancer therapy describe an initial burning or tingling sensation followed by intolerance to food.

In chemotherapy-related mucositis, the clinical early sign is erythema: although it can occur in any region of the mouth, it is frequently localized on non-keratinized areas such as the inner surfaces of the cheeks and lips, soft palate, lateral and bottom surface of the tongue and the floor of the mouth.

In contrast, radiation-induced mucositis involves the tissues limited to the exposed field, including hard palate and gingiva, and it begins to manifest at cumulative radiation dose about 10 Gy, with erythema or mucosal white discoloration due to transient hyperkeratinization.

Ulcerative lesions occur at 7–14 days after chemotherapy or at cumulative radiation dose of 30–50 Gy.

Mucosa ulcerative breakdown is always a potential focus for localized infections that, especially in the neutropenic child, offer an easy access to the bloodstream for the oral flora and allow to disseminate life-threatening infections.

Pain associated with ulcerative mucositis can inhibit patients from eating, swallowing and drinking and requires analgesic management with topical anaesthetics such as viscous lidocaine followed with non-steroidal anti-inflammatory agents. Supportive parenteral nutrition, consequently longer hospitalization and additional hospital charges are more commonly required with lower quality of life. Ulcers, pseudo-membranes and pain cause drooling in children who cannot swallow normally.

In addition, severe mucositis often compromises the care rates and can result in interruption or modification of anticancer treatment planning, as dose reduction and/or treatment discontinuous are necessary in order to heal oral lesions in children.

Mucositis can not only prevent the oral intake of food and liquid, but it can also lead to oropharyngeal airway embarrassment secondary to swelling, bleeding and a decreased ability to protect the airway. Reduced pharyngeal reflex results in a significant risk of compromised airway and aspiration pneumonia and anoxia-induced brain injury.

Life-threatening infections, total parenteral nutrition, days of fever, antibiotic and narcotic analgesic use, 100-day mortality and higher cost of care are clearly related to the severity of mucositis in childhood.

There are multiple scoring methods to grade mucositis. Objective, subjective and a combination of both findings have been used to measure the severity of mucositis.

Furthermore, a lot of age-related inabilities to explain and describe subjective symptoms require careful exams and an expert and suitable team of investigators.

13.5.1.2 Oral Infections

With the complete ablation of the immune system and compromise of mucosal barriers, children are at risk for all types of oral infections.

Viral—Herpes group viruses (*HSV*, *CMV*) and adenovirus.

Fungal—*Candida*, *Aspergillus*, and *Mucor*.

Bacterial—Gram + oral flora (*Streptococcus* spp., *Staphylococcus* spp.) and opportunistic and acquired Gram organisms (e.g., *E. coli*, *Enterobacter*, *Pseudomonas*, *Neisseria*, *Klebsiella*, *Serratia*, *Fusobacterium*).

Bacterial infections most commonly involve gingival tissues, though any mucosal surface is potentially at risk. Oral mucosal infections may cause fevers and can result in systemic bacteremia.

A specialist in infectious diseases is usually involved when treatment protocols are drawn up.

Secondary infection and bleeding can also be associated with exfoliation of primary teeth and eruption of permanent teeth.

HSV causes most of the oral infections in children with cancer. The clinical features of HSV oral infection are oral and extra-oral ulcers with erythema and crusts. Often, oral ulcers can be confused with recurrent aphthous stomatitis or traumatic lesions; consequently, it's always important to suspect it, in particular in the primary infection. It is not unusual to see the sudden emergence of herpetic stomatitis in children with cancer, and it is consequently important to be vigilant and alert to the possibility of these infections.

Oral fungal infections often develop in children undergoing chemoradiotherapy, especially during severe immunosuppression and neutropenia.

Prevention of fungal colonization and control of local infection may be of critical importance in avoiding systemic candidiasis.

13.5.1.3 Salivary Gland Dysfunction

Salivary gland dysfunction is related to toxicity from conditioning regimens prior to HSCT and during chemoradiotherapy. Clinical features include parotitis, viscous saliva, hyposalivation and xerostomia. In paediatric patients, xerostomia remains the most involved dysfunction, because of the importance of saliva in maintaining oral health. Oral dryness worsens the quality of life causing changes in taste and difficulty in chewing, swallowing and speaking. Chemotherapy-induced xerostomia is transient and self-limiting, usually resolving in 48 h.

Despite the severe damage caused by radiation to the salivary glands, some patients nevertheless improve their salivary function within 2–12 months after the end of the therapy. When the radiation beam directly involves parotids glands, xerostomia and hyposalivation are persistent. In paediatric patients, decreased salivary flow leads to modified oral bacteria favouring caries-related microflora and opportunistic infections, especially during periods of neutropenia.

13.5.1.4 Taste Dysfunction

Cancer therapy is a frequent cause of loss of taste or altered sense of taste: sweet, sour, bitter and salty are affected. These sequelae may cause serious discomfort to the patients, reducing nutritional supply and interfering with physiological growth and weight. Children usually recover their sense of taste between 1 and 3 months after cancer therapy ends.

Furthermore several food-related problems are common in children undergoing antineoplastic therapy, due to mucositis, nausea and inappetence, with consequent lower food intakes.

13.5.1.5 Oral Haemorrhage

Oral bleeding ranges from 6% to 42% in children undergoing cancer therapy and can vary between minor gingival oozing and frank bleeding. The most common risk factors are thrombocytopenia, coagulopathies, mucosal infections, trauma (especially on tongue and lips), mobile primary teeth, orthodontic appliances and poor oral hygiene. With severe thrombocytopenia in the presence of mucosal breakdown or infection, oral bleeding can be clinically problematic. When platelet counts above 20,000/mm^3 can be maintained, the incidence and severity of oral bleeding are decreased, and spontaneous bleeding is rare at 50,000/mm^3.

13.5.2 Long-Term Complications

13.5.2.1 Dental Developmental Abnormalities

Dental anomalies such as microdontia, hypodontia, enamel hypoplasia, over-retention of primary teeth, enlarged pulp chamber and delayed or arrested root development, root stunting and agenesis are well-known long-term effects of antineoplastic therapy in survivors of childhood cancer.

Chemoradiotherapy administered during odontogenesis might affect developing teeth with consequently dental anomalies.

These sequelae may be related to the child's age at the beginning of cancer therapy (the risk increases when cancer therapy starts before 5 years), the stage of tooth development and the type, intensity and frequency of treatment protocols used.

Children who underwent cancer therapy with mixed dentition have a higher incidence of dental anomalies, probably due to the effect of therapeutic damage on rapid odontogenic changes during this period.

Dental abnormalities caused by radiation are limited to the irradiated area; high-dose radiation during very early phases of tooth development may destroy the cells of the tooth germ and can lead to complete dental agenesis. In contrast, less drastic complications like microdontia, enamel hypoplasia and defective calcification and stunted or tapering roots occur with a lower dose or when radiotherapy starts at a later stage of dental development. Root defects can result when crown formation has been completed.

Radiotherapy-related damages occur simultaneously in the bone, periodontal ligament and pulp.

Whereas radiation damages cells only in the path of its beam, chemotherapy provokes systemic effects, interfering with the cell cycle and with intracellular metabolism of rapidly dividing cells in the whole body.

Developing odontogenic cells may be susceptible to chemotherapy damages causing disturbances in dental development as crown hypoplasia, microdontia, enlarged pulp chamber and root anomalies (conical roots and short V-shaped) mostly of the lower incisors and premolars.

Short half-life of chemotherapeutic agents causes usually localized dental defects, while complete dental agenesis is rare, and it may result when repetitive and intensive chemotherapy is used.

In children undergoing chemoradiotherapy, eruption of teeth can be delayed, and the frequency of impacted maxillary canines appears to be increased.

With shortened root length, alveolar processes can be consequently shortened, leading to decreased vertical dimension of the mandible and the lower third of the face.

Additionally, damage to jaw growth centres by conditioning regimens can lead to decreased size and mobility of jawbones, and their extent can be appreciated by a cephalometric analysis.

Cancer therapy may be associated with an increase of enamel hypoplasia and white spot lesions caused by interferences with ameloblasts during dental crown formation.

13.5.2.2 Dental Caries

Children during cancer treatment are at high risk of dental caries resulting from multiple factors.

The damage caused by chemotherapeutic agents and radiation on salivary glands reduce the salivary flow and cause oral environment changes favouring caries-related microflora.

Using sugary drinks to relieve oral dryness, in addition to taking sugary syrups, can increase the risk of tooth decay.

Cancer therapy-induced enamel defects (white spots, hypo-mineralization) increase the risk of dental caries especially in children treated in early years of their lives (3–5 years). In survivors, severe radiation tooth damages rapidly develop into decay.

During nausea and vomiting, acids coming from the stomach increase the risk of developing decay, and children must rinse their mouth with water after each emesis episode.

Poor oral hygiene, carbohydrate-rich diet, long hospitalization and psychological factors are well-known causes of predisposition for dental decay.

13.5.2.3 Oral GvHD

While the frequency of GvHD is usually lower in paediatric patients than in adult population who underwent HSCT, the oral cavity can be involved with both acute and chronic forms of the disease. Oral GvHD usually presents as part of multi-system involvement, but in numerous patients it is the first or only manifestation of disease. Clinically the most common presentation is a combination of mucosal erythema, atrophy and lichenoid changes appearing as hyperkeratotic striae, papules and plaque. The oral manifestations of acute (30 days post HSCT) and chronic (100 days post-HSCT) GvHD are extremely similar, characterized by pseudomembranous ulcerative lesions. In addition to oral mucosal lesions, GvHD affects salivary glands and can cause xerostomia. Mucoceles also result from mucosal and ductal damage to minor salivary glands by lymphocytes.

One of the most serious oral complications long-term survivors of HSCT are facing is secondary oral malignancy such as squamous cell carcinoma and lymphomas. GvHD appears to be a significant risk factor for this complication.

13.6 Guidelines for Management

The management guidelines are summarized in Table 13.1.

13.6.1 Oral Mucositis

In the absence of effective measures for preventing oral mucositis, its management in children is mostly palliative and focuses primarily on reduction of factors that will increase injury and irritation of the oral mucosa, in limiting hospital stays and costs of care and in improving quality of life.

Good oral hygiene protocols should be applied during and after chemoradiotherapy motivating the children and their caregivers to maintain an appropriate level of oral hygiene.

Recent strategies for preventing and treating cancer therapy-related oral mucositis in children suggest oral cryotherapy for short serum half-life chemotherapeutic agents because the intake of ice reduces the absorption of mucotoxic agents through local vasoconstriction.

Benzydamine oral rinses, antimicrobial gel and hyaluronic acid with verbascoside rinses promoting a rapid re-epithelialization are suggested. Chlorhexidine is not recommended in childhood mucositis.

Table 13.1 Oral complication management

Mucositis	Prevention strategies Oral hygiene (with extreme caution) to reduce bacterial colonization Reduction of any activities that may injure and irritate oral mucosa Symptoms management (PAIN) Bland rinses (0.9% saline, sodium bicarbonate) Topical anaesthetics (2% lidocaine, benzocaine, etc.) Mucosal coating agents (hyaluronic acid, verbascoside) Anti-inflammatory mouth rinses (ibuprofen, ketoprofen, nimesulide) Benzydamine HCl Prostaglandins, growth factors: KGF-1, -2, TGFβ, HeNe laser Lip care: keep lips moist with lip save lipsticks or lanolin or vitamin E and ointments Low level laser therapy (LLLT) Ozone therapy
Infections	
Bacterial (*streptococci*, *pseudomonas*, *Klebsiella*, *Enterobacter*, *E. coli*, *Serratia*, *fusobacterium*, normal oral flora)	Identification of causative organisms by appropriate oral cultures: Systemic antibiotics (as indicated by culture and sensivity results) Topical agents: antiseptic agents (chlorhexidine, povidone-iodine) Broad-spectrum antibiotics (neomycin/bacitracin/polymyxin, tetracycline solution) Oral or intravenous antibiotic
Viral (*HSV*, *CMV*, *VZV*, *adenovirus*)	HSV and VZV: oral or intravenous acyclovir, oral valacyclovir GMV: ganciclovir
Fungal (*Candida*, *aspergillus*, *Mucor*)	Antifungal prophylaxis protocols (oral or i.v. fluconazole, amphotericin, etc.) Topical oral treatment: nystatin and amphotericin (rinse), miconazole (gel), clotrimazole (troches) For invasive fungal infections: systemic antifungals, surgical resection
Haemorrhage	Trauma prevention Identify site—reduce risk factors Direct pressure packs Topical haemostatic agents (thrombin, collagen clot forming) Tranexamic acid as mouth rinse Topical vasoconstrictors (epinephrine, ice chips) Antifibrinolytic agents: aminocaproic acid Platelet transfusion
Xerostomia	Oral hygiene and fluoride rinses Salivary gland stimulation with sugar-free candies and gum (especially lemon flavoured products) Artificial saliva Sialogogues (pilocarpine, bethanechol)
GVHD	Topical steroids: dexamethasone, halobetasol, clobetasol, betamethasone Prevention/treatment of oral infections (bacterial, fungal, viral) Management of xerostomia
Taste dysfunction	Improve food aroma and visual appeal Zinc sulphate (oral)

The use of topical anaesthetics, recommended for pain, should be supervised in children, to avoid the risk of swallowing with consequent loss of gag reflex.

Furthermore, periodically delivered photobiomodulation using low level laser therapy (LLLT) has been proven effective of reducing the average severity of oral mucositis and the related pain.

Ozone therapy can be also effective to reduce pain, being a versatile bio-oxidative therapy with immunostimulant, analgesic and antimicrobial properties.

13.6.2 Infections

Treatment of documented oral bacterial infection is directed by the result of laboratory test for antibiotic sensitivity. A combination of topical and systemic antibiotic can be used if bacteria demonstrate sensitivity to the chosen drug. Because HSV infection is often a reactivation of the virus in previously infected children, oral or intravenous acyclovir, or more recently oral valacyclovir, is used prophylactically to prevent HSV reactivation in seropositive patients. Intravenous acyclovir is utilized to treat documented infection. Systemic antifungal prophylaxis protocols routinely use systemic azoles, especially fluconazole, with or without additional topical agents for documented oral infection. However, a combined topical/systemic approach is definitely warranted to reduce the risk of systemic spread of infection. Invasive *Candida* and filamentous fungi (*Aspergillus*, *Mucor*, etc.) are treated with aggressive systemic antifungal and surgical resection.

13.6.3 Oral Haemorrhage

Oral bleeding is initially managed with direct pressure packs. Subsequently, topical haemostatic agents (thrombin, collagen clot-forming agents, etc.), tranexamic acid as mouthwashes and topical vasoconstrictors (epinephrine or ice chips) can be used alone or in combination. More severe or persistent bleeding requires systemic therapy including administration of platelets or antifibrinolytic agents and dental cares.

13.6.4 Xerostomia

Management of xerostomia remains primarily symptomatic. Salivary flow rate can be stimulated by sucking or chewing a sugar-free gum, in addition to artificial saliva or simply frequent rinses with fresh water. Sialogogues can be effective in preventing and treating xerostomia. Oral lubricants such as bicarbonate mouthwashes and use of salivary substitutes can also be effective. To moist dry lips, lipsticks or lanolin creams and ointments may be helpful.

In order to reduce the risk of dental decay in children with xerostomia, intensive oral care, frequent topical fluoride applications, sugar-free diet and fissure sealants can be suggested. In addition, the high risk of oral candidiasis needs antifungal therapy when indicated by documented overgrowth and/or infection.

13.6.5 Trismus

Fibrosis of the masticator muscles due to high doses of radiation to the head and neck may lead to development of trismus. In order to prevent and ameliorate this condition, daily stretching oral exercises and physical therapy during and after radiation (3–6 months) are recommended.

13.6.6 Oral GVHD

Patients with oral GvHD must carry out careful and effective oral hygiene. Oral GvHD is best managed with successful systemic therapy. The primary goal of topical therapy for oral GvHD is to reduce symptoms. Topical oral steroids (rinses, creams or gels) can be applied to help resolve ulcers as well as to help reduce symptoms (burning, sensitivity, etc.) and can reduce mucosal inflammation and mucocele. Topical cyclosporine in rinses or muco-adherent gels has been reported to help oral GvHD.

13.6.7 Taste Dysfunction

Current protocols focus on improving smell and eye appeal of food and acceptable texture. It's recommended to choose foods typically preferred by children and adolescents (snacks and liquid nutritional supplements) when easily available. Zinc supplements have been reported to be effective in helping the recovery of the sense of taste, following head and neck radiation.

13.7 Specific Management Including Follow-Up and Referral

13.7.1 Role of Paediatric Dentistry: Oral Care

Oral health-care providers play an important role in the assessment and management of paediatric patient undergoing cancer therapy.

Stabilization of oral and dental infections prior to treatment and conditioning can reduce the incidence and severity of oral and/or systemic complications.

In fact cancer therapy-induced immunosuppression represents a high risk for opportunistic infections coming from oral cavity. A pre-cancer therapy evaluation is essential to decrease oral problems during and after treatment, and cooperation with the child's physician is suggested in order to coordinate the timing of oral care.

Paediatric dentists and dental hygienists should support the oncology team by providing basic oral care, implementing oral hygiene, delivering emergency dental treatment and assisting or managing oral complications from cancer therapy.

Before the beginning of the treatment, the dental team should identify and eliminate all active and potential oral infections or trauma sources. In particular, dental caries should be treated whenever possible prior to cancer therapy; while permanent restorations are best, temporary materials can stabilize teeth safely till definitive filling is possible. Incipient caries may be stopped through topical fluorides, remineralizing solutions and sealants. Teeth with endodontic infections or abscesses need to be treated urgently by endodontic therapy or extraction. Non-restorable teeth with deep decay or with significant periodontal disease including pericoronitis or mobile primary teeth should be extracted. Surgical procedures and dental extraction must be as atraumatic as possible and primary closure obtained whenever possible to promote rapid healing.

In the presence of documented infections, antibiotic treatment is indicated.

Orthodontic appliances and space maintainers should be removed as they can abrade oral mucosa and increase the risk of severe mucosal trauma and microbial invasion into deeper tissues and to prevent accumulation of plaque around brackets and wires.

Therefore, all dental treatment must be completed before the patient becomes immunosuppressed.

During immunosuppression, no elective dental care but only dental emergency that requires an acute care must be provided.

Continued follow-up of patients after therapy facilitates earlier diagnosis.

Once the patient has recovered sufficiently following the end of the therapy and is immunologically stable, restorative dentistry and orthodontic care (at least 2 years) can be resumed.

The ultimate goals of the dental care team's coordinated efforts are to reduce the incidence and frequency of oral complications, improve patient comfort and help reduce the overall cost of care.

13.7.2 Oral Hygiene Measures and Management

Motivating patients and parents to maintain an appropriate level of oral hygiene is mandatory during cancer therapy.

Strategies to remove dental plaque from the teeth and gums are critically important for children's health and to reduce the risk of oral complications.

Children should be encouraged to use extra-soft nylon toothbrushes to reduce the risk of trauma to gingival and other soft tissue, while complete and atraumatic brushing should be always supervised by either professional staff or parents.

Toothpicks and water irrigation devices should be used carefully to avoid tissue trauma.

Careful flossing technique once a day should be done only in older trained children. In addition, fluoridated toothpaste, fluoride varnish and neutral fluoride rinses or gels are recommended for high caries risk patients during all phases of cancer treatment.

Useful solutions include 0.9% saline solution, sodium bicarbonate solutions and combination of saline and sodium bicarbonate solutions. Patients should be encouraged to rinse/swish and spit out 8/12 mouthfuls at frequent intervals throughout the day.

Topical oral antifungal prophylaxis appears to have variable efficacy in preventing fungal colonization and infection in immunosuppressed patients.

Additionally, non-prescription mouthwashes or medications containing alcohol and flavouring agents should be avoided. These agents increase stinting and burning and interfere with such patients' ability to comply with the protocol.

Frequent dental visits, with a complete oral examination and the application of prevention protocols, could decrease or eliminate the need for invasive dental procedures in children with cancer.

13.7.3 Role of Parents

The experience of a child diagnosed with cancer is a devastating situation and a severe source of stress for parents. Most of them complain about fatigue, sleep disturbances, hypervigilance, difficulty concentrating, guilt, anger, uncertainty about child's future, inability to meet each other's emotional needs within the family, difficulty in child's care (cleaning, eating, rearing) and financial strain. In addition, symptoms of post traumatic stress disorder are not uncommon and can continue years after the treatment ended. These conditions, usually more severe for mothers than for fathers and more common when the child is under 5 years old, influence parental well-being, which is in turn one of the most important factors to promote child well-being. Higher levels of parenting stress, overprotection and perception of child vulnerability often lead to ineffective child-rearing practices and following child behavioural problems. When a child is ill, parents often focus exclusively on child's demands ignoring their own wants or needs.

Parents of children with cancer need concrete services such as babysitting, financial support, help in food preparation and cleaning, transportation, assistance with household management and psychological, social and school support. Open communication between parents and medical staff and gaining information about child's disease help parents to fortify and to take a sense of control.

Through the Internet or support groups, parents can also connect to other families with the same cancer experience. These intensive comparisons, access to research literature and the discussion with family experts can help parents to get through this situation.

Bibliography

1. Abramoff MM, Lopes NN, Lopes LA, Dib LL, Guilherme A, Caran EM, Barreto AD, Lee ML, Petrilli AS. Low-level laser therapy in the prevention and treatment of chemotherapy-induced oral mucositis in young patients. Photomed Laser Surg. 2008;26(4):393–400. https://doi.org/10.1089/pho.2007.2144.
2. Amadori F, Bardellini E, Conti G, Pedrini N, Schumacher RF, Majorana A. Low-level laser therapy for treatment of chemotherapy-induced oral mucositis in childhood: a randomized

double-blind controlled study. Lasers Med Sci. 2016;31(6):1231–6. https://doi.org/10.1007/s10103-016-1975-y. Epub 2016 Jun 6.
3. Bardellini E, Amadori F, Majorana A. Oral hygiene grade and quality of life in children with chemotherapy-related oral mucositis: a randomized study on the impact of a fluoride toothpaste with salivary enzymes, essential oils, proteins and colostrum extract versus a fluoride toothpaste without menthol. Int J Dent Hyg. 2016a;14(4):314–9.
4. Bardellini E, Amadori F, Schumacher RF, D'Ippolito C, Porta F, Majorana A. Efficacy of a solution composed by verbascoside, polyvinylpyrrolidone (PVP) and sodium hyaluronate in the treatment of chemotherapy-induced oral mucositis in children with acute lymphoblastic leukemia. J Pediatr Hematol Oncol. 2016b;38(7):559–62.
5. Bardellini E, Amadori F, Schumacher RF, Foresti I, Majorana A. A new emerging oral infection: Raoultella planticola in a boy with haematological malignancy. Eur Arch Paediatr Dent. 2017;18(3):215–8.
6. Brennan MT, von Bültzingslöwen I, Schubert MM, Keefe D. Alimentary mucositis: putting the guidelines into practice. Support Care Cancer. 2006;14:573–9.
7. Cruz LB, Ribeiro AS, Rech A, Rosa LG, Castro CG Jr, Brunetto AL. Influence of low-energy laser in the prevention of oral mucositis in children with cancer receiving chemotherapy. Pediatr Blood Cancer. 2007;48(4):435–40.
8. Cubukçu CE, Sevinir B. Dental health indices of long-term childhood cancer survivors who had oral supervision during treatment: a case-control study. Pediatr Hematol Oncol. 2008;25:638–46.
9. De Castro JF, Abreu EG, Correia AV, da Mota Vasconcelos Brasil C, da Cruz Perez DE, de Paula Ramos Pedrosa F. Low-level laser in prevention and treatment of oral mucositis in pediatric patients with acute lymphoblastic leukemia. Photomed Laser Surg. 2013;31(12):613–8. https://doi.org/10.1089/pho.2012.3327. Epub 2013 Nov 21.
10. De Koning BA, Philipsen-Geerling B, Hoijer M, Hählen K, Büller HA, Pieters R. Protection against chemotherapy induced mucositis by TGF-beta(2) in childhood cancer patients: results from a randomized cross-over study. Pediatr Blood Cancer. 2007;48(5):532–9.
11. Gobbo M, Verzegnassi F, Ronfani L, Zanon D, Melchionda F, Bagattoni S, Majorana A, Bardellini E, Mura R, Piras A, Petris MG, Mariuzzi ML, Barone A, Merigo E, Decembrino N, Vitale MC, Berger M, Defabianis P, Biasotto M, Ottaviani G, Zanazzo GA. Multicenter randomized, double-blind controlled trial to evaluate the efficacy of laser therapy for the treatment of severe oral mucositis induced by chemotherapy in children: laMPO RCT. Pediatr Blood Cancer. 2018;65(8):e27098.
12. Graber CJ, de Almeida KN, Atkinson JC, Javaheri D, Fukuda CD, Gill VJ, Barrett AJ, Bennett JE. Dental health and viridans streptococcal bacteremia in allogeneic hematopoietic stem cell transplant recipients. Bone Marrow Transplant. 2001;27:537–42.
13. Guo L, Shi W. Salivary biomarkers for caries risk assessment. J Calif Dent Assoc. 2013;41(2):107–18.
14. Hegde AM, Joshi S, Rai K, Shetty S. Evaluation of oral hygiene status, salivary characteristics and dental caries experience in acute lymphoblastic leukemic (ALL) children. J Clin Pediatr Dent. 2011;35(3):319–23.
15. Lark RL, McNeil SA, Vander Hyde K, et al. Risk factors for anaerobic bloodstream infections in bone marrow transplant recipients. Clin Infect Dis. 2001;33:338–43.
16. Lauritano D, Petruzzi M, Di Stasio D, Lucchese A. Clinical effectiveness of palifermin in prevention and treatment of oral mucositis in children with acute lymphoblastic leukaemia: a case-control study. Int J Oral Sci. 2014;6(1):27–30. https://doi.org/10.1038/ijos.2013.93. Epub 2013 Dec 20.
17. Lucchese A, Matarese G, Ghislanzoni LH, Gastaldi G, Manuelli M, Gherlone E. Efficacy and effects of palifermin for the treatment of oral mucositis in patients affected by acute lymphoblastic leukemia. Leuk Lymphoma. 2016;57(4):820–7. https://doi.org/10.3109/10428194.2015.1081192. Epub 2015 Nov 20.

18. Majorana A, Amadori F, Bardellini E, Campus G, Conti G, Strohmenger L, Schumacher RF, Polimeni A. Taste dysfunction in patients undergoing hematopoietic stem cell transplantation: clinical evaluation in children. Pediatr Transplant. 2015;19(5):571–5.
19. Marron A, Carratalà J, González-Barca E, Fernández-Sevilla A, Alcaide F, Gudiol F. Serious complications of bacteremia caused by viridans streptococci in neutropenic patients with cancer. Clin Infect Dis. 2000;31:1126–30.
20. McGuire E. Breastfeeding and high maternal body mass index. Breastfeed Rev. 2013;21:7–14.
21. McLaren L, Patterson S, Thawer S, Faris P, McNeil D, Potestio M, Shwart L. Measuring the short-term impact of fluoridation cessation on dental caries in Grade 2 children using tooth surface indices. Community Dent Oral Epidemiol. 2016;44:274–82.
22. Moynihan PJ, Kelly SA. Effect on caries of restricting sugars intake: systematic review to inform WHO guidelines. J Dent Res. 2014;93(1):8–18.
23. Newton JT. Interdisciplinary health promotion: a call for theory-based interventions drawing on the skills of multiple disciplines. Community Dent Oral Epidemiol. 2012;40:49–54.
24. Ritter AV, Preisser JS, Puranik CP, Chung Y, Bader JD, Shugars DA, Makhija S, Vollmer WM. A predictive model for root caries incidence. Caries Res. 2016;50:271–8.
25. Suma Sogi HP, Hugar SM, Nalawade TM, Sinha A, Hugar S, Mallikarjuna RM. Knowledge, attitude, and practices of oral health care in prevention of early childhood caries among parents of children in Belagavi city: a questionnaire study. J Family Med Prim Care. 2016;5:286–90.

Oral Graft-Versus-Host Disease

14

Alessandro Villa and Amal Bajonaid

14.1 Introduction

Hematopoietic stem cell transplantation (HSCT) is considered the treatment of choice for a variety of benign and malignant conditions including chronic leukemia, non-Hodgkin lymphoma, bone marrow failure, thalassemia, aplastic anemia, and many others. Stem cells can be obtained from the bone marrow (BM), peripheral blood (PB), or umbilical cord blood (UCB). In autologous HCT the hematopoietic cells are derived from the patient with the disorder, while in allogeneic HCT the hematopoietic cells are obtained from a genetically similar donor. The number of patients receiving bone marrow transplantation is increasing. Worldwide, there are more than 40,000 hematopoietic cell transplantations performed each year. The number of long-term survivors is also increasing with recent advancements in the field, such as refinement in human leukocyte antigen matching, improvement in supportive care, and management of complications following transplantation.

Graft-versus-host disease (GVHD) is a serious complication following both allogeneic and autologous HSCT, which accounts for up to 10% of the mortality following transplantation. GVHD is an immune mediated disease in which immune cells

A. Villa (✉)
Department of Orofacial Sciences, University of California San Francisco, San Francisco, CA, USA
e-mail: alessandro.villa@ucsf.edu

A. Bajonaid
Division of Oral Medicine and Dentistry, Brigham and Women's Hospital and Dana Farber Cancer Institute, Boston, MA, USA

Department of Oral Medicine Infection and Immunity, Harvard School of Dental Medicine, Boston, MA, USA

Department of Diagnostic Dental Sciences, College of Dentistry, Jazan University, Jazan, Saudi Arabia
e-mail: abajonaid@bwh.harvard.edu

R. Nair (ed.), *Orofacial Supportive Care in Cancer*,
https://doi.org/10.1007/978-3-030-86510-8_14

transplanted from a non-identical donor recognize the recipient's tissue antigens as foreign and initiate an immune reaction which results in GVHD.

In this chapter, we provide an overview on the prevalence, pathobiology, clinical presentation, and management of oral GVHD.

14.2 Epidemiology and Pathobiology of GVHD

Graft-versus-host disease has been classified into acute (aGVHD) and chronic (cGVHD) based upon the time of onset (Fig. 14.1). Acute GVHD refers to clinical manifestations arising within 100 days following transplantation, while chronic GVHD is usually diagnosed 100 days post-transplantation. However, the clinical characteristics of both aGVHD and cGVHD may also be seen outside these periods. As such, the National Institutes of Health (NIH) consensus criteria for GVHD diagnosis refer to the clinical presentation of acute and chronic GVHD rather than the time of onset (Table 14.1).

Acute GVHD and chronic GVHD have different clinical manifestations and pathophysiologies. Acute GVHD typically involves the skin, the gastrointestinal tract, and the liver. On the other hand, chronic GVHD affects also other organs including the lung, oral cavity, genitalia, muscles, and joints. Clinical features of aGVHD and cGVHD are presented in (Table 14.2).

Several factors are involved in the development and severity of GVHD and include:

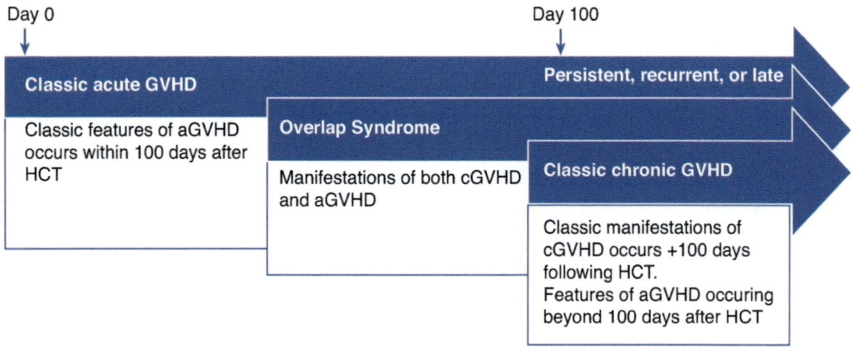

Fig. 14.1 Timeline of acute and chronic GVHD

Table 14.1 Acute and chronic GVHD

Acute GVHD	
Classic acute	Signs and symptoms of aGVHD occur within 100 days following the transplantation
Late onset, persistent, recurrent	Clinical manifestations of aGVHD that occur, persist, or recur beyond 100 days after transplantation
Chronic GVHD	
Classic chronic	Clinical manifestations of chronic GVHD that occurs beyond 100 days following transplantation
Overlap syndrome	Clinical manifestations of both aGVHD and cGVHD at any point in time following hematopoietic stem cell transplantation

Table 14.2 Clinical manifestation of acute and chronic GVHD

Affected organ	aGVHD	cGVHD
Skin	Maculopapular rash Pruritus	Lichen planus-like features, poikiloderma, scleroderma-like features
Oral cavity	Diffuse ulceration, erythema, mucositis, crusting of lips	Lichen planus-like features, mucoceles, xerostomia, skin sclerosis resulting in restriction of mouth opening
Gastrointestinal tract	Diarrhea Nausea and vomiting	Esophageal web, or stricture
Genitalia Male	Not affected	Phimosis, scarring, lichen planus-like features
Female	Not affected	Lichen planus-like manifestation, vaginal ulcerations and stenosis
Liver	Hyperbilirubinemia, cholestatic	Jaundice, elevated liver function test
Lung	Not affected	Bronchiolitis obliterans, pleural effusion
Kidney	Not affected	Nephrotic syndrome
Muscles/joints	Not affected	Myositis, joint stiffness

The degree of disparity in human leukocyte antigen (HLA) between the donor and the recipient.
Sex mismatch between the donor and the recipient.
Type of conditioning regimen.
Source of the transplanted progenitor cells.
Type and properties of the transplanted T cells.

The incidence of acute GVHD depends on several factors, one of which is the degree of HLA disparity. GVHD in matched related donor HSCT patients has an incidence of 20–50%, 70% in matched unrelated donors, and up to 80–90% in mismatched unrelated donors. Acute GVHD is characterized by an exaggerated inflammatory response, which leads to activation of antigen-presenting cells (APCs). Tissue destruction caused by the conditioning regimen causes cytokine activation and leads to the release of tumor necrosis factor-alpha (TNF-alpha), interleukin-6 (IL-6), and interleukin-1 (IL-1); these cytokines are responsible for the upregulation of expression of major histocompatibility complex (MHC) antigen and cell surface adhesion molecules on the host cells. The immune response is propagated by damage of intestinal epithelium which causes release of bacteria and alteration in the intestinal microbiome. Other soluble inflammatory mediators associated with exaggeration of the immune response are danger-associated molecular patterns (DAMPs) and pathogen-associated molecular patterns (PAMPs). The release of these cytokines activates host APCs, which presents alloantigens that are recognized by the donor T cells. Donor APCs could also contribute to GVHD; once they recognize an alloantigen, they release certain cytokines which result in the production of interleukin-2 (IL-2) and interferon-gamma (IFN-gamma). The release of IL-2 further amplifies the immune response through the activation of T cells and natural killer (NK) cells. Of note, the role of INF-gamma is thought to be protective through promoting the graft-versus-leukemia effect.

Chronic GVHD develops in 30–70% of patients who have undergone allogeneic HSCT. Chronic GVHD is often characterized by fibrosis with less inflammation compared to the acute disease. cGVHD is initiated by an innate immune response as a result of tissue damage following conditioning regimen (first phase). It is characterized by antigen presentation and activation of T cells, endothelial cells, and fibroblasts. In the second phase, the adaptive immune response plays a major role. T cell receptor and B cell receptor activate T cells and B cells, respectively, by recognizing the peptides presented by APCs. The activation of B cell results in somatic hypermutation and production of immunoglobulin isotype-switched antibodies, which have the potential to promote cutaneous cGVHD. Activation of T cell receptors results in expansion and polarization of T cells into type 1, 2, and 17 helper T cells; these autoreactive and alloreactive helper T cells escape immune regulation and produce IL-17A which maintains inflammation. Another product of the helper T cells is IL-21 which leads to germinal center formation that is not balanced by sufficient follicular regulatory T cells. Thymic epithelium is lost due to thymic injury caused by the conditioning regimen and alloreactive T cells; these events lead to overall depletion of the regulatory T cell population. The third phase includes activation of fibroblasts by platelet-derived growth factor alpha (PDGF-alpha) and transforming growth factor beta (TGF-beta), resulting in increased production of extracellular matrix (ECM) which leads to sclerosis. Pathogenic immunoglobulin deposition in various organs leads to fibrosis and organ damage.

GVHD may also occur following autologous transplantation in 5–10% of the cases (auto-GVHD). Rates as high as 30–80% have been reported following induction with cyclosporine-based therapy or interleukin-2 (IL-2). The pathobiology of autologous GVHD is still under investigation but is thought to be the result of elimination of peripheral immunoregulatory cells and failure to inhibit the deletion of autoreactive T cells in the affected tissue.

14.3 Acute Graft-Versus-Host Disease

The clinical manifestations of aGVHD typically involve the skin, GI tract, and liver. It presents with diarrhea, skin rash, and elevated bilirubin and is associated with recurrent infections. Mortality risk is variable and depends on the stage and grade of aGVHD.

Staging and grading of acute GVHD depend on the extent of involvement of the upper and lower GI tract, skin, and liver (for additional details, please refer to Tables 14.3 and 14.4).

The diagnosis of acute GVHD is generally based on the history and clinical presentation in patients with skin rash, diarrhea, and hyperbilirubinemia in the first several weeks and up to 100 days after transplantation.

Several regimens have been described for the prevention of aGVHD; the prophylactic approach to aGVHD is generally based on immunosuppression. The conventional regimens for aGVHD prevention include a combination of two drugs: a calcineurin inhibitor and methotrexate or mycophenolate mofetil (MMF); the most commonly used regimen includes a combination of calcineurin inhibitor (cyclosporine or tacrolimus) and a short course of methotrexate. The combination of

Table 14.3 Staging of acute GVHD

Clinical stage	Lower GI tract	Upper GI tract	Skin (% rash of body surface area)	Liver (bilirubin level in mg/dl)
1	Diarrhea <500 mL/day	Nausea and vomiting	<25%	2–3
2	Diarrhea 500–1000 mL/day		25–50%	3–6
3	Diarrhea 1000–1500 mL/day		Generalized erythroderma	6–15
4	Diarrhea >1500 mL/day		Bullae/desquamation	>15

From: Nassereddine S, Rafei H, Elbahesh E, Tabbara I. Acute Graft Versus Host Disease: A Comprehensive Review. Anticancer Res. 2017;37(4):1547–55

Table 14.4 Grading of acute graft-versus-host disease

Overall clinical grade	Lower GI	Upper GI	Skin	Liver
I	0	0	1–2	0
II	1	1	3	1
III	2–3		–	2–4
IV	4		4	–

From: Nassereddine S, Rafei H, Elbahesh E, Tabbara I. Acute Graft Versus Host Disease: A Comprehensive Review. Anticancer Res. 2017;37(4):1547–55

calcineurin inhibitor with mycophenolate mofetil was found to be associated with less mucositis and rapid neutrophil engraftment. Many new preventive strategies remain under investigation.

Treatment of aGVHD depends on the severity of the disease. Management of stages I and II can range from observation to prescription of a topical corticosteroid for the skin involvement. Disease of stage II to IV can be further managed by prescription of systemic corticosteroid. The median time for resolution of aGVHD is 30–42 days. The treatment generally consists of continuing the established immunosuppressive prophylaxis and the addition of methylprednisolone, with a starting dose of 2 mg/kg/day for grades III and IV and 0.5–1 mg/kg/day for grade II aGVHD. For steroid refractory cases, other management options include antithymocyte globulin, MMF, cyclosporine alone, infliximab, daclizumab, vilizumab, anti-CD5-specific immunotoxin, and pentostatin.

14.4 Oral Acute GVHD

Oral cavity involvement is not common in aGVHD. Oral aGVHD presents as mucosal erythema, ulceration, painful desquamative gingivitis, and crusting of the lips (Fig. 14.2). The clinical manifestation of oral aGVHD may be mistaken for mucositis induced by the conditioning regimen or recrudescent herpes simplex virus (HSV) infection as a result of immune suppression. However, oral mucositis typically develops and resolves shortly after the conditioning regimen and before

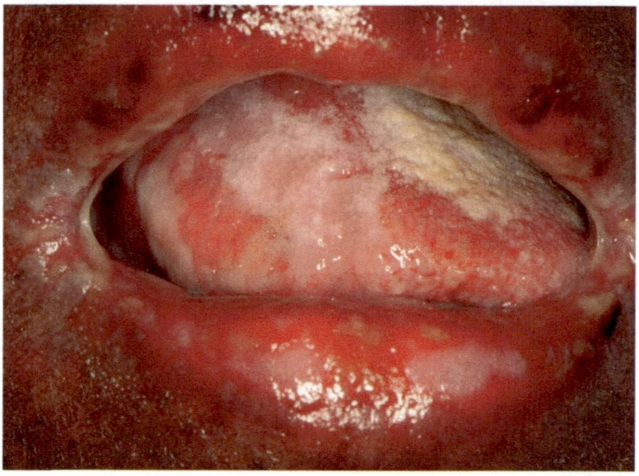

Fig. 14.2 Oral acute GVHD: severe erythema, ulceration, and crusting of the upper and lower lips

engraftment, while aGVHD tends to persist over time. Diagnosis is usually made based on the clinical findings. Oral viral culture may be helpful to rule out recrudescent HSV infection.

14.5 Chronic Graft-Versus-Host Disease

Chronic GVHD may affect the skin, lungs, gastrointestinal tract, kidneys, liver, musculoskeletal system, joints, oral cavity, genitalia, ocular tissue, hair, and nails. Chronic disease is often characterized by fibrosis with minimal inflammation. The clinical features of chronic GVHD are summarized in Table 14.1. Chronic GVHD has three clinical patterns of onset: de novo (no prior acute GVHD), progressing directly from acute GVHD, and quiescent onset which follows complete resolution of acute GVHD. The NIH consensus criteria for diagnosis and staging of chronic GVHD have multiple aspects; first, it classifies the clinical manifestations into four categories:

1. *Diagnostic signs*: these are signs sufficient to establish the diagnosis of cGVHD.
2. *Distinctive signs*, which are seen in chronic GVHD, but are not sufficient alone to establish the diagnosis.
3. *Common signs*, seen in both acute and chronic GVHD.
4. *Other* features or unclassified entities.

The second aspect of the NIH criteria for diagnosis is the severity score for cGVHD. The severity of cGVHD is scored for each involved organ system individually: the skin, oral cavity, eyes, GI tract, liver, lungs, genital tract, and fasciae or joints. The third aspect of the NIH diagnostic criteria is the global severity of cGVHD which is classified into mild, moderate, and severe based on the cumulative severity score of the involved organs.

The prophylactic regimen used for chronic GVHD differs from the one used for acute GVHD. Paradoxically, GVHD prophylaxis with calcineurin inhibitors and following withdrawal may promote the development of cGVHD manifestations by blocking the peripheral regulatory T cell function and thymic central tolerance. Depletion of alloreactive T cells through anti-T cell globulin and high-dose cyclophosphamide has been shown to reduce the incidence of cGVHD. The use of monoclonal antibody (e.g., rituximab) in the post-transplant period has been associated with reduced incidence of cGVHD as well.

Treatment of cGVHD depends on the organ involved and the severity of symptoms. In mild disease (specific to certain organs), patients may benefit from supportive care and topical treatment specific to the organ affected, such as the use of topical corticosteroid for the management of mild skin disease. For patients with moderate to severe disease, systemic glucocorticoids are the standard first-line treatment. The addition of calcineurin inhibitor (cyclosporine) to prednisone was demonstrated to be beneficial by reducing steroid exposure; the addition of cyclosporine is reserved for steroid refractory disease (patients with progressive disease after 2 weeks of prednisone or lack of response after 4–6 weeks). Other treatments include immunomodulatory therapy such as extracorporeal photopheresis, mTOR inhibitors, thalidomide, hydroxyl-chloroquine, and cytotoxic agents such as methotrexate and MMF.

14.6 Oral Chronic Graft-Versus-Host Disease

The oral cavity is affected in 70% of the patients with cGVHD. The clinical presentation of oral cGVHD can be broadly divided into three categories:

1. Oral mucosal disease
2. Salivary gland dysfunction
3. Sclerotic changes

The spectrum of oral manifestations in cGVHD includes reticular white lichen planus-like changes with erythema and minimal ulceration that affects both the keratinized and non-keratinized mucosa (Fig. 14.3). Patients typically complain of sensitivity to spicy, acidic food or strongly flavored products. Salivary gland involvement results in alteration of the quality and quantity of saliva, with hyposalivation and reduction in the immune components of saliva. Patients report xerostomia, difficulty chewing, speaking, and swallowing. Rampant caries and secondary recurrent candidiasis may be seen in patients with severe oral dryness. Involvement of the minor salivary glands results in multiple superficial mucoceles typically seen on the soft palatal mucosa.

One of the late complications of long-standing cGVHD is the sclerotic changes that present as fibrosis and limitation in mobility, with subsequent trismus secondary to cutaneous and muscle fibrosis (Table 14.5).

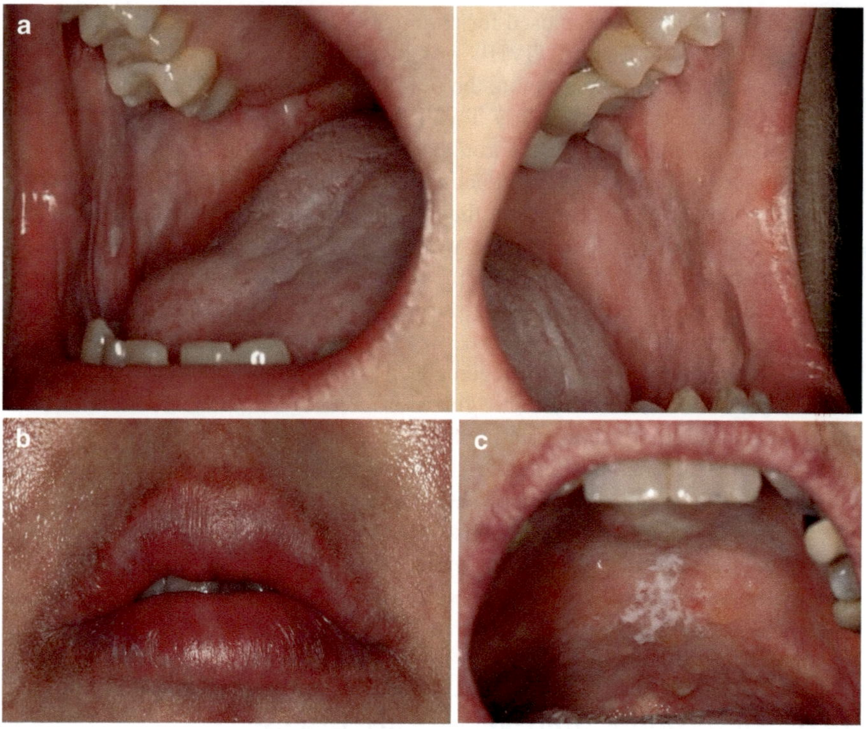

Fig. 14.3 (**a**) Oral chronic GVHD: bilateral white reticular changes of the buccal mucosa. (**b**) Oral chronic GVHD: diffuse erythema of the upper and lower lips. (**c**) Oral chronic GVHD: multiple mucoceles of the hard palpatal mucosa and soft palate with diffuse white reticulations

Table 14.5 Manifestations of oral chronic GVHD

	Signs	Symptoms
Oral mucosal disease	Lichen planus-like lesions	Sensitivity to spicy, salty, and acidic food and carbonated or hot drinks Sensitivity to other products such as strongly flavored toothpaste and mouthwashes Usually minimal discomfort at rest
Salivary gland dysfunction	Hyposalivation (as a consequence: recurrent candidiasis, rampant caries) Multiple superficial mucoceles on the palatal mucosa	Xerostomia, difficulty chewing, swallowing, and speaking
Sclerotic changes	Trismus Limitation in range of motion of the jaw Loss of vestibular depth Gingival recession	Compromised chewing and speaking

Table 14.6 The NIH scoring system for oral chronic GVHD

Lichen planus-like features present: Yes/No	Score 0	Score 1	Score 2	Score 3
	No symptoms	Mild symptoms with disease signs, but not limiting oral intake	Moderate symptoms with disease signs and partial limitation of oral intake	Severe symptoms with disease signs and major limitation of oral intake
Abnormality present but explained entirely by non-GVHD documented cause (specify):				

From: Jagasia MH, Greinix HT, Arora M, Williams KM, Wolff D, Cowen EW, et al. National Institutes of Health Consensus Development Project on Criteria for Clinical Trials in Chronic Graft-versus-Host Disease: I. The 2014 Diagnosis and Staging Working Group report. Biol Blood Marrow Transplant. 2015;21(3):389–401 e1

Mouth

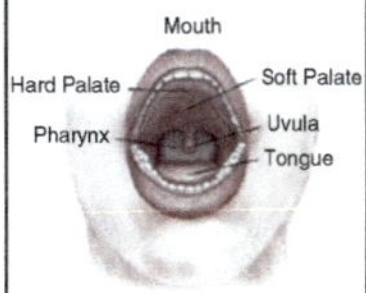

Mucosal change	No evidence of cGVHD		Mild		Moderate		Severe	
Erythema	None	0	Mild erythema or moderate erythema (<25%)	1	Moderate (≥25%) or Severe erythema (<25%)	2	Severe erythema (≥25%)	3
Lichenoid	None	0	Hyperkeratotic changes (<25%)	1	Hyperkeratotic changes (25-50%)	2	Hyperkeratotic changes (>50%)	3
Ulcers	None	0	None	0	Ulcers involving (≤20%)	3	Severe ulcerations (>20%)	6
Mucoceles*	None	0	1-5 mucoceles	1	6-10 scattered mucoceles	2	Over 10 mucoceles	3
			*Mucoceles scored for lower labial and soft palate only				**Total score for all mucosal changes**	

Fig. 14.4 NIH oral GVHD clinical scoring instrument. (From: Treister NS, Stevenson K, Kim H, Woo SB, Soiffer R, Cutler C. Oral chronic graft-versus-host disease scoring using the NIH consensus criteria. Biol Blood Marrow Transplant. 2010;16(1):108–14)

The NIH classifies oral cGVHD into mild, moderate, and severe. Mild disease is characterized by classic oral signs, without limitation of oral intake; moderate disease causes partial limitation of oral intake; and severe disease inflicts major limitation of oral intake (Table 14.6). The NIH oral cGVHD clinical scoring instrument is used for the documentation of clinical severity of the hyperkeratotic changes, erythema, ulceration, and mucoceles (Fig. 14.4).

According to the NIH diagnostic criteria for oral cGVHD, the presence of lichen planus-like features is sufficient to establish the diagnosis of oral chronic GVHD. Other clinical manifestations of oral CGVHD such as xerostomia, mucoceles, mucosal atrophy, ulcers, and pseudomembrane are distinctive features (seen in cGVHD but not sufficient alone to establish the diagnosis); and gingivitis, mucositis, and erythema are considered common features (seen in both acute and chronic GVHD). Diagnosis is generally based on history and clinical presentation, when there's at least on diagnostic feature, or at least one distinctive feature supported by pertinent laboratory evidence such as biopsy of the mucosa or salivary gland.

14.7 Management of Oral GVHD

The management of both acute and chronic oral GVHD is generally the same, with the exception that cGVHD may require treatment for longer time, generally years after transplantation. As with the systemic management described, the first-line

Table 14.7 Topical agents for oral GVHD

	Treatment	Instructions
Localized oral mucosal lesions	Fluocinonide gel 0.05% Clobetasol gel 0.05% Betamethasone dipropionate 0.05% gel	Apply 2–4 times/day Up to 6 times (on gauze if appropriate); no food or drink for 20 min after Gels may be applied directly to the dried mucosa on gauze and held in place for 10–15 min
Localized refractory symptomatic ulcer	Triamcinolone acetonide 40 mg/mL 5–10 mg/cm^2	Intralesional steroid injection for refractory or large ulcers
Generalized/difficult-to-access oral mucosal lesions	Dexamethasone solution 0.5 mg/5 mL Clobetasol 0.05% solution Budesonide 3 mg/10 mL Tacrolimus solution 5 mg/mL	Use four times per day. Swish for 5 min then spit. Avoid food/drinks/brushing teeth for 10–15 min after using the medication
Lip lesions	Tacrolimus 0.1% ointment Desonide cream 0.05%	Apply 2–4 times per day

treatment for oral GVHD is topical corticosteroid therapy. Topical corticosteroids may be prescribed to support systemic therapy in refractory oral GVHD or as the sole therapy in cases limited to the oral cavity (Table 14.7). Effectiveness of the topical therapy depends on the potency of the medication, the form in which it is applied, the frequency, and duration of application, as well as patient's compliance. The application of topical medications is also affected by tissue penetration and the presence of saliva. Steroids in the form of solutions are generally prescribed in case of extensive oral disease; while gels, ointments, and creams are used for localized lesions; gels are preferred over creams and ointments due to their hydrophilic nature. Based on the NIH ancillary therapy and supportive care guidelines, initial therapy for most patients is with dexamethasone solution 0.5 mg/5 mL; patients are instructed to swish/gargle for 4–6 min then spit, 4–6 times per day, and to avoid eating or drinking for 10–15 min using the medication.

To maximize tissue contact and penetration of the topical gel, ointment, or cream, the tissue should be dried with gauze before applying the medication; if it is challenging to keep the area dry, patients are instructed to apply the gel on a piece of gauze and place it on the affected area for several minutes. Other topical steroids with higher potency may also be prescribed (e.g., clobetasol). Involvement of the lips requires special attention because the long-term use of potent topical steroid may cause irreversible atrophy of the lip vermilion. Tacrolimus 0.1% ointment or 0.05% desonide cream is the treatment of choice in cases of lip involvement. Intralesional steroid (triamcinolone acetonide 40 mg/mL) injections may be used for refractory and painful ulcerative lesions. Topical anesthetics (such as 2% viscous lidocaine or Magic mouthwash) may help relieve oral symptoms until ulcers heal.

Patients with chronic GVHD are at higher risk for developing candidiasis because of immunosuppression and salivary gland dysfunction and may require antifungal therapy. To prevent the development of candidiasis, patients may be given topical antifungals (e.g., nystatin suspension) which can be used concomitantly with the topical steroid.

Patients with salivary gland cGVHD involvement usually complain of xerostomia and generalized oral burning sensation. Stimulation of salivary flow can be achieved with sugar-free candies and gums for patients with mild hyposalivation. Patients with severe hyposalivation may require prescription sialogogue therapy (such as pilocarpine or cevimeline) in the absence of contraindications such as pulmonary GVHD. Another complication of hyposalivation is rampant dental caries in the cervical and interproximal surfaces. Topical fluoride 1.1% is prescribed for the prevention of dental caries in the form of paste or gel and can be applied directly to the teeth with soft custom-made dental trays. Calcium- and phosphate-based remineralizing agents can also be used before the application of topical fluoride.

Nonpharmacologic phototherapy such as the use of psoralen UV-A (PUVA), extracorporeal photopheresis, low-level laser therapy, and carbon dioxide laser has shown beneficial results in refractory cases, but data are limited, and further studies are needed to determine their efficacy.

14.8 Long-Term Complications of Oral GVHD

Patients with oral chronic GVHD are at risk of development of late complications. Fibrosis of the skin and oral mucosa along with trismus result in limited mouth opening with difficulties in eating and speaking. These patients may benefit from long-term physical therapy and passive stretching jaw exercises to increase the range of motion; passive stretching can be done manually or with commercially available devices (Dynasplint, Dynasplint Systems, Inc., Severna Park, MD, and TheraBite, Atos Medical Inc., West Allis, WI). In some cases, surgical intervention may be needed to release some of the fibrotic bands and improve mouth opening.

Patients with a history of oral GVHD should be monitored periodically due to a higher risk of oral squamous cell carcinoma. Patients who receive an allogeneic transplant for dyskeratosis congenita or Fanconi anemia are at increased risk for developing malignancies whether they developed cGVHD or not, and hence they must be carefully monitored for early signs of malignancy.

Chronic GVHD has a significant impact on patients' quality of life. The major aspects of social and emotional well-being are affected by the long-term complications seen in cGVHD. Long-term survivors may suffer from deterioration in oral health secondary to chronic immune suppression and xerostomia. Great emphasis should be directed towards preventing oral infections and dental caries. Periodic follow-ups are essential to assess oral health. Oral cancer screening is an important aspect of care in long-term survivors. Greater efforts in interdisciplinary management may facilitate early diagnosis and management and lead to improved outcome and quality of life.

Bibliography

1. Barbash B, Kramer S, Tzimas D, Saitta P. Graft-versus-host disease of the upper gastrointestinal tract after an autologous stem cell transplant. ACG Case Rep J. 2014;2(1):55–7.
2. Batra A, Cottler-Fox M, Harville T, Rhodes-Clark BS, Makhoul I, Nakagawa M. Autologous graft versus host disease: an emerging complication in patients with multiple myeloma. Bone Marrow Res. 2014;2014:891427.
3. Carpenter PA, Kitko CL, Elad S, Flowers ME, Gea-Banacloche JC, Halter JP, et al. National Institutes of Health consensus development project on criteria for clinical trials in chronic graft-versus-host disease: V. The 2014 Ancillary Therapy and Supportive Care Working Group report. Biol Blood Marrow Transplant. 2015;21(7):1167–87.
4. Cutler C, Nekhlyudov L, Rosmarin A. The approach to hematopoietic cell transplantation survivorship. UpToDate; 2017.
5. Cornell RF, Hari P, Drobyski WR. Engraftment syndrome after autologous stem cell transplantation: an update unifying the definition and management approach. Biol Blood Marrow Transplant. 2015;21(12):2061–8.
6. Cutler C, Miklos D, Kim HT, Treister N, Woo SB, Bienfang D, et al. Rituximab for steroid-refractory chronic graft-versus-host disease. Blood. 2006;108(2):756–62.
7. DePalo J, Chai X, Lee SJ, Cutler CS, Treister N. Assessing the relationship between oral chronic graft-versus-host disease and global measures of quality of life. Oral Oncol. 2015;51(10):944–9.
8. Filipovich AH, Weisdorf D, Pavletic S, Socie G, Wingard JR, Lee SJ, et al. National Institutes of Health consensus development project on criteria for clinical trials in chronic graft-versus-host disease: I. Diagnosis and staging working group report. Biol Blood Marrow Transplant. 2005;11(12):945–56.
9. Holmberg L, Kikuchi K, Gooley TA, Adams KM, Hockenbery DM, Flowers ME, et al. Gastrointestinal graft-versus-host disease in recipients of autologous hematopoietic stem cells: incidence, risk factors, and outcome. Biol Blood Marrow Transplant. 2006;12(2):226–34.
10. Ion D, Stevenson K, Woo SB, Ho VT, Soiffer R, Antin JH, et al. Characterization of oral involvement in acute graft-versus-host disease. Biol Blood Marrow Transplant. 2014;20(11):1717–21.
11. Jagasia MH, Greinix HT, Arora M, Williams KM, Wolff D, Cowen EW, et al. National Institutes of Health consensus development project on criteria for clinical trials in chronic graft-versus-host disease: I. The 2014 Diagnosis and Staging Working Group report. Biol Blood Marrow Transplant. 2015;21(3):389–401.e1.
12. Kharfan-Dabaja MA, Mhaskar AR, Djulbegovic B, Cutler C, Mohty M, Kumar A. Efficacy of rituximab in the setting of steroid-refractory chronic graft-versus-host disease: a systematic review and meta-analysis. Biol Blood Marrow Transplant. 2009;15(9):1005–13.
13. Korngold R, Antin JH. Biology and management of acute graft-versus-host disease. Cancer Treat Res. 2009;144:257–75.
14. Kuten-Shorrer M, Woo SB, Treister NS. Oral graft-versus-host disease. Dent Clin N Am. 2014;58(2):351–68.
15. Lee SJ, Vogelsang G, Flowers ME. Chronic graft-versus-host disease. Biol Blood Marrow Transplant. 2003;9(4):215–33.
16. Mawardi H, Elad S, Correa ME, Stevenson K, Woo SB, Almazrooa S, et al. Oral epithelial dysplasia and squamous cell carcinoma following allogeneic hematopoietic stem cell transplantation: clinical presentation and treatment outcomes. Bone Marrow Transplant. 2011;46(6):884–91.
17. Mawardi H, Hashmi SK, Elad S, Aljurf M, Treister N. Chronic graft-versus-host disease: current management paradigm and future perspectives. Oral Dis. 2018;25(4):931–48.
18. Motta A, Zhan Q, Larson A, Lerman M, Woo SB, Soiffer RJ, et al. Immunohistopathological characterization and the impact of topical immunomodulatory therapy in oral chronic graft-versus-host disease: a pilot study. Oral Dis. 2018;24(4):580–90.

19. Nassereddine S, Rafei H, Elbahesh E, Tabbara I. Acute graft versus host disease: a comprehensive review. Anticancer Res. 2017;37(4):1547–55.
20. Teshima T, Reddy P, Zeiser R. Reprint of: Acute graft-versus-host disease: novel biological insights. Biol Blood Marrow Transplant. 2016;22(3 Suppl):S3–8.
21. Treister N, Chai X, Kurland B, Pavletic S, Weisdorf D, Pidala J, et al. Measurement of oral chronic GVHD: results from the chronic GVHD consortium. Bone Marrow Transplant. 2013;48(8):1123–8.
22. Treister N, Duncan C, Cutler C, Lehmann L. How we treat oral chronic graft-versus-host disease. Blood. 2012;120(17):3407–18.
23. Treister N, Li S, Lerman MA, Lee S, Soiffer R. Narrow-band UVB phototherapy for management of oral chronic graft-versus-host disease. Photodermatol Photoimmunol Photomed. 2015;31(2):75–82.
24. Treister NS, Stevenson K, Kim H, Woo SB, Soiffer R, Cutler C. Oral chronic graft-versus-host disease scoring using the NIH consensus criteria. Biol Blood Marrow Transplant. 2010;16(1):108–14.
25. Wolff D, Gerbitz A, Ayuk F, Kiani A, Hildebrandt GC, Vogelsang GB, et al. Consensus conference on clinical practice in chronic graft-versus-host disease (GVHD): first-line and topical treatment of chronic GVHD. Biol Blood Marrow Transplant. 2010;16(12):1611–28.
26. Zeiser R, Blazar BR. Pathophysiology of chronic graft-versus-host disease and therapeutic targets. N Engl J Med. 2017;377(26):2565–79.

15 Dental Diseases and Management

Leah M. Bowers and Michael T. Brennan

15.1 Introduction

Dental disease in the oncology setting includes unique pathoses such as radiation caries and cGVHD-related dental decay as well as other more commonly seen diseases such as periodontitis. Due to their distinctive and often aggressive behavior, each of these diseases must be managed proactively and preventive strategies implemented.

Treating such dental diseases presents a number of challenges for the clinician. There may be limitations in treatment options, high risk of treatment failure, and lack of patient compliance. Their management may require a team of clinicians and must consider the patient's medical complexity.

Many of the changes that occur in the oral environment following cancer therapy are permanent, and therefore life-long close clinical follow-up is necessary. Recently, with the increase in human papillomavirus (HPV)-associated head and neck cancers (HNC), patients may face an extended period at risk of the late effects of therapy since these cancers tend to affect a relatively younger, healthier population and have an improved survival rate.

This chapter will discuss the current knowledge, clinical presentation, preventive strategies, and management of dental diseases in the patient following completion of radiation therapy.

L. M. Bowers
Department of Stomatology, Division of Oral Medicine, College of Dental Medicine, Medical University of South Carolina, Charleston, SC, USA

M. T. Brennan (✉)
Department of Oral Medicine, Atrium Health's Carolinas Medical Center, Charlotte, NC, USA
e-mail: mike.brennan@atriumhealth.org

R. Nair (ed.), *Orofacial Supportive Care in Cancer*,
https://doi.org/10.1007/978-3-030-86510-8_15

15.2 Definitions

Radiation caries (RC), also known as "radiation-related" or "radiation-associated" caries, refers to the unique and aggressive form of dental decay observed in patients treated with radiation therapy (RT) to the head and neck. It is a complex and multifactorial disease resulting from both direct and indirect radiation-induced damage.

The term "cGVHD-related caries" has been proposed to describe the pattern of dental decay observed in patients following allogeneic hematopoietic cell transplantation (alloHCT) who develop chronic graft-versus-host disease (cGVHD).

Periodontitis is a host-driven inflammatory response to bacterial biofilm in the subgingival environment resulting in the progressive destruction of the supporting tissues of the teeth, namely, the gingiva, periodontal ligament and alveolar bone, and the cementum.

15.3 Current Knowledge

15.3.1 Radiation Caries

Radiation caries (RC) is likely a product of radiation's direct effect on the dental hard tissues and damage to the surrounding structures and tissues including the salivary glands.

Both adults and children subject to RT of the head and neck have a higher prevalence of dental caries, with the greatest risk of development of RC occurring in the first year following completion of RT. Walker et al. found that with every month since completion of RT, there was a 6% increase in the odds of having moderate/severe tooth damage.

The effect of RT on the overall structural integrity of the dental hard tissues is proportional to dose. Walker et al. stratified tooth damage into three categories: "minimal" damage seen below 30 Gy, 2–3 times increased damage at 30–60 Gy, and 10 times increased damage at a critical threshold of 60 Gy and above.

Between 30 and 60 Gy, enamel shear fracture is observed at loading and flexure sites. At doses in excess of 60 Gy, there is decreased dentin and enamel hardness and elastic modulus and tensile strength and increased susceptibility to enamel shear fracture. There is also a reduction in bond strength between enamel and dentin.

The effect of radiation on the mechanomorphological properties of enamel may be dependent upon the unique characteristics of the individual enamel layer. Dehydration and decarboxylation (particularly at the inner enamel) may result in increased brittleness, while demineralization (especially of the middle and outer enamel layers) may result in increased softness. These factors combined lead to increased susceptibility of enamel loss by shear fracture.

Enamel craze lines (ECLs), incomplete fractures confined to the enamel extending from the cervical region to the incisal/occlusal surfaces, may be one of the first signs of weakening of tooth structure in irradiated teeth and can lead to delamination and dentin exposure. ECLs may harbor bacteria and other biofilm components which may encourage dental decay. In RT-exposed teeth, ECLs occur with greater frequency and are of larger size.

The dentin-pulp complex in irradiated teeth appears to retain the capacity to react against external injury such as caries. Histologic studies indicate that there is normal odontoblast function with deposition of reactionary dentin and intratubular dentin in RC, and the overall pulpal micromorphology remains intact, although it may appear hypocellular. Radiation also does not appear to significantly impair dentin bonding strength which supports the use of restorative procedures employing conventional adhesive protocols.

During and following RT, there tends to be a shift in the oral microbial population favoring cariogenic bacteria as well as other pathologic changes in flora composing the supra- or subgingival biofilms such as proliferation of obligate anaerobes and microaerophilic bacteria. This is attributed to, in part, by a reduction in radiosensitive cells involved in local immunity which would normally subdue these populations. Studies have indicated that there can be a persistent increase in acidogenic microorganisms up to 4 years after RT.

In vitro studies in primary teeth indicate that RT causes a reduction in surface hardness, alters mineral and organic composition, and promotes morphological changes in enamel and dentin. Certain features of primary teeth such as the thinner and higher numerical density of rods, abundant microporosities, exposed prisms, and major carbonate incorporation, result in an increased susceptibility to development and progression of caries compared to the permanent dentition.

The effect of RT on tooth formation is dependent upon the stage of development at the time of exposure. If a sufficient dose of radiation is applied prior to calcification, this may result in destruction of the tooth bud. If the developing tooth is exposed during calcification, this may result in tooth malformation or arrest of growth.

Hyposalivation due to RT is believed to significantly contribute to development of RC as radiation affects both the major and minor salivary glands, associated nerves, and endothelium. Salivary gland tissue is highly radiosensitive despite being well differentiated and having a relatively lower cellular proliferation rate.

Hyposalivation and the increased viscosity of saliva associated with RT also result in decreased oral clearance and increased plaque retention, further contributing to the risk of dental decay. Attendant radiation mucositis may impair the patient's ability to comfortably maintain optimal oral hygiene adding to the increased risk of RC.

RT is also associated with a decrease in salivary pH and buffering capacity, both of which can promote an increase in acidophilic and cariogenic cocci and yeasts. The acidic milieu of RT-associated hyposalivation also promotes demineralization and is associated with an additional decrease in enamel and dentin hardness and elasticity. The compromised enamel, along with newly exposed dentin, may allow for greater penetration of acidic saliva favoring even more demineralization.

Enhanced risk of dental caries may also be due to changes in diet during and after RT. During treatment, there may be an emphasis on prevention of weight loss; thus, patients may be counselled to eat frequent small, calorie-dense meals and/or use liquid food supplements containing refined carbohydrates. The higher frequency of intake may promote dental decay. Following completion of cancer therapy, a patient may be unable to return to a regular diet. Some factors that may influence dietary choices include persistent radiation mucositis, dysgeusia or hypogeusia, radiation fibrosis of the muscles of mastication, lack of functional dentition or surgery that impairs mastication.

15.3.2 "cGVHD-Related Caries"

Chronic graft-versus-host disease (cGVHD) affecting the oral mucosa and/or salivary glands following allogeneic hematopoietic cell transplantation (alloHCT) can cause significant morbidity in the oral cavity. There have been a few reports of rampant dental caries developing as a complication of salivary gland cGVHD in patients following alloHCT.

cGVHD-related caries tend to develop within 1 year of transplant and, like RC, progress swiftly. Hyposalivation is the primary shared complication between cGVHD-related caries and RC and could, at least in part, explain some similarities.

Salivary gland involvement of cGVHD can affect both the major and minor glands resulting in a diminished salivary flow rate and elevated salivary concentrations of sodium and magnesium ions, lysozyme, epidermal growth factor, total protein, albumin, and IgG and decreased levels of IgM and IgA. These changes result in decreased cleansing ability, reduced antimicrobial activity, compromised buffering capacity, and a decreased rate of enamel and dentin remineralization.

Oral mucosal involvement of cGVHD may manifest as painful ulcerations hindering optimal oral hygiene and influencing dietary choices. This combined with the aforementioned changes in saliva may also contribute to the development of cGVHD-related caries.

15.3.3 Effect of Radiation Therapy on the Periodontium

Both the direct and indirect effects of high-dose RT on the periodontium are detrimental, resulting in an increased risk of periodontal attachment loss, tooth loss, and osteoradionecrosis (ORN). Some patients who receive RT develop periodontitis in the irradiated bone which can be particularly severe in a patient with poor oral hygiene. Worsening of pre-existing periodontal disease following RT for HNC is also commonly reported.

RT appears to have a dose-dependent effect on periodontal status. High-dose RT can result in localized alterations in cellularity, vascularity, and a reduced healing and remodeling capacity of the periodontium. The radiated periodontal ligament may show diminished vascularity and cellularity, and there may be a thickening, rupturing, and disorientation of Sharpey's fibers.

Additional factors may contribute to the increased risk of periodontal disease in patients who received RT for HNC. Hyposalivation and qualitative changes in saliva may result in a diminishment of saliva's protective factors. Reduced host defense mechanisms with respect to plaque caused by RT may further foster attachment loss. Studies have reported variable changes in periodontal pathogens, both increases and no significant changes, in patients who received head and neck RT. Additional studies therefore are required to determine the effect of RT on periodontal flora and its clinical significance.

Following RT, increases in gingival recession have been attributed to a reduction in blood flow to the gingiva and an alteration in immune response. This recession may lead to dental root exposure and dentin hypersensitivity, increased difficulty in maintaining optimal oral hygiene, thereby increasing the risk of RC.

There is a dose-dependent increase in the prevalence of periapical periodontitis in irradiated bone. This is attributed to the sequela of RC extending into the root canal system leading to pulpal necrosis, bacterial ingress into the periradicular tissues, inflammation, and localized bone destruction. Irradiated pulp may be more prone to necrosis as a consequence of dental caries due to its relative hypocellularity.

There may also be a change in the composition of microflora associated with infected root canals in irradiated patients. The microflora represent greater variety, with species such as *Lactobacillus*, *Capnocytophaga*, *Actinomyces*, *Selenomonas*, and *Propionibacterium* present exclusively or more often in patients treated with RT. The effect of radiation on the incidence and severity of periapical pathology and overall outcome of root canal therapy, however, have yet to be definitively determined.

15.4 Clinical Presentation

15.4.1 Radiation Caries

RC is unique in its presentation, severity, and progression. It is a rapidly developing and aggressive form of dental decay which can quickly result in the loss of dentition if not treated definitively and in the absence of preventive measures.

RC differs clinically from caries in non-irradiated patients in myriad ways. It has a predilection for cuspal, incisal, and cervical regions (sites usually considered resistant to decay), and often affects the facial and incisal surfaces of canine teeth and incisors (Fig. 15.1).

New lesions representing RC often develop on the incisal or occlusal surfaces and progress into irregularly shaped erosions. Mechanical changes within the tooth, namely, a decrease in the elastic modulus and increased stiffness, coupled with occlusal loading forces, result in increased wear of the incisal and occlusal regions.

Initial enamel loss may also occur near the dentin-enamel junction (DEJ) leading to partial or total enamel delamination exposing dentin that is vulnerable to subsequent decay. As demineralization progresses, enamel is lost at the most susceptible

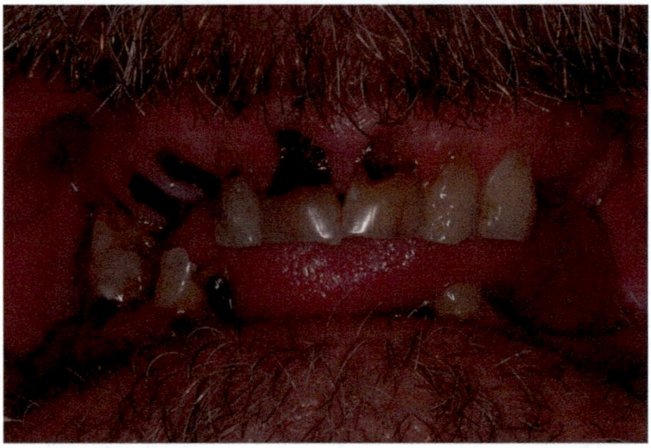

Fig. 15.1 Extensive dental caries in a 63-year-old male 14 months post-RT for HPV-related tonsillar squamous cell carcinoma

sites of loading and flexure, principally the cervical region, in a circumferential pattern. Further progression results in a decrease in the overall integrity of the tooth, which may lead to catastrophic fracture and gross loss of tooth structure.

Early manifestations of RC also include enamel craze lines (ECLs) extending from the cervical region to the incisal/occlusal surfaces, and diffuse brown spotting of the enamel smooth surfaces representing demineralization. Due to the unremitting nature of RC, these brown discolorations should be considered incipient decay and treated accordingly. In addition to frank radiation caries and loss of tooth structure, the remaining non-carious enamel and dentin may become significantly discolored.

Interestingly, RC, even when extensive, is not always associated with pain typically accompanying extensive dental decay. A patient with RC may be asymptomatic or experience only mild pain even when the dental pulp is involved.

15.4.2 cGVHD-Related Caries

Similar to RC, the dental caries associated with cGVHD after alloHCT has a tendency to progress at an alarming rate once established. These lesions favor the cervical and interproximal regions of both dental crowns and roots; areas where plaque tends to accumulate due to the lack of salivary flow.

Early lesions may occur along the cervical margins and appear white and chalky; indicative of demineralization. There may also be areas of widespread brown discoloration of smooth surfaces without cavitation. With progression, these early lesion can develop into frank cavitations eventually resulting in extensive loss of tooth structure.

Most notably among reports on patients with cGVHD-related caries is the startling onset and seemingly relentless progression of decay. The decay often appeared within the first year after alloHCT, and despite restorative intervention and preventive protocols, dental decay recurred and progressed often resulting in complete loss of multiple crowns.

15.4.3 Periodontitis

Periodontitis in patients who have received RT tends to be more aggressive but otherwise may be clinically indistinguishable from periodontitis in radiation-naïve patients. Radiographically, a subclinical widening of the periodontal ligament space along the mandibular teeth roots in the absence of adjacent bone destruction has been reported in patients treated with RT for HNC. It is believed that this represents a radiographic marker of irradiated bone only and therefore requires no treatment.

While an increase in periapical periodontitis in patients with a history of radiation to the tooth-bearing areas is reported, periapical inflammation may not present in the same manner as in non-irradiated patients. A radiographically detectable periapical lesion may not develop in areas exposed to higher doses of radiation due to its effect on the component cells including osteoclasts, osteoblasts, mononuclear and polymorphonuclear leukocytes, and fibrovascular elements.

15.5 Prevention and Specific Management

15.5.1 Radiation Caries

In the absence of preventive measures, breakdown of the dentition due to RC often begins within the first year and can become severe at an alarming rate. Without intervention, complete edentulism may result within a few years.

Several strategies can be employed to diminish the risk of development of RC. Among them, a comprehensive dental assessment prior to cancer treatment has been shown to be the most effective. As the effects of RT on salivary flow and composition are likely to be permanent, patients with a history of head and neck RT are at a life-long increased risk for demineralization and dental caries. Therefore, adherence to life-long preventive regimens and an increased frequency of recall appointments are recommended.

The risk of caries correlates with the RT dose received by the parotid glands. Parotid gland-sparing intensity-modulated radiation therapy (IMRT) and contralateral submandibular gland (CSMG) transfer, done separately or combined, are two techniques employed to diminish post-RT hyposalivation and xerostomia. Both have been shown in prospective clinical trials to result in decreased xerostomia and improved quality of life. To minimize damage to the parotid glands, the recommended mean dose to a single parotid gland is <20 Gy and <26 Gy to both glands. Where possible, RT planning should also seek to limit the mean dose to the dentition to less than 60 Gy to minimize collateral damage.

More recent efforts have focused on reducing the dose to the submandibular glands as they are recognized to contribute significantly to the patient's oral comfort. The submandibular glands are responsible for up to 90% of unstimulated flow (resting state), which has more of an influence on xerostomia than the stimulated flow. In addition, salivary mucins expressed from the submandibular and minor salivary glands act as lubricants and as a selectively permeable barrier of mucosal membranes. Their presence helps maintain tissue hydration and an overall sense of comfort.

The submandibular salivary gland tissue may be more radioresistant than that of the parotid. Studies have indicated that there is an exponential decrease in salivary flow as the mean dose to these glands exceeds a threshold of 39 Gy. If this threshold is not exceeded, there may be a gradual improvement in salivary output in the 2 years following completion of RT.

Surgical transfer of the contralateral submandibular gland to the non-irradiated submental space, with shielding of the transferred gland during receipt of RT, has also been employed. This procedure has been reported to spare approximately 30% of pre-treatment stimulated salivary function. The surgical complexity, additional surgical risk, and cost, however, limit this treatment option for most HNC patients.

Following completion of RT, there should be an emphasis on promoting an increase in salivary flow rates since this is correlated with a lower risk of RC. There is often a concomitant increase in salivary pH and buffering capacity that accompanies an increase in stimulated salivary flow rate. An increase in stimulated salivary secretion rate in excess of 1.0 ml/min and buffering capacity of $\geq$6.0 also promotes a re-establishment of microflora associated with oral health. Without intervention, the greatest increase in both unstimulated and stimulated salivary flow appears to occur between 1 and 2 years following completion of RT.

Dry mouth management can include the use of sugar-free chewing gums, mints, or candies and the use of muscarinic-cholinergic agonists (e.g., pilocarpine, cevimeline) to stimulate the remaining salivary gland tissue where appropriate. The use of xylitol-containing products may also be useful as xylitol is a sugar alcohol that inhibits *Streptococcus mutans*. Other modalities that can be used include oral mucosal lubricants, saliva substitutes, and acupuncture. Patients should be encouraged to remain well hydrated and frequently sip water throughout the day to moisten the oral tissues (please see Chap. 7).

15.5.2 Hygiene

Maintaining optimal oral hygiene is an important component in the prevention of dental disease, particularly in the post-RT setting. Patient instruction on oral hygiene maintenance, especially with respect to minimizing plaque accumulation, is fundamental. Recommended practices include brushing at least twice a day and at least daily use of interdental devices such as floss or interproximal brushes.

The antiseptic chlorhexidine used as a mouth rinse can reduce cariogenic microbial load and is effective as a chemical plaque control agent. It can be especially helpful in patients with high levels of *Streptococcus mutans* ($\geq 10^6$ colony forming units per ml saliva).

Accommodations may need to be made for patients who are not able to engage in routine oral hygiene practices. This may be due to persistent oral mucositis (either in association with RT or cGVHD), trismus following RT and/or a limited oral opening due to reconstructive surgery. Softer, smaller toothbrushes, floss aids, and non-irritating hygiene products, for example, may be employed. Such patients will also likely benefit from more frequent in-office dental cleanings and recall appointments with a review of home oral hygiene practices at each appointment.

15.5.3 Dietary and Other Considerations

Dietary counseling should be an integral part of cancer patient management. Coordination between the patient's dietitian and dental care team should occur to establish clear recommendations. From a caries prevention standpoint, dentists often advise against between-meal snacking, frequent intake of easily fermentable carbohydrates and sticky foodstuffs with low oral clearance; this may contradict recommendations from their dietitian leading to confusion for the patient.

Attention should be paid to avoid prescription or recommendation of medicines compounded with sucrose or other sugars. If such medicines are within the patient's established regimen and there is no viable substitute, the patient should be advised to gently rinse the mouth with water (if appropriate) following use. Patients should also be counselled to avoid acidic beverages which may promote dental erosion especially in those with compromised salivary flow. It may also be necessary to counsel patients to avoid excess alcohol consumption and tobacco use.

In patients experiencing frequent vomiting due to chemotherapy or otherwise, measures should be taken to prevent dental erosion. Patients should be counselled to rinse the mouth gently with water or a dilute solution of baking soda following vomiting and avoiding brushing the teeth immediately after vomiting. Consideration for fabrication of mouth guards to protect the teeth from acidic vomitus should also be made if vomiting is experienced frequently and for a prolonged period. Topical fluoride application can also protect against enamel erosion and therefore an appropriate frequency for application should be established with the patient.

15.5.4 Fluoride

Fluoride reduces enamel and dentin demineralization in the presence of acids produced by cariogenic bacteria, promotes remineralization of early enamel caries, and can inhibit cariogenic bacterial activity in dental plaque. Use of various high-potency fluoridated products therefore is a crucial part of a long-term post-cancer therapy dental regimen. As there is no appreciable difference in the efficacy of various high-potency fluoridated products, the patient can be involved in deciding which method is most likely to result in long-term compliance.

Emphasis should be on frequency of application, especially in the presence of hyposalivation, and should continue for the remainder of the patient's life. Daily application of a prescription neutral 1.1% sodium fluoride for at least 1–2 min using custom trays has been shown to significantly diminish the odds of developing moderate/severe dental damage. These custom-made dental trays are often recommended and fabricated, but compliance typically diminishes significantly with time. The patient should also undergo a professional application of fluoride with appropriate regularity.

In the presence of lesions of demineralization, remineralizing products, such as those containing calcium and phosphate, may be of benefit. Increased salivary calcium and phosphate levels can reduce enamel solubility, enhance remineralization, and thereby may be protective against caries development. Casein phosphopeptide-amorphous calcium phosphate (CPP-ACP) complex is reported to have anti-cariogenic effects, can reduce enamel demineralization, and can promote remineralization by buffering free calcium and phosphate ions. ACP can be incorporated into plaque and dental surfaces and maintains a state of supersaturation with respect to tooth enamel. Remineralizing products can be applied to cleansed teeth just prior to the application of a high-potency fluoridated product.

15.5.5 Dental Restorations

RC is associated with a very high rate of recurrent decay and early restoration failure. Silva et al. concluded that this early restoration failure is due to same etiological factors leading to restoration failure in decay not associated with RT; that is, incomplete removal of diseased dental hard tissue. They suggested that complete caries removal may be more challenging in irradiated patients due to the presence of "soft dentinal caries" and difficulty in achieving "proper anatomical shape" in cavity preparation. They speculated that recurrent decay may be multifactorial: due to changes in salivary composition and quantity, bacterial colonization, age, dental hygiene, fluoride bioavailability, and the quality of restorations—factors similarly cited as causes of recurrent decay in non-irradiated patients.

Silva et al. also suggested that to prevent residual and recurrent decay, care must be taken to ensure complete removal of soft dentinal caries, to avoid equivocal anatomical forms of cavity preparations and restorations, even when access is difficult, and to use restorative materials that release fluoride.

In the post-RT setting, where direct dental restorations are concerned, composite resins, resin-modified glass ionomer cements (RM-GICs), and amalgam restorations are preferred over conventional GICs. RM-GICs, in particular, provide a number of advantages. They are chemically bonded to tooth structure, and their elastic modulus can offset fatigue stress caused by tensile forces that are transferred to the vulnerable cervical region of the tooth. They have a coefficient of thermal expansion similar to that of tooth structure which leads to improved retention. They are able to release fluoride to the restored tooth and the oral environment, thereby preventing recurrent decay and potentially remineralizing early lesions, and they are "rechargeable" upon additional fluoride exposure.

15.5.6 Silver Diamine Fluoride

Thirty-eight percent silver diamine fluoride (SDF) is a colorless solution that combines the remineralizing potential of a high concentration of fluoride (44,800 ppm) with antibacterial silver ions. Its relative ease of use, safety, and effectiveness make it a potential adjunctive treatment in a patient's caries management program.

Although clinical trials using SDF on patients after cancer treatment have not been performed, its use among patients with a high caries risk is well established. It has been shown to be effective in prevention and arrest of root caries in elderly adults who often have hyposalivation accompanied by xerostomia. It is also effective in management of dentin hypersensitivity.

SDF should not be used on lesions suspected of having pulpal involvement, however, because it will not prevent further progression of the infection into surrounding tissues. SDF also darkens carious lesions which may not be esthetically acceptable to the patient. As it has no effect on composite bonding to non-carious dentin using either self-etch or full etch systems and appears to be compatible with GIC, it may be used in conjunction with conventional restorative procedures.

15.5.7 "cGVHD-Related Caries"

Interestingly, in studies reporting on patients who developed extensive cGVHD-related dental decay, all patients underwent pre-transplant dental examination and had any existing dental decay addressed, yet they still developed rampant dental disease. Therefore, in addition to a comprehensive pre-transplant dental examination and treatment, patients should be counselled on caries-preventive strategies and taught to identify early signs of decay.

As this pattern of dental decay appears to have a predilection for interproximal surfaces, bitewing radiographs, along with a comprehensive clinical exam, performed no later than 6 months following transplant, are advised. These patients should also be closely followed after alloHCT for development of hyposalivation, xerostomia and oral mucositis. A recall schedule of appointments every 3 months for at least the first year following transplant should also be established. During these appointments, the patient should also undergo a professional application of fluoride and a review of home oral hygiene and dietary recommendations.

Dental treatment during the first year after transplant will require consultation with the patient's care team as the immune system undergoes reconstitution. Due to the relative paucity of reported cases, there are no guidelines for treatment of cGVHD-related dental decay. Given the tendency of this form of dental decay to disseminate widely and rapidly, areas of dental decay and demineralization should be addressed promptly and definitively and a protocol for preventive therapy established. With respect to direct dental restorations, conventional GICs may provide some distinct advantages in these cases. Conventional GICs are capable of greater fluoride release than RM-GICs and composite resins, thereby providing superior protection against secondary caries. In the presence of hyposalivation, conventional GICs may also provide better resistance against abrasion and erosion over RM-GICs.

15.5.8 Periodontitis

Periodontal therapy initiated prior to, during, and after head and neck radiation and anti-neoplastic chemotherapy has been shown to result in an improvement in the periodontal health in cancer patients. However, periodontal disease is likely to progress in the post-treatment period if the patient does not adhere to an appropriate periodontal maintenance schedule.

Patients should undergo a comprehensive periodontal assessment at most 3 months following completion of RT and may undergo non-surgical periodontal therapy (i.e., scaling and root planing) in the absence of contraindications (e.g., persistent oral mucositis or sub-optimal blood counts). Patients should return for re-evaluation and a professional dental cleaning at least every 3 months, or sooner if problems arise, especially during the first year after RT. This recall frequency may be increased in a patient who is unable to maintain optimal oral hygiene.

Bibliography

1. Almstahl A, Wikstrom M, Fagerberg-Mohlin B. Microflora in oral ecosystems and salivary secretion rates—a 3-year follow-up after radiation therapy to the head and neck region. Arch Oral Biol. 2015;60(9):1187–95.
2. Brennan MT, et al. Dental disease before radiotherapy in patients with head and neck cancer: Clinical Registry of Dental Outcomes in Head and Neck Cancer Patients. J Am Dent Assoc. 2017;148(12):868–77.
3. Crystal YO, Niederman R. Evidence-based dentistry update on silver diamine fluoride. Dent Clin N Am. 2019;63(1):45–68.
4. De Felice F, et al. Treatment improvement and better patient care: which is the most important one in oral cavity cancer? Radiat Oncol. 2014;9:263.
5. Deasy JO, Moiseenko V, Marks L, Chao KS, Nam J, Eisbruch A. Radiotherapy dose-volume effects on salivary gland function. Int J Radiat Oncol Biol Phys. 2010;76(3 Suppl):S58–63.
6. Marangoni-Lopes L, Rovai-Pavan G, Steiner-Oliveira C, Nobre-Dos-Santos M. Radiotherapy reduces microhardness and mineral and organic composition, and changes the morphology of primary teeth: an *in vitro* study. Caries Res. 2018;53(3):296–304.
7. Murdoch-Kinch CA, Kim HM, Vineberg KA, Ship JA, Eisbruch A. Dose-effect relationships for the submandibular salivary glands and implications for their sparing by intensity modulated radiotherapy. Int J Radiat Oncol Biol Phys. 2008;72(2):373–82.
8. Silva AR, Alves FA, Berger SB, Giannini M, Goes MF, Lopes MA. Radiation-related caries and early restoration failure in head and neck cancer patients. A polarized light microscopy and scanning electron microscopy study. Support Care Cancer. 2010;18(1):83–7.
9. Sroussi HY, et al. Common oral complications of head and neck cancer radiation therapy: mucositis, infections, saliva change, fibrosis, sensory dysfunctions, dental caries, periodontal disease, and osteoradionecrosis. Cancer Med. 2017;6(12):2918–31.
10. Treister N, Duncan C, Cutler C, Lehmann L. How we treat oral chronic graft-versus-host disease. Blood. 2012;120(17):3407–18.
11. Walker MP, Wichman B, Cheng AL, Coster J, Williams KB. Impact of radiotherapy dose on dentition breakdown in head and neck cancer patients. Pract Radiat Oncol. 2011;1(3):142–8.

Interpretation of Investigations 16

Ian Olver

16.1 Introduction

The investigations pertinent to patients with orofacial cancers commence with those used to diagnose the disease from the presenting symptoms. These are then repeated to follow the progress of the cancer, both to document its response to treatment and if in remission to diagnose relapse. This group of investigations is important in supportive care because a new presenting symptom could represent a change in the underlying cancer, the immediate or late side effects of the treatment, or a comorbid illness or side effect of a supportive care drug or medication unrelated to the cancer. Investigations specifically informing supportive care are those investigating the toxicities of treatment.

My approach to discussing the investigations is to follow an optimal care pathway for people with head and neck cancers. I am using a pathway produced by the Australian Government's National Cancer Expert Reference Group [1].

16.2 Supportive Care

Supportive care encompasses the management of the symptoms of cancer and the acute and late side effects of treatment from diagnosis through treatment, posttreatment survivorship, and end-of-life care. Clinicians are often expert at managing the side effects of their treatment modality, while allied health practitioners attend to emotional, social, existential issues, and lifestyle factors like diet and exercise that are so important to well-being on treatment and beyond. It encompasses alleviating both the

I. Olver (✉)
Medical Oncology, Faculty of Health and Medical Sciences, University of Adelaide, Adelaide, SA, Australia
e-mail: Ian.olver@adelaide.edu.au

R. Nair (ed.), *Orofacial Supportive Care in Cancer*,
https://doi.org/10.1007/978-3-030-86510-8_16

symptoms of the cancer and the side effects of treatment. It includes addressing physical, psychosocial, and spiritual needs. If these can be anticipated, then prophylactic management is ideal (such as giving antiemetics prior to chemotherapy).

Patients are often in the best position to articulate those needs, so increasingly data collection during treatment includes patient reported outcomes. There are often differences between patients, particularly in the extent of the information about their cancer and its treatment that they want.

Supportive care can be delivered by all members of the multidisciplinary team throughout treatment and follow-up. Palliative care clinicians have particular expertise at managing the symptoms at the end-of-life, but their expertise can be useful for difficult cancer-related symptoms earlier.

Patients often feel well supported if they observe that their care is well coordinated and they receive all of the information that they need to make treatment decisions and understand in advance what adverse effects may ensue.

Research into the best way of delivering supportive care and in new anti-cancer and supportive care treatment investigations and treatments ideally should be regarded as part of routine care, offering the patients further alternatives to the current standard practice.

16.3 Tests at Diagnosis

There are no population screening tests for orofacial cancer, but these cancers may be detected early by opportunistic observation by dentists and medical practitioners when patients, particularly those at high risk of head and neck cancer, present for routine care. Risk factors include patients over 40 who are male and with pre-existing oral cancer, exposed to human papilloma virus or Epstein Barr virus, and with a history of high tobacco usage and consumption of alcohol.

The patients often present with symptoms that can range from lumps in the neck that are growing, to hoarseness, difficulty swallowing, or ulceration or lesions or conditions on the oral mucosa. In general, patients with suspected head and neck cancer should be referred early to the appropriate specialist. Certainly nothing more substantive than a fine needle aspiration (FNA) of a suspicious lump or lesion and some scans should be attempted prior to that referral.

16.3.1 Fine Needle Aspiration

Whereas the use of FNA in head and neck cancer has been well documented, for example, for lymph nodes and parotid tumors, it is not as well documented for oral and maxillofacial tumors [2, 3]. In parotid tumors the reported sensitivity varies widely between 41% and 100% and the specificity between 86% and 100% [4]. In salivary gland masses, a meta-analysis shows a sensitivity of 94% and a specificity of 98% [5]. FNA and cytology are very accurate and cost-effective for diagnosing oromaxillary lesions. In a study of 50 patients, the rate of obtaining unsatisfactory specimens was 4%. The sensitivity ranged from 77.7% to 75% with a specificity of

100% [6]. In another study of 229 intraoral lesions, there was a 13.1% incidence of obtaining an inadequate specimen, but the diagnostic accuracy when compared with subsequent biopsy was 94.9% with a sensitivity of 93.2% and a specificity or 96.8% [7]. Moreover, neck node FNA where human papillomavirus 16 is detected strongly indicates that the primary site is the oropharynx [8]. FNA is used in these cancers instead of core biopsy because of the belief that the tumor could spread along the core needle track, despite little evidence for this.

16.4 Clinical Investigation, Endoscopy, and Biopsy

The clinical examination will start by taking a history. From the supportive care viewpoint, in addition to the physical symptoms, this should elicit psychosocial issues. Also, patients who are heavy alcohol drinkers and tobacco users may tolerate their treatment better and decrease their chance of relapse if strategies to reduce alcohol consumption and smoking cessation strategies, including nicotine replacement therapy, are considered. Tobacco use may be monitored by the measurement of cotinine, a metabolite of nicotine, in plasma, saliva, or urine, and it has a high sensitivity and specificity for tobacco use in the absence of nicotine replacement therapy and a long enough half-life to detect tobacco use a few days after cessation [9].

A thorough examination of the head and neck by a specialist including indirect laryngoscopy and palpation of the neck for any lumps that could be involved lymph nodes is supplemented by an endoscopy. The whole area must be visualized as it is probable that there is a field change in the mucosa that can be associated with multiple lesions. The endoscopy is usually performed through the nose but can be done trans-orally with wide opening of the mouth so that the lateral and anterior oropharynx, posterior hypopharynx, and post-cricoid area are adequately visualized [10]. Suspicious lesions can then be biopsied.

Ideally scans to determine the extent of disease should be done prior to a biopsy so that no distortion is caused by the swelling associated with a biopsy.

In addition to a biopsy of a suspicious lesion seen on clinical examination or on scans, either from a potential primary site or lymph nodes, there have also been trials of a sentinel lymph node (SLN) biopsy in early oral squamous cell carcinoma to try to avoid the morbidity of a neck dissection for T1 and T2 cancers with clinically uninvolved nodes. A meta-analysis of the literature up until September 2016 included 66 studies involving 3566 patients in this category. The SLN could be identified in 96.3% cases and the sensitivity was 0.87 with a negative predictive value of 0.98. The sensitivity increased with the use of immunohistochemistry. This suggests that SLN biopsy could replace elective neck dissection in these patients [11].

16.4.1 Staging Scans

A combination of scans for head and neck cancer is required to determine the extent and spread of the disease and subsequently for surveillance [12].

16.4.2 Radiographs or X-Rays

A chest X-ray is sometimes done as a quick test when head and neck cancer is found, to see whether there are any obvious metastases to the chest or even synchronous or metachronous primary lung cancers. It may also reveal information about concomitant illnesses like chronic airways disease or scarring from old infections. An orthopantomogram is a panoramic or rotating X-ray that images the upper and lower jaw to evaluate the teeth prior to treatment with radiotherapy or chemotherapy. It may also detect cancer.

16.4.3 Ultrasound

An ultrasound often supplements other scans in head and neck cancer. It can be useful to rapidly image lymph nodes in the neck, thyroid gland, and salivary glands, although it is difficult to visualize the deep lobe of the parotid gland. It can be used to guide fine needle aspiration of tumors such as in salivary glands [5]. It is harmless for patients but the images can vary as they are operator dependent and may not visualize structures adjacent of bone or air because sound is not transmitted through these.

16.4.4 Computed Tomography (CT) Scan

CT scan enhanced by iodinated contrast material is the major scanning modality used in imaging primary head and neck cancer. Usually the neck and chest are imaged. It is a relatively cheap modality and is good spatially, but soft tissue resolution is not as good as that of bone. It is not as good as MRI in avoiding the streaking from metal artifacts such as amalgam, but with dual-energy CT and software iterative metal artifact reduction algorithms, the distortion is being reduced [13]. Since oral cavity cancers have been reported as having bone invasion in up to 56% cases, CT is good for picking cortical erosion but MRI better at detecting bone marrow invasion, so the two tests complement each other in this situation [12, 14]. Newer techniques such as perfusion CT scans maybe helpful in determining recurrent disease [15].

16.4.5 Magnetic Resonance Imaging (MRI)

MRI is particularly useful for imaging soft tissues in the oral cavity, tonsils, and base of tongue and is particularly more sensitive than CT for smaller tumors and where streaking can occur from the amalgam used for dental fillings and the beam hardening from the adjacent bone, mandible, and maxilla [16]. For smaller tumors images can be enhanced with contrast such as gadolinium. MRI is superior to CT for imaging soft tissues and perineural spread. MRI is also superior to CT in distinguishing between benign and malignant salivary gland tumors with 70% sensitivity and 73% specificity for detecting malignancy [17]. If head and neck cancers recur, it is likely to be in the first 2–3 years, and the recurrence will usually be at the site of surgery or at the margins where it can be difficult to choose between postoperative change and recurrence. A PET scan may be positive, and techniques such as MR perfusion scanning may help determine whether a change in architecture represents recurrence or not [18].

Exposing the patients to magnetic fields avoids the toxic effects of radiation.

16.4.6 Positron Emission Tomography (PET) or PET-CT

PET is a functional image made because cancer cells use more energy than surrounding cells and so take up a radiolabeled sugar ^{18}F-fluorodeoxyglucose (FDG) which is detected by a scanner to image the body. Combining with a CT gives both information about the functional and anatomic location of the tumor. In general, it has been found that a high pretreatment metabolic tumor volume is associated with a worse overall survival [19]. In T3 or N1 disease, PET scans may detect more nodal or distant involvement that will upstage the disease and may as a result change the treatment plan [20]. FDG-PET/CT may not be helpful in distinguishing benign from malignant salivary tumors as many salivary tumors that are benign are FDG avid. It is a useful scan for detecting metastases but not if the primary is not FDG avid, as is the case with adenoid cystic carcinoma [21].

Where cancer is diagnosed in cervical nodes and the site of the primary is unknown, which occurs in 2–9% of head and neck squamous cell carcinomas, the detection rate of the primary by FDG-PET/CT from a meta-analysis was 37% [22, 23]. In head and neck cancers which have no clinical or radiological evidence of neck nodes, a neck dissection will detect any small volume involvement of neck nodes. PET will not be better than a neck dissection so would not be helpful in N0 and stage I or II disease but may upstage stage III or IV disease [24].

16.5 HPV- and EBV-Associated Head and Neck Cancers

In addition to environmental carcinogens in tobacco smoke, alcohol and air pollutants, and oncogenic viruses, the human papilloma virus (HPV) and the Epstein-Barr virus (EBV) contribute to the incidence of head and neck cancer [25].

16.5.1 HPV

E6 and E7 are two viral oncogenes expressed due to HPV infection which are part of triggering malignant transformation mainly in the tonsils and base of tongue. HPV-associated oropharyngeal cancer in the USA and Western Europe now represents 70–80% of the cancers in those sites. Most of these are due to the HPV-16 genotype [26]. Non-oropharyngeal cancers can be associated with HPV with most studies giving estimates of between 4% and 8% [27, 28].

Clinically the oropharyngeal cancers associated with HPV occur at a younger age, are predominantly in males, and are at earlier stage, and although they often have more lymph node involvement, they have a better prognosis than non-HPV oropharyngeal cancers and less second cancers [29].

The definitive diagnosis is the detection of HPV DNA by polymerase chain reaction or in situ hybridization. The p16 protein, which is a tumor suppressor, is overexpressed in cancers associated with HPV. Either the HPV status can be measured or p16 protein measured by immunohistochemistry can be used as a surrogate marker [26, 30]. When both are used, 10% of p1-positive patients were negative for HPV and 7% negative for p16 were positive for HPV. Being HPV positive and having a high p16 is associated with a better prognosis [31].

It is important to identify this subset of cancers because they may respond as well to less intense treatment. More recent studies are focused on using oral rinses or blood to test for HPV DNA or serological assays for HPV proteins to monitor for residual disease or recurrence [32].

16.5.2 EBV

EBV is associated with nasopharyngeal cancer particularly in Southeast Asia and the south of China. It is an aggressive cancer which tends to metastasize early to lymph nodes and beyond to the liver. High levels of EBV DNA as detected by in situ hybridization of the non-polyadenylated EBER RNAs are found in the plasma, and this is being explored as a marker for recurrence [33–35].

16.6 Investigations for Supportive Care

Some investigations will be required to determine the appropriate supportive care for a patient during the treatment phase and beyond. This will include investigations of nutritional status, dental and oral investigations, and investigations of swallowing difficulties if that is a presenting symptom.

In the area of psychosocial support, in addition to clinical psychological evaluation, there are objective tests to assess the likelihood of suffering what is being called "financial toxicity" as a result of the cost of treatments or job loss.

16.7 Investigating Nutritional Status

The quality of life and outcomes of head and neck cancer have been related to the patients' nutritional status [36]. The need for nutritional support is very much part of supportive care for these patients, and therefore they will need serial investigations to evaluate their nutritional status. The clinical assessment will reveal any difficulty in swallowing and signs of weight loss. Three screening and assessment tools that have been validated in patients with cancer are the Subjective Global Assessment (SGA) tool which is based on history and examination, the Patient-Generated SGA (PG-SGA), and the Malnutrition Screening Tool [37]. Measuring height and weight is important, but weight change and body mass index less than 18.5 kg/sq m may suggest undernutrition. Triceps skinfold thickness assesses fat stores and hand grip strength assesses muscle function.

Biochemistry should include urea and electrolytes which may indicate fluid status. Refeeding syndrome after starvation is characterized by hypophosphatemia but can also include hypomagnesaemia, hypokalemia, and changes in glucose, protein, and fat metabolism [38]. Albumin may not be a good indicator of the nutritional state because it can be affected by many other conditions such as sepsis and has a long half-life. Pre-albumin with a shorter half-life may be better. However, it has been reported that a low pretreatment serum albumin is associated with six times the chance of cancer progression and worse progression-free and overall survival in patients with squamous cell head and neck cancer who receive definitive treatment [39]. However, other studies have shown that nutritional status is not correlated with surgical results or complications [40].

16.7.1 Oral Health

The investigation of the oral cavity is mainly a clinical investigation by the general practitioner and dentist looking for ulceration, masses in the mucosa or tongue, erythematous patches or leukoplakia on the mucosa, or infections such as candida, which can be painful or even bleeding. The dentist should investigate any unexplained loose teeth. Dental care should continue throughout treatment and survivorship [41].

16.7.1.1 Swallowing

Patients diagnosed with head and neck cancer may experience swallowing and speech problems due to the cancer-causing obstruction, pain, or loss of coordination of swallowing [42, 43]. Aspiration is particularly a problem with hypopharyngeal or laryngeal cancers. The pharyngeal phase of swallowing is affected by tumors in the above sites as well as the base of the tongue [44].

A scale for recording swallowing dysfunction is the Swallowing Performance Status Scale (SPSS). This is a 7-point scale which grades swallowing from normal to severe dysfunction with aspiration [45]. An objective measure to visualize neuromuscular activity and patterns of swallowing is videofluoroscopic analysis and oropharyngeal motility [46].

Tests should be done pretreatment, but often surgery will also impact on swallowing. For example, if less than 50% of the tongue is resected, patients can regain a high degree of swallowing function. The extent of resection and the reconstruction will determine how well speech can be regained [47].

Radiotherapy postoperatively can worsen swallowing outcomes, and xerostomia reduces the ability to chew food. The dry mouth and post-radiation fibrosis can have adverse outcomes for both swallowing and speech [48].

Speech pathologists use tests like the Frenchay Dysarthria Assessment (FDA) which looks at respiration and movement of the tongue, lip, and palate and the ability to sustain vowel sounds and how intelligible the speech is [49]. Patients can then be supported by exercises to increase the range of movement and strength of the tongue and lips, or if speech is totally compromised, portable synthetic speech devices are provided [50]. Swallowing can be managed by teaching patients to compensate for the changed tissue by changing posture, increasing sensory input with the swallow, modifying food volume and speed of eating and its viscosity, or using intraoral prostheses [50].

16.7.1.2 Pain

It is estimated that up to 70% of patients experience pain from head and neck cancer at and after diagnosis [51]. There are many methods for scoring pain. In head and neck cancer, it can be due to the underlying disease and the treatment. For example, mucositis is associated with radiation therapy. In a study of neuropathic and nociceptive pain in head and neck cancer patients who received radiotherapy, the assessment of pain used a well-validated and reliable tool, the McGill Pain Questionnaire [52, 53]. The localization of pain was measured as the number of pain sites on a body map and the intensity of pain by a 0–5 least to worst verbal scale. Pain quality was assessed by descriptors ranging from sensory and affective to miscellaneous and total pain. The pain pattern was measured by nine descriptors including intermittent, continuous, and brief. This illustrates the range of investigations required to characterize pain. The outcome of the study was that the most common neuropathic descriptors were aching and burning; nociceptive words were dull, sore, tender, and throbbing; and affective descriptors were tiring and annoying. Both nociceptive and neuropathic pain were reported, with neuropathic pain descriptors reported by 73% of patients. Continuous pain was reported by 57% of patients and both continuous and intermittent by 79%.

There are other pain assessment tools, and an interesting study comparing three of them found no differences in the mean pain intensity scores between using the Numeric Rating Scale, the Faces Pain Scale, or the Visual Analogue Scale [54]. The vital concept here is the importance of the proper investigation of pain due to the disease and its treatment, as part of good supportive care in head and neck cancer.

16.8 Measuring Distress

Distress can be caused by physical symptoms such as pain or psychosocial and spiritual experiences that are unpleasant. Distress can occur at both the time of diagnosis and treatment but also can continue through the survivorship phase and at the end-of-life [55]. Distress compromises quality of life and can be associated with poorer survival and poor adherence to treatment [56].

The simplest screening tool for distress is the Distress Thermometer, a visual analogue scale where patients rate their distress as between 0 and 10, that is, no distress to extreme distress [56]. In a study with head and neck cancer patients, the greatest distress was during treatment, and it correlated with pain, mucositis, and difficulty swallowing. With radiotherapy, skin and mucosal toxicity contributed to the distress as the treatment continued. Quality of life was compromised with increasing distress [57].

Overall distress and social and emotional distress correlated with anxiety and depression and spiritual and existential distress occurred in half of the patients, particularly later in treatment.

16.8.1 Psychological Well-Being

Depression has been estimated to occur in a range from 6% to 48% in patients with head and neck cancer, although it is greater in studies using self-report questionnaires as compared to those using diagnostic interviews [58]. A common measure of anxiety and depression is the Hospital Anxiety and Depression Scale (HADS) [59]. The scale is a self-report scale which excludes somatic symptoms. It has been validated, and normative data in a nonclinical sample has been generated [60].

In a study using the HADS, Functional Assessment of Cancer Therapy-Head and Neck (FACT-H+N) was used to measure quality of life. This is a 39-item scale which measures physical, functional, social/family, and emotional well-being, and its validity and reliability have been confirmed [61]. Depression was found to increase from pretreatment to posttreatment, and posttreatment depression was predicted by the treatment including chemotherapy and the occurrence of pretreatment depression. Anxiety, however, reduced after treatment, and again posttreatment anxiety was predicted by pretreatment anxiety and was more likely in males [62].

In a study evaluating the impact of depression on the health-related quality of life (HRQOL) of patients with head and neck cancer, a Structured Clinical Interview of the Diagnostic and Statistical Manual of Mental Disorders (DSM)-IV (SCID) was used [63]. This is a clinician-administered semi-structured interview. In this study one of the many tools to measure quality of life was used: the European Organisation for Research and Treatment of Cancer (EORTC) Quality of Life Questionnaire (QLQ) module for head and neck cancer [64]. Anxiety was highest pretreatment and then declined, whereas depression peaked at 3 months. Several symptoms related to depression included loss of the senses, speech, libido, dry mouth, and weight loss. Depressed patients used more analgesics and nutritional supplements, and loss of social contacts and social eating predicted depression.

Psychological distress and fatigue have been associated with self-reported cognitive decline after therapy in patients treated for cancer. Subjective cognitive decline does not always correlate with altered objective tests of cognitive dysfunction, but it is often associated with anxiety and depression [65]. Cognitive dysfunction was originally thought to be associated with receiving chemotherapy but has been reported more generally after therapy. Objective cognitive decline can be measured by cognitive function tests such as Cogstate, a web-based test involving card shuffling and a computer keyboard to measure reaction times [66]. Ongoing studies are exploring prediction of this side effect and strategies for management which would be part of supportive care to maximize quality of life.

16.8.2 Spiritual Well-Being

All of us at some time question the meaning and purpose of our lives, often in the context of illness. These are spiritual questions. Faced with a life-threatening illness, we can seek peace to counter our existential distress, and this impacts our quality of life. Religion is just one path to expressing our spirituality. There are several scales of spiritual well-being, but one tool for investigating this is the Functional Assessment of Chronic Illness Therapy-Spiritual Wellbeing (FACIT-Sp) with its three domains of meaning peace and faith [67]. When correlated with a quality of life assessment, peace accounted for 3% of the prediction of quality of life and meaning 1.3% [68].

Given the independent contribution of spiritual well-being to quality of life, it is important that spiritual well-being is investigated. The FACIT-Sp is a well-validated scale.

16.9 Financial Toxicity

Financial toxicity is a relatively new term to describe the unintended potential economic harm or damage of cancer and its treatment. It refers to situations of grossly compromising a patient's finances in situations such as having to pay for very high-cost drugs or losing a job as a result of cancer and finding it difficult to re-enter the workforce. There is the objective component of how poor the financial situation has become and the subjective component known as financial distress which encompasses the reaction to the state of personal finances [69].

Scales have been developed to investigate this toxicity. One scale grades the financial burden and assesses the availability of income and liquid assets to cover medical bills [70]. A comprehensive score for financial toxicity (COST) considers both the objective burden and subjective distress [71].

It may be possible to predict who are most likely to experience financial toxicity, and it should be investigated as a social impact of head and neck cancer and its treatment.

16.10 Investigations Associated with Systemic Therapy

The investigation of the local therapies of surgery and radiotherapy is covered under the imaging techniques above. The systemic therapies include chemotherapy and immunotherapy.

16.10.1 Chemotherapy

With chemotherapy drugs it is important to monitor complete blood examination since nadir counts occur 10–14 days post-therapy and with neutropenia there is the risk of infection. If thrombocytopenia is severe, bleeding may result. Electrolytes and renal and liver function also require monitoring since many drugs can impair organ function which should be routinely measured while on therapy. In addition, it is important to monitor for specific toxicities known to occur with specific drugs [72].

A common drug used in combination in head and neck cancer is cisplatin. This can cause renal dysfunction, and renal function should be assessed regularly with serum creatinine and creatinine clearance. Ototoxicity can also be cumulative, and a hearing test looking for high-frequency hearing loss will alert the clinician to the early sings of this side effect. Cumulative doses may result in anemia which will be diagnosed on the full blood examination. Other side effects such as nausea and vomiting and peripheral neuropathy are clinically detected.

Specific side effects which should be monitored in addition to the routine standard tests with 5-fluorouracil (5FU) are mouth ulcers and diarrhea which may be dose limiting. Rash is a clinical diagnosis. If patients experience severe toxicity, they probably have a deficiency in dihydropyrimidine dehydrogenase (DPD) which is involved in the catabolism of the drug and should be measured in this circumstance before continuing therapy [73].

The taxane, paclitaxel, is given with a premedication to avoid hypersensitivity reactions. It can cause profound myelosuppression which will be detected on a full blood examination and in addition to clinical observations of hair loss, neuropathy, mucositis, and diarrhea, arthralgias and myalgias can occur. Docetaxel can have similar effects but can be also associated with injection site reactions, and care must be taken with liver impairment.

16.10.2 Immunotherapy and Targeted Agents

Afatinib is a small molecule and a second-generation tyrosine kinase inhibitor, taken by mouth, which was initially used to treat lung cancer with mutations in the epidermal growth factor receptor (EGFR) gene but also HER2 gene and is active against mutations such as T790M. It has been shown to improve progression-free survival in subtypes of head and neck cancer resistant of platinum which have biomarkers including those which demonstrate that the tumor is p16-negative and EGFR amplified [74].

Although still requiring more clinical trials, the point to be made here about the investigations is that before using this drug the biomarkers which predict its efficacy should be measured. For example, in lung cancer, where it has been listed by the Australian Pharmaceutical Benefits Scheme [75], the conditions of approval are that tumors must have EGFR exon 19 deletions or L858 substitution mutations. This introduces the concept of companion diagnostics for these targeted therapies to ensure that the tumors have the appropriate targets measured.

The side effects do not need special tests beyond the routine blood tests, they need monitoring as the toxicities are clinically diagnosed, including diarrhea and mucositis, skin rash, and paronychia.

More recent treatments have included antibodies and immunotherapeutic agents which have a different spectrum of toxicities, which need to be investigated if they occur. Cetuximab is a monoclonal antibody targeted at the epidermal growth factor receptor (EGFR) and is used for head and neck cancer in combination with radiotherapy or cisplatin regimens. It can be associated with an acneiform rash and nail changes which are apparent clinically as are other side effects such as fatigue, nausea, vomiting, and diarrhea. In monitoring electrolytes and hematology tests, it should be noted that administration of the drug may be associated with low magnesium, potassium, and calcium, and it can cause anemia [76].

Pembrolizumab and nivolumab are antibodies targeting the PD-1 protein on immune T cells which prevents them from attacking the cancer. PD-1 on T cells and PDL-1 on tumors need to be measured before this class of drugs known as checkpoint inhibitors are used [77]. The most remarkable side effects of these drugs are autoimmune side effects including pneumonitis, colitis, hepatitis, arthritis, encephalitis, cardiac inflammation, and inflammation in the endocrine organs including thyroid, pituitary, and adrenal glands. This means that investigations while receiving these drugs will have to include endocrine function tests. These side effects can be managed by steroids and ceasing the drugs. Skin rashes and pruritus also occur [78].

16.11 Conclusions

Investigations are primarily used to diagnose and stage head and neck cancers, choose and monitor treatment, and detect progression or relapse. However, it is also vital to target investigations at the supportive care of the patients to assess physical symptoms and side effects of treatment and psychosocial and spiritual well-being to allow optimization of quality of life during treatment and in posttreatment survival.

Bibliography

1. National Cancer Expert Reference Group. Optimal care pathway for people with head and neck cancers. www.cancer.org.au/ocp. Last accessed 2018.
2. Al-Khafaji BM, Nestok BR, Katz RL. Fine-needle aspiration of 154 parotid masses with histological correlation: ten-year experience at the University of Texas M.D. Anderson Cancer Centre, Cancer 1998;84:153–9.
3. Shakeel MK, Daniel MJ, Srinivasan SV, Koliyan R, Kumar JV. Comparative analysis of detecting cervical lymph node metastasis with fine needle aspiration cytology. J Natl Sci Biol Med. 2015;6(Suppl S1):1–7.
4. Ghantous Y, Naddaf R, Barak M, Abd-Elrazik M, Ein-Naaj I. The role of fine needle aspiration in the diagnosis of parotid gland tumours: correlation with preoperative computerised tomography tumour size. J Craniofac Surg. 2016;27:192–6.
5. Kim HJ, Kim JS. Ultrasound-guided core biopsy in salivary glands: a meta-analysis. Laryngoscope. 2018;128:118–25.

6. Singh S, Garg N, Gupta S, Marwah N, Kalra R, Singh V, et al. Fine needle aspiration cytology in lesions of oral and maxillofacial region: diagnostic pitfalls. J Cytol. 2011;28:93–7.
7. Khan N, Afroz N, Haider A, Hassan MJ, Hashmi SH, Hasan S. Role of fine needle aspiration, imprint and scrape cytology in the evaluation of intraoral lesions. J Cytol. 2013;30:263–9.
8. Begum S, Gillison ML, Nicol TL, Westra WH. Detection of human papillomavirus-16 in fine-needle aspirates to determine tumour origin in patients with metastatic squamous cell carcinoma of the head and neck. Clin Cancer Res. 2007;13:1186–91.
9. SRNT Subcommittee on Biochemical Verification. Biochemical verification of tobacco use and cessation. Nicotine Tob Res. 2002;4:149–59.
10. Hamada K, Ishihara R, Yamasaki Y, Akasaka T, Arao M, Iwatsubo T, et al. Transoral endoscopic examination of head and neck region. Dig Endosc. 2018;30:516–21.
11. Liu M, Wang SJ, Yang X, Peng H. Diagnostic efficacy of sentinel lymph node biopsy in early oral squamous cell carcinoma: a meta-analysis of 66 studies. PLoS One. 2017;12:e0170322. https://doi.org/10.1371/journal.pone.0170322.
12. Seeburg DP, Baer AH, Aygun N. Imaging of patient with head and neck cancer. From staging to surveillance. Oral Maxillofacial Surg Clin N Am. 2018; https://doi.org/10.1016/j.coms.2018.06.004.
13. Bongers MN, Schabel C, Thomas C, Raupach R, Notohamiprodjo M, Nikolaou K, Bamberg F. Comparison and combination of dual-energy-and iterative-based metal artifact reduction on hip prosthesis and dental implants. PLoS One. 2015;10(11):e0143584. https://doi.org/10.1371/journal.pone.0143584. eCollection 2015.
14. Handschel J, Naujokas C, Depprich RA, Kübler NR, Kröpil P, Kuhlemann J, et al. CT-scan is a valuable tool to detect mandibular involvement in oral cancer patients. Oral Oncol. 2012;48:361–6.
15. Garcia MR, Passos UL, Ezzedine TA, Zuppani HB, Gomes RL, Gebrim EM. Postsurgical imaging of the oral cavity and oropharynx: what radiologists need to know. Radiographics. 2015;35:804–18. (erratum in Radiographics 2015;35:1624)
16. Sarrion Pérez MG, Bagan JV, Jiménez Y, Margaix M, Marzal C. Utility of imaging techniques in the diagnosis of cancer. J Craniomaxillofac Surg. 2015;43:1880–94.
17. Christe A, Waldherr C, Hallett R, Zbaeren P, Thoeny H. MR imaging of parotid tumours: typical lesion characteristics in MR imaging improve discrimination between benign and malignant disease. AJNR Am J Neroradiol. 2011;32:1202–7.
18. Choi SH, Lee JH, Choi YJ, Park JE, Sung YS, Kim N, et al. Detection of local tumour recurrence after definitive treatment of head and neck squamous cell carcinoma: histogram analysis of dynamic contrast-enhanced T1-weighted perfusion MRI. AJR Am J Roentgenol. 2017;208:42–7.
19. Bonomo P, Merlotti A, Olmetto E, Bianchi A, Desideri I, Bacigalupo A, et al. What is the prognostic impact of FDG PET in locally advanced head and neck squamous cell carcinoma treated with concomitant chemo-radiotherapy? A systematic review and meta-analysis. Eur J Nucl Med Mol Imaging. 2018; https://doi.org/10.1007/s00259-018-4065-5. [Epub ahead of print].
20. National Comprehensive Cancer Network Head and neck cancers (Version 2.2017). Last accessed Oct 2017.
21. Park HL, Yoo IR, Lee N, Yoon H, Choi EK, Choi HS, et al. The value of F-18 FDG PET for planning treatment and detecting recurrence in malignant salivary gland tumors: comparison with conventional imaging studies. Nucl Med Mol Imaging. 2013;47:242–8.
22. Kwee TC, Kwee RM. Combined FDG-PET/CT for the detection of unknown primary tumors: systematic review and meta-analysis. Eur Radiol. 2009;19:731–44.
23. Lee JR, Kim JS, Roh JL, Lee JH, Baek JH, Cho KJ, et al. Detection of occult primary tumors in patients with cervical metastases on unknown primary tumors: comparison of 18(F) FDG PET/CT with contrast-enhanced CT or CT/MR imaging-prospective study. Radiology. 2015;274:764–71.
24. Fleming AJ Jr, Smith SP Jr, Paul CM, Hall NC, Daly BT, Agrawal A, et al. Impact of [18F]-2-fluorodeoxyglucose-positron emission tomography on previously untreated head and neck cancer patients. Laryngoscope. 2007;117:1173–9.

25. Ngan H-L, Wang L, Lo K-W, Lui VWY. Genomic landscapes of EBV-associated head and neck cancer. Cancers. 2018;10 https://doi.org/10.3390/cancers10070210.
26. Vokes EE, Agrawal N, Seiwert TY. HPV-associated head and neck cancer. J Natl Cancer Inst. 2015;107:djy344. https://doi.org/10.1093/jnci/djv344.
27. Castellsaguè X, Alemany L, Quer M, Halec G, Quirós B, Tous S, et al. HPV involvement in head and neck cancers: comprehensive assessment of biomarkers in 3680 patients. J Natl Cancer Inst. 2016;108:djv403. https://doi.org/10.1093/jnci/djv403.
28. Chakravarthy A, Henderson S, Thirdborough SM, Ottensmeier CH, Su X, Lechner M, et al. Human papillomavirus drives tumour development throughout the head and neck: improved prognosis is associated with an immune response largely restricted to the oropharynx. J Clin Oncol. 2016;34:4132–41.
29. O'Sullivan B, Huang SH, Su J, Garden AS, Sturgis EM, Dahlstrom K, et al. Development and validation of a staging system for HPV-related oropharyngeal cancer by the International Collaboration on Oropharyngeal Cancer Network for Staging (ICON-S): a multicenter cohort study. Lancet Oncol. 2016;17:440–51.
30. Shi W, Kato H, Perez-Ordonez B, Pintilie M, Huang S, Hui A, et al. Comparative prognostic value of HPV16 E6 mRNA compared with in situ hybridization for human oropharyngeal squamous carcinoma. J Clin Oncol. 2009;27:6213–21.
31. Weinberger PM, Yu Z, Haffy BG, Kowalski D, Harigopal M, Brandsma J, et al. Molecular classification identifies a subset of human papillomavirus-associated oropharyngeal cancers with favorable prognosis. J Clin Oncol. 2006;24:736–47.
32. Mirghani H, Lang Kuhs KA, Waterboer T. Biomarkers for early identification of recurrences in HPV-driven oropharyngeal cancer. Oral Oncol. 2018;82:108–14.
33. Lo YMD, Chan LYS, Chan ATC, Leung SF, Lo KW, Zhang J. Quantitative and temporal correlation between circulating cell-free Epstein-Barr virus DNA and tumour recurrence in nasopharyngeal carcinoma. Cancer Res. 1999;59:5452–5.
34. Tsao SW, Tsang CM, Lo KW. Epstien-Barr virus infection and nasopharyngeal carcinoma. Philos Trans R Soc Lond Ser B Biol Sci. 2017;372(1732):20160270. https://doi.org/10.1098/rstb.2016.0270.
35. Young LS, Dawson CW. Epstein-Barr virus and nasopharyngeal carcinoma. Chin J Cancer. 2014;33:581–90.
36. Talwar B, Donnelly R, Skelly R, Donaldson M. Nutritional management in head and neck cancer: United Kingdom National Multidisciplinary Guidelines. J Laryngol Otol. 2016;130(Suppl S2):S32–40.
37. Ottery FD. Definition of standardized nutritional assessment and interventional pathways in oncology. Nutrition. 1996;12(Suppl 1):S15–9.
38. Mehanna HM, Moedina J, Travis J. Refeeding syndrome: what it is, and how to prevent and treat it. BMJ. 2008;336:1495–8.
39. Lim WS, Roh JL, Kim SB, Choi SH, Nam SY, Kim SY. Pretreatment albumin level predicts survival in head and neck squamous cell carcinoma. Laryngoscope. 2017;127:E437–42.
40. Matthews TW, Lampe HB, Dragosz K. Nutritional status in head and neck cancer patients. J Otolaryngol. 1995;24:87–91.
41. Epstein JB, Barasch A. Oral and dental health in head and neck cancer patients. In: Maghami E, Ho AS, editors. Multidisciplinary care of the head and neck cancer patients. Switzerland: Springer; 2018. p. 43–57.
42. Muz J, Mathog RH, Hamlet SL, Davis LP, Kling GA. Objective assessment of swallowing function in head and neck cancer patients. Head Neck. 1991;13:33–9.
43. Stenson KM, MacCracken E, List M, Haraf DJ, Brockstein B, Weichselbaum R, et al. Swallowing function in patients with head and neck cancer prior to treatment. Arch Otolaryngol Head Neck Surg. 2000;126:371–7.
44. Logeman JA, Bytell DE. Swallowing disorder in three types of head and neck surgical patients. Cancer. 1979;44:597–601.
45. Karnell MP, MacCracken E. A database information storage and reporting system for videofluorographic oropharyngeal motility (OPM) swallowing evaluations. Am J Speech Lang Pathol. 1994;3:25–32.

46. Humphries B, Mathog R, Rosen R, Miller P, Nelson R. Videofluoroscopic and scintigraphic analysis of dysphagia in the head and neck cancer patient. Laryngoscope. 1987;97:25–32.
47. Lazarus CL. Management of swallowing disorders in head and neck cancer patients: optimal patterns of care. Semin Speech Lang. 2000;21:293–309.
48. Pauloski BR, Rademaker AW, Logemann JA, Colangelo LA. Speech and swallowing in irradiated and nonirradiated postsurgical oral cancer patients. Otolaryngol Head Neck Surg. 1998;118:616–24.
49. McKinstry A, Perry A. Evaluation of speech in people with head and neck cancer: a pilot study. Int J Lang Commun Discord. 2003;38:31–46.
50. Perry A, Frowen J. Speech and swallowing function in head and neck cancer patients: what do we know? Cancer Forum. 2006;30:178–83.
51. Van Cleave J, DiMaria C, DiMaria S, Liang EW, Long C, Fu C. Pain and function in head and necks cancer: a systematic literature review. J Pain. 2017;18(Suppl 4):S82.
52. Epstein JB, Wilkie DJ, Fischer DJ, Kim Y-O, Villines D. Neuropathic and nociceptive pain in head and neck cancer patients receiving radiation therapy. Head Neck Oncol. 2009;1:26. https://doi.org/10.1186/1758-3284-1-26.
53. Melzak R. The McGill pain questionnaire: major properties and scoring methods. Pain. 1975;1:277–99.
54. Rodriguez CS, McMillan S, Yarandi H. Pain measurement in older adults with head and neck cancer and communication impairments. Cancer Nurs. 2004;27:425–33.
55. Carlson LE, Waller A, Mitchell AJ. Screening for distress and unmet needs in patients with cancer: review and recommendations. J Clin Oncol. 2012;30:1160–77.
56. Tuinman MA, Gazendam-Donofrio SM, Hoekstra-Webers JE. Screening and referral for psychological distress in oncologic practice: use of the distress thermometer. Cancer. 2008;113:870–8.
57. Lewis S, Salins N, Kadam A, Rao R. Distress screening using distress thermometer in head and neck cancer patients undergoing radiotherapy and evaluation of causal factors predicting occurrence of distress. Indian J Palliat Care. 2013;19:88–92.
58. Archer J, Hutchison I, Korszun A. Mood and malignancy: head and neck cancer and depression. J Oral Pathol Med. 2008;37:255–70.
59. Hermann C. International experiences with the hospital anxiety and depression scale – a review of validation data and clinical results. J Psychosom Res. 1997;42:17–41.
60. Crawford JR, Henry JD, Crombie C, Taylor EP. Normative data for the HADS from a large non-clinical sample. Br J Clin Psychol. 2001;40:429–343.
61. List MA, D'Antonio LL, Cella DF, Siston A, Mumby P, Haraf D, et al. The performance status scale for head and neck cancer patients and the functional assessment of cancer therapy-head and neck scale. A study of utility and validity. Cancer. 1996;77:2294–301.
62. Neilson KA, Pollard A, Boonzaier AM, Corry J, Castle DJ, Mead KR, et al. Psychological distress (depression and anxiety) in people with head and neck cancers. Med J Aust. 2010;193:S48–51.
63. First MB, Gibbon M, Spitzer RL, JBW W. User's guide for the structural clinical interview for DSM-IV axis I disorders: SCID-I. Washington: American Psychiatric Press; 1997. Clinical versions.
64. Wu Y-S, Lin P-T, Chien C-Y, Fang F-M, Chiu N-M, Hung C-F, et al. Anxiety and depression in patients with head and neck cancer: 6-month follow-up study. Neuropsychiatr Dis Treat. 2016;12:1029–36.
65. O'Farrell E, Smith A, Collins B. Objective-subjective disparity in cancer-related cognitive impairment: does the use of change measures help reconcile the difference? Psycho-Oncology. 2017;26:1667–74.
66. Darby D, Maruff P, Collie A. Repeated administration of a cognitive test battery in mild cognitive impairment. Neurology. 2002;59:1042–6.
67. Peterman AH, Fitchett G, Brady MJ, Hernandez L, Cella D. Measuring spiritual wellbeing in people with cancer: The Functional Assessment of Chronic Illness Therapy-Spiritual Wellbeing scale (FACIT-Sp). Ann Behav Med. 2002;24:49–58.

68. Whitford HS, Olver IN. The multidimensionality of spiritual wellbeing: peace, meaning and faith and their association with quality of life and coping in oncology. Psycho-Oncology. 2012;21:602–10.
69. Carrera P, Olver I. The financial hazard of personalised medicine. Support Care Cancer. 2015;23:3399–401.
70. Carrera O, Ormond M. Current practice in and considerations for personalised medicine in lung cancer: from the patient's molecular biology to patient values and preferences. Maturitas. 2015;82:94–9.
71. De Souza JA, Yap BJ, Wroblewski K, Blinder V, Araújo FS, Hlubocky FJ, et al. Measuring financial toxicity as a clinically relevant patient-reported outcome: the validation of the Comprehensive Score for Financial Toxicity (COST). Cancer. 2017;123:476–84.
72. Remesh A. Toxicities of anticancer drugs and its management. Int J Basic Clin Pharmacol. 2012;1:2–12.
73. Baek JH, Kim JG, Lim SN, Kim DH, Sohn SK, Hong YJ, et al. Unpredicted severe toxicity after 5-Fluorouracil treatment due to dihydropyrimidine dehydrogenase deficiency. Korean J Int Med. 2006;21:43–5.
74. Cohen EEW, Lictra LF, Burtness B, Fayette J, Gauler T, Clement PM, et al. Biomarkers predict enhanced clinical outcomes with afatinib versus methotrexate in patients with second-line recurrent and/or metastatic head and neck cancer. Ann Oncol. 2017;28:2526–32.
75. The Pharmaceutical Benefits Scheme. Afatinib. http://www.pbs.gov.au/info/industry/listing/elements/pbac-meetings/psd/2013-07/afatinib-second-third-line. Accessed 12 Sept 2018.
76. Specenier P, Vermorken J. Cetuximab: its unique place in head and neck cancer treatment. Biologics. 2013;7:77–90.
77. Udall M, Rizzo M, Kenny J, Doherty J, Dahm S, Robbins P, et al. PD-L1 diagnostic tests: a systematic literature review of soring algorithms and test-validation metrics. Diagn Pathol. 2018;13:12. https://doi.org/10.1186/s13000-018-0689-9.
78. Marshall HT, Djamgoz MBA. Immuno-oncology: emerging targets and combination therapies. Front Oncol. 2018;19:315. https://doi.org/10.3389/fonc.2018.00315.

Photobiomodulation and Light Therapy in Oncology

17

Mechanisms and Positive or Negative Effects on Cancer

Michael R. Hamblin

17.1 Introduction

Nearly all patients with advanced head and neck cancer (HNC) suffer complications from treatment with radiation therapy (RT) or chemoradiotherapy (CRT) [1]. CRT is currently the standard of care with or without surgery in advanced HNC. Typically, there is an increased frequency and severity of side effects, particularly when chemotherapy (CT) is combined with accelerated or hyperfractionated RT regimens. It is now recognized that organ preservation in HNC treatment is not synonymous with function preservation, and effects on quality of life (QoL) must be considered in cancer treatment planning and extending survival [2, 3].

RT to the head and neck, with or without CT, damages adjacent tissues within the radiation field despite continuing efforts to minimize these effects [1]. Furthermore, targeted therapies whether they are administered as single agents, or combined with RT or CRT, may generate additional symptoms [4–6]. Acute complications in the orofacial region and neck include oral mucositis (OM), pain, dysphagia, infections, salivary changes, dysgeusia, and dermatitis. Common chronic complications are hyposalivation and xerostomia, mucosal infections, mucosal atrophy, neuropathies including mucosal pain, dysgeusia, tooth decalcification and rampant caries, progression of periodontitis, soft tissue and/or bone necrosis, mucocutaneous and muscular fibrosis, dysphagia, trismus, lymphedema, dermatitis, and voice and speech alterations. The severity of complications varies depending upon the type and site of the tumor, mode and intensity of therapies involved, and individual patient characteristics. Orofacial and neck complications are associated with morbidity and

M. R. Hamblin (✉)
Laser Research Centre, University of Johannesburg, Doornfontein, Johannesburg, South Africa

Radiation Biology Research Center, Iran University of Medical Sciences, Tehran, Iran

R. Nair (ed.), *Orofacial Supportive Care in Cancer*,
https://doi.org/10.1007/978-3-030-86510-8_17

mortality and increased use of health-care resources and costs and may compromise patient adherence to cancer therapy protocols resulting in suboptimal outcomes. Most patients develop multiple complications, which result in a significant burden of illness with negative impact on QoL [1, 7–9].

Supportive care addressing these complications must continue from the initial diagnosis of HNC, through treatment and survival. However, many interventions have limitations and are primarily palliative in nature [10].

17.2 Photobiomodulation or Low-Level Laser Therapy

Among the presently available supportive care measures, low-level laser therapy (PBM) now known as photobiomodulation (PBM) has shown significant promise. PBM refers to the use of light therapy that may control pain, stimulate tissue regeneration, and reduce inflammation. These treatments were originally referred to as "low-level laser" because the light was of relatively low intensity compared with other forms of medical laser treatment, which were used for ablation, cutting, and coagulation. However, at the 2014 joint North American Association for Laser Therapy (NAALT) and World Association for Laser Therapy (WALT) conference, a consensus committee convened to discuss the diverse nomenclature, false positive database results, and inappropriate emphasis on the word "laser." PBM was accepted as the preferred name with the following definition: "The therapeutic use of light [e.g. visible, near infrared (NIR), infrared (IR)] absorbed by endogenous chromophores, triggering non-thermal, non-cytotoxic, biological reactions through photochemical or photophysical events, leading to physiological changes."

These photobiological reactions have been shown to occur in various tissues (skin, mucosa, muscle, tendon, ligament, cartilage, bone, nerve, lymph, brain, blood components, and blood vessels). Systematic reviews have suggested efficacy of PBM for OM management in hematopoietic stem cell transplant (HSCT) recipients and in HNC patients [11–16]. Whereas in most studies PBM is applied intra-orally on the oral mucosal tissues, studies indicate that it may also be administered extra-orally, with a resultant effect on structures at risk for OM. Transcutaneous PBM may enhance the ease of delivery and possibly the efficacy of treatment [14, 17]. In addition, new-generation PBM devices consisting of a cluster of laser or light-emitting diode (LED) beams, instead of a single laser beam, provide exposure of larger fields, and when used with appropriate parameters, the light is able to penetrate into tissues sufficiently to activate cellular processes [18]. This finding suggests that extra-oral administration of PBM (with or without concurrent use of intra-oral PBM) and taking advantage of advances in PBM technology enable the light to reach other anatomical structures of the head and neck at risk for RT- and CRT-induced complications. This may broaden the range of indications for PBM for the prevention and treatment of cancer treatment-induced complications.

A task force consisting of an international multidisciplinary panel of clinicians and researchers with expertise in the area of supportive care in cancer and/or PBM clinical application and dosimetry was formed. The mission of this group is to aid in the design of PBM study protocols, identify validated outcome measures, and test the efficacy and safety of proposed protocols for the management of complications related to cancer therapy.

The goals of the present chapter are to (1) discuss PBM mechanisms and safety issues; (2) identify selected oral, oropharyngeal, facial, and neck complications of treatment for HNC, in which PBM may have potential for prophylaxis and/or treatment; (3) propose PBM parameters for prophylaxis and therapy to mitigate these complications based on current evidence and knowledge; (4) address the possibility that PBM could exacerbate cancer and speculate whether instead it could be used a treatment for cancer; and (5) discuss directions of future research related to the use of PBM in HNC.

17.2.1 Mechanisms of Action of PBM

PBM has been consistently shown in laboratory studies to have distinct biological effects and has a dose-dependent mechanism of action at the cellular level [19, 20]. Since the introduction of PBM in 1967, over 400 randomized, double-blinded (some placebo-controlled) clinical trials have been published for multiple applications. The first clinical application of PBM was for enhancement of wound healing [21]. A meta-analysis including animal and human studies concluded that PBM was an effective tool for accelerating wound repair and tissue regeneration [22]. It has been shown that PBM influences different phases of wound healing including (1) the inflammatory phase, in which immune cells migrate to the site of tissue injury; (2) the proliferative phase, which includes stimulation of fibroblasts and macrophages as well as other repair components; and (3) the remodeling phase, consisting of collagen deposition and rebuilding of the extracellular matrix at the wound site [23].

Although the complex biological mechanisms underlying the therapeutic effects of PBM have not been completely elucidated and may vary among different cell types and tissue states (healthy versus stressed or hypoxic), laboratory and clinical studies suggest that PBM significantly reduces inflammation and prevents fibrosis [24–29]. Moreover, PBM, when delivered appropriately, reduces pain and improves optimal function [19, 30–32]. In addition, in vivo studies show that PBM is neuroprotective and may benefit neurodegenerative diseases and neurotrauma [33, 34].

Current data suggest that PBM acts predominantly on cytochrome c oxidase (CCO) in the mitochondrial respiratory chain by facilitating electron transport resulting in an increased transmembrane proton gradient that drives adenosine triphosphate (ATP) production [35]. ATP is the universal energy source in living cells essential for all biologic reactions, and even a small increase in ATP levels can enhance bioavailability to power the functions of cellular metabolism [36]. In addition, the absorption of red or NIR light may cause a short, transient burst of reactive oxygen species (ROS) that is followed by an adaptive reduction in oxidative stress. See Fig. 17.1 for a schematic illustration of the cellular and molecular mechanisms of PBM.

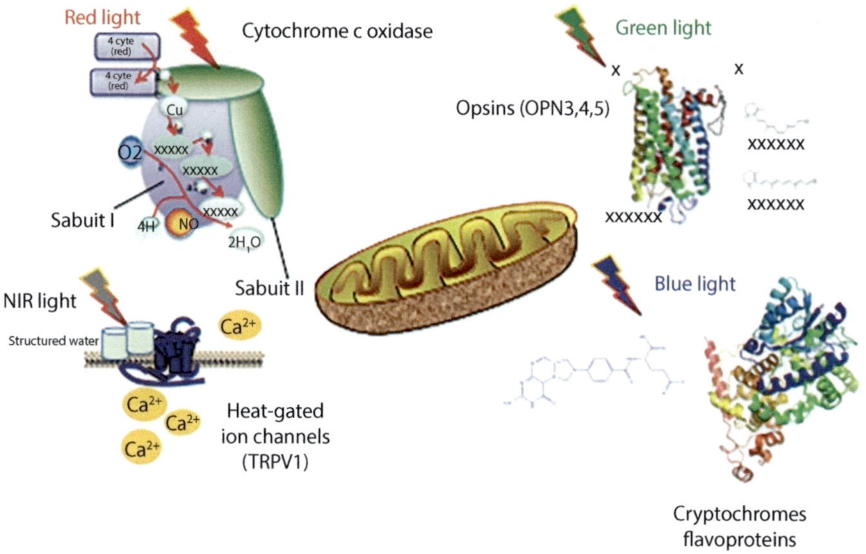

Fig. 17.1 Cellular and molecular mechanisms of photobiomodulation

A low concentration of ROS activates many cellular processes, since ROS activates transcription factors including nuclear factor kappa B (NF-κB), resulting in the upregulation of stimulatory and protective genes [37]. These genes generate growth factors belonging to the fibroblast growth factor family, cytokines, and chemokines that are involved in tissue repair.

In hypoxic or otherwise stressed cells, mitochondria produce nitric oxide (mtNO), which binds to CcO and displaces oxygen [38]. This binding results in inhibition of cellular respiration, decreased ATP production, and increased oxidative stress (a state that develops when the levels of ROS exceed the defense mechanisms), leading to the activation of intracellular signaling pathways, including several transcription factors [39]. These include redox factor-1 (Ref-1), activator protein-1 (AP-1), NF-κB, p53, activating transcription factor/cAMP-response element-binding protein (ATF/CREB), hypoxia-inducible factor (HIF)-1, and HIF-like factor [40]. These transcription factors induce downstream production of both inflammatory mediators, such as tumor necrosis factor-alpha (TNF-α), interleukin [IL]-1 and IL-6, cyclooxygenase (COX)-2, and prostaglandin E2 (PGE-2) [39, 41, 42], and anti-inflammatory mediators [transforming growth factor (TGF)-beta, IL-10]. There is evidence suggesting that when PBM is administered with appropriate parameters to stressed cells, NO is dissociated from its competitive binding to CcO, ATP production is increased, and the balance between pro- and antioxidant mediators is restored, resulting in a reduction of oxidative stress [43]. For example, PBM has been shown to attenuate the production of ROS by human neutrophils [44]. Silveira et al. [45] reported that PBM reduced ROS in an animal model of traumatic tissue injury, whereas a study in a model of acute lung inflammation found PBM to reduce the generation of TNF-α and to increase IL-10 [46]. In addition, NO is a potent vasodilator [47] and can increase the blood supply to the laser-illuminated tissue. PBM-mediated vascular regulation increases tissue oxygenation and also allows for greater traffic of immune cells, which may contribute to the promotion of wound repair and regeneration [39].

Analgesic effects are probably induced by additional mechanisms rather than by the increased ATP/reduced oxidative stress model. PBM with a relatively high power density (>300 mW/cm^2), when absorbed by nociceptors, has an inhibitory effect on A and C neuronal pain fibers. This slows neural conduction velocity, reduces amplitude of compound action potentials, and suppresses neurogenic inflammation [32].

Virtually all conditions modulated by PBM (e.g., ulceration, inflammation, edema, pain, fibrosis, neurological and muscular injury) are thought to be involved in the pathogenesis of (C)RT-induced complications in patients treated for HNC. For example, in an animal model of OM, it was demonstrated that PBM decreased COX-2 expression [48] and decreased the number of neutrophils in the inflammatory infiltrate [49]. Moreover, in the chronic sequelae of (C)RT, an excessive fibroblastic response was hypothesized to be related to acute oxidative injury, with resulting cell damage, ischemia, and an ongoing inflammatory response resulting in fibrosis [50]. The critical difference between normal wound healing and fibrosis development appears to be that, in fibrosis, signaling pathways escape normal cellular regulation [51]. Reduction of fibrosis could be mediated by the beneficial effects of PBM on the oxidant/antioxidant balance [52], downregulation of TGF-β, and inhibition of excessive fibroblast proliferation [53].

Although most studies have demonstrated efficacy in management of both acutely and chronically affected tissues, not all PBM investigations have yielded positive outcomes. As discussed below, these divergent results may be attributed to several factors, including dosimetry. It has been observed that increasing the overall dose of PBM may have a counterproductive effect compared with the benefit obtained with lower doses [54].

17.2.2 PBM Parameters

PBM parameters have been mostly studies using the red and NIR wavelength range of 600–1100 nm, with a power density of between 5 and 150 mW/cm^2, and are typically applied for 30–60 s per point, or for up to 10 min over a large area. The therapeutic effect is anticipated to be dictated by the energy density measured in J/cm^2. Evidence can be found in the literature for parameters as widely divergent as 0.1–12 J/cm^2. Commonly reported PBM devices include helium–neon (HeNe) gas laser, gallium arsenide (GaAs), neodymium-doped yttrium aluminum garnet (Nd:YAG), gallium aluminum arsenide (GaAlAs), indium gallium aluminum phosphide (InGaAlP) diode lasers, and non-thermal, non-ablative carbon dioxide (CO_2) lasers, and recently LED arrays have become significantly more common.

The PBM effects on the exposed tissues depend on cell type, redox state of the cell, irradiation parameters (wavelength, power density), and time of exposure [14, 54]. A biphasic dose response has been shown, which underlines that there are optimal irradiation and dose parameters, although these will vary according to the depth of the pathology below the mucosal surface or skin. Doses lower than the optimal value may have a diminished effect, while doses higher than optimal can have negative therapeutic outcomes [39, 54].

Thus for PBM to be effective, the irradiation parameters, including the energy delivered, power density, pulse structure, delivery to the appropriate anatomical location, appropriate treatment timing, and repetition, need to be within the biostimulatory dose windows [13, 39, 54–56].

For example, a study in which PBM was not found effective in reducing severe OM in HNC patients treated with CRT may have used too low a dose of energy [57].

Titrating adequate doses and defining the other required PBM parameters according to evidence gathered in a systematic way for each indication is a prerequisite for a successful use of this technique. Without standardization in beam measurement, dose calculation, and the correct reporting of these parameters, studies will not be reproducible, and outcomes will not be consistent. A common misconception is that wavelength and energy (in J) or energy density (J/cm^2) are all that is necessary in order to replicate a successful treatment, and that it does not matter what the original power, power density, and duration parameters are [58, 59].

A checklist to help researchers understand and report all the necessary parameters for a reproducible scientific study has been developed (Table 17.1) [59]. It is not uncommon to find discrepancies between the specifications provided by a device manufacturer and the actual performance of the device [60]. Therefore, device maintenance including power measurements should be carried out regularly during research trials and also in clinical practice.

Table 17.1 Necessary parameters for a reproducible scientific study

Manufacturer
Model identifier
Year produced
Number & type of emitters [laser or LED]
Wavelength and bandwidth [nm]
Pulse mode [CW or Hz, duty cycle]
Beam spot size at target [cm2]
Irradiance at target [mW/cm2]
If pulsed peak irradiance [mW/cm2]
Exposure duration [s]
Radiant exposure [J/cm2]
Radiant energy [J]
Number of points irradiated
Area irradiated [cm2]
Application technique [contact or distance]
Number and frequency of treatment sessions
Total radiant energy over entire treatment course [J]

17.3 Potential Effects of PBM on Cancer Cells and Tumors

Since its first use clinically in the late 1960s, the potential for PBM to impact cancer risk or development, as well as possible uses in directly combating cancer itself, has been studied sporadically. However, the potential effects of PBM on tumor, including tumor protection, tumor promotion, no (direct) effects, or beneficial effects, require ongoing studies before definitive conclusions can be made.

17.3.1 Effects on Molecular Pathways and Tumor Cells In Vitro

A vast amount of progress has been made in the past decade to advance our understanding of the molecular biology which drives squamous cell carcinoma of the head and neck (HNSCC) and the mechanism of action of PBM. Activation of the PI3K/AKT/mTOR pathway is associated with many of the activities that may be associated with PBM's favorable impact on wound healing: cell survival, migration, proliferation, and angiogenesis. Yet PI3K/AKT/mTOR signaling is also among commonly dysregulated pathways associated with cancer, including HNSCC [61], and its activation has been reported to promote the acquisition of epithelial-mesenchymal transition, cancer stem cell phenotypes, and cancer radioresistance [62]. Conversely, inhibition of the pathway has been viewed as a potential strategy to increase radiation sensitivity of tumor cells [63]. Recently reported data suggest that the migration of oral keratinocytes noted to occur following PBM is attributable to activation of the AKT/mTOR signaling pathway [64]. Consequently, the observation reported by Sperandio et al. [65] that PBM modified the expression of proteins related to the progression and invasion of oral cancer cell lines suggests that PBM activation of the Akt/mTOR signaling pathway may not be desirable. The lack of data obtained from in vivo models or patients leaves open the question of the breadth of PBM effects on malignant cells and nonmalignant tissue. For example, assuming Akt/mTOR is activated by PBM, would tumor tissue be affected if it was distant from the site of phototherapy application, i.e., treating the mouth for OM in an individual being treated for a hypopharyngeal cancer?

TGF-β may play contradictory roles relative to tumor behavior [66]. While its tumor suppressive effects are notable in the early stages of carcinogenesis, it may promote growth and spread of established tumors. Through serine/threonine kinases and Smad effectors, TGF-β can act as a tumor suppressor by inhibiting proliferation and inducing apoptosis [67]. Conversely, it may be overproduced by human tumors and is associated with induction of epithelial-mesenchymal transition, the prelude to tumor invasiveness, angiogenesis, suppression of elements of immune surveillance, and recruitment of signaling pathways that may facilitate metastases [68]. Additionally, it appears that TGF-β1 signaling may enhance tumor progression by altering the surrounding stroma through Smad signaling [69]. Thus, the observation that PBM stimulates TGF-β/smad signaling pathway [70] could be viewed as a double-edge sword depending on when and what tissue was exposed [71].

Mitogen-activated protein kinase (MAPK) pathways play a significant role in cancer [72]. Among the MAPK pathways, perhaps the best studied relative to cancer is the ERK pathway. ERK signaling is associated with a number of tumor behaviors. Of relevance to HNC is a correlation of its expression with increased epithelial growth factor receptor (EGFR) [73]. The ERK pathway also impacts vascular epithelial growth factor (VEGF) expression and its consequent angiogenesis. While angiogenesis may be desirable from a wound healing perspective, the finding that PBM stimulates EGFR and VEGF production through ERK signaling may be a concern in a tumor environment [74, 75].

The biological robustness of PBM is borne out by the observations of its ability to stimulate a range of biological processes including upregulation of heat shock proteins (HSP) [76] and microRNAs [77]. Relative to the current discussion, HSP is essential for cancer survival and has been identified as a potential target for anti-cancer therapy. While the number of miRNAs that are upregulated following PBM is substantial, of particular note is the finding that mi126 is among the list as endogenous mi126 has been reported to be associated with metastatic progression [78].

While the information above raises questions about possible undesirable effects of PBM on tumor progression and response to anti-cancer treatment, some observations suggest that PBM might favorably impact tumor behavior through its effects on vimentin expression, MyD88-dependent signaling, reduction in TLR-4, and down-regulation of NF-κB [33]. Furthermore, upregulation of ATP signaling by PBM may promote apoptosis, as well as differentiation of tumor cells, thereby slowing down tumor proliferation [35, 79].

The lack of consistent findings and/or the latitude of interpretation of the clinical significance of these findings hampers meaningful conclusions. The molecular mechanisms outlined above indicate the need to continue study addressing the molecular pathways affected by PBM.

The effects of PBM on cell proliferation and differentiation have been investigated in vitro using malignant cell lines, which have generated conflicting data across a range of different tumor cell lines and PBM parameters [80–84]. For example, Kreisler and coworkers reported proliferation of laryngeal carcinoma cells after 809 nm GaAlAs laser irradiation at energy densities between 1.96 and 7.84 J/cm^2 [81]. Werneck and coworkers also found increased cell proliferation of HEp2 carcinoma cells after PBM exposure at different wavelengths (685 and 830 nm) and doses [85]. In a study comparing PBM administered to normal osteoblasts and to osteosarcoma cells with a range of different wavelengths and doses, only 10 J/cm^2 from an 830 nm laser was able to enhance osteoblast proliferation, whereas energy densities of 1, 5, and 10 J/cm^2 from a 780 nm laser decreased proliferation. Osteosarcoma cells were unaffected by 830 nm laser irradiation, whereas 670 nm laser had a mild proliferative effect [86]. An in vitro study compared the effects of different doses of PBM at various wavelengths on human breast carcinoma and melanoma cell lines [87]. Although certain doses of PBM increased breast carcinoma cell proliferation, multiple exposures had either no effect or showed negative dose response relationships. PBM (wavelength 660 nm) administered in low doses (1 J/cm^2) increased in vitro proliferation and potentially increased invasive potential of tongue SCC cells [88]. Similarly, another in vitro study suggested that

PBM (660 or 780 nm, 40 mW, 2.05, 3.07, or 6.15 J/cm^2) may stimulate oral dysplastic and oral cancer cells to a more aggressive behavior [65].

In contrast, a decreased mitotic rate was found in gingival squamous cell carcinoma (SCC) after PBM at 805 nm and energy density of 4 and 20 J/cm^2 [83], whereas no effect on cell proliferation or protein expression of osteosarcoma cells was found when PBM was administered with a wavelength of 830 nm [89]. PBM (808 nm; 5.85 and 7.8 J/cm^2) had an inhibitory effect on the proliferation of a human hepatoma cell line [90], and Sroka et al. [91] reported that glioblastoma/astrocytoma cells exhibited a slightly decreased mitotic rate after PBM at 805 nm and 5–20 J/cm^2. Similarly, 808 nm laser irradiation with an energy density of more than 5 J/cm^2 inhibited cell proliferation of glioblastoma cells in vitro [92]. Moreover, Al Watban et al. [93] observed growth inhibition of cancer cell lines at relatively high cumulative PBM doses. This prompted Crous and Abrahamse [94] to hypothesize that PBM may have a therapeutic potential in lung cancer.

It seems unlikely that PBM has carcinogenic effects on normal cells. The non-ionizing wavelengths of the red and NIR spectrum used in PBM are far longer than the safety limit of 320 nm for DNA damage [95]. No signs of malignant transformation in non-malignant epithelial cells and fibroblasts were observed following exposure to PBM with a wavelength of 660 nm, 350 mW for 15 min during 3 consecutive days [96]. In addition, no malignant transformation of normal breast epithelial cells was detected in an in vitro study comparing the effects of different doses and wavelengths of PBM during multiple exposures [87].

The results from these studies suggest that different tumor cells have distinct responses to specific PBM parameters and doses. In part, these differences may be also explained by variations in the cellular microenvironment, since these have been shown to affect cellular signal transduction pathways to PBM exposure [97]. The microenvironment of tumor cells varies among in vitro studies and differs significantly from that found in animal models. Moreover, this difference implies that the potential of PBM to enhance proliferation of tumor cells in vitro does not necessarily translate into harmful effects of PBM in cancer patients.

17.3.2 Can PBM Make Cancer Worse in Animal Models?

PBM (660 nm, 30 mW, 424 mW/cm^2, 56.4 J/cm^2, 133 s, 4 J) applied to chemically induced SCC in hamster cheek pouch tissue, increased tumor growth [98]. PBM at a dose of 150 J/cm^2 appeared safe, with only minor effects on B16F10 melanoma cell proliferation in vitro, and had no significant effect on tumor growth in vivo. Only a high power density (2.5 W/cm^2) combined with a very high dose of 1050 J/cm^2 could induce melanoma tumor growth in vivo [99]. In a mouse model to study PBM effects on UV-induced skin tumors, the experimental mice received full-body 670 nm PBM delivered twice a day at 5 J/cm^2 for 37 days, whereas controls received sham PBM [100]. No enhanced tumor growth was observed, whereas there was a small but significant reduction in tumor area in the PBM group, potentially related to a local photodynamic effect or PBM-induced antitumor immune activity.

Current evidence suggests that PBM in the red or NIR spectrum, with an energy density of 1–6 J/cm^2 is safe and effective, which suggests that it should not be withheld from HNC patients. However, the potential effect on dysplastic and malignant cells has not been definitively resolved. Virtually all studies have focused on cell-based assays rather than conventional xenograft or orthotopic animal models. And the results of in vitro investigations have been largely dependent on the experimental design and selection of target cells. Key biologic effects of wavelength, energy density, and time/duration of exposure are important measures of PBM characteristics that must be recognized and evaluated. As robust evidence for the lack of malignant cell protection or enhancement of tumor growth has not been published, vigilance remains warranted.

17.3.3 Can PBM Directly or Indirectly Attack Cancer?

When we consider the possibility that PBM can have a beneficial effect on cancer, it is important to realize that there are three possible ways by which this may happen (Fig. 17.2). The first involves the direct effect of the light on the tumor cells themselves and may be thought of as a deliberate use of the biphasic dose response curve to "overdose" the cancer cells [101]. This possible methodology has been championed by Da Xing's laboratory in China [102]. They call this approach "high fluence low-power laser irradiation, HF-LPLI," and this group often uses a 632 nm HeNe

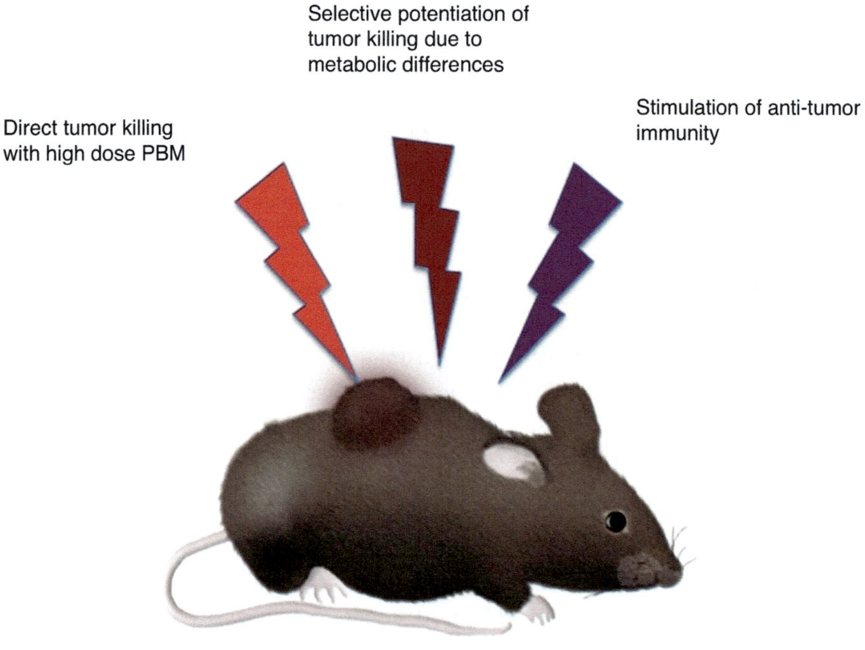

Fig. 17.2 Possible mechanisms by which PBM could be applied against cancer

laser delivering 1200 J/cm^2 at 500 mW/cm^2, over 40 min [103]. After publishing several in vitro papers, they carried out an in vivo study in BALB/c mice bearing EMT6 breast tumors [104]. A single dose of 1200 J/cm^2 caused complete regression of tumors, which did not occur in rho-zero EMT6 tumors (lacking functional mitochondria). Moreover, since EMT6 tumors are known to be immunogenic, the mice that were cured of cancer showed some long-term immunological memory.

The second method relies on taking advantage of a differential effect of PBM between malignant cancer cells compared to the effects seen on healthy normal cells. This involves combining PBM with an additional cytotoxic anti-cancer therapy, so that it increases the killing of cancer cells, while at the same time protecting normal healthy cells. While this may appear "too good to be true," there are some scientific reasons why it may in fact be the case. These considerations are related to the Warburg effect, by which the mitochondria of cancer cells change their metabolism to carry out aerobic glycolysis instead of oxidative phosphorylation [105]. This phenomenon occurs due to the rapid growth of tumor cells outpacing the development of a sufficient blood supply, forcing the cancer cells to become tolerant to chronic hypoxia. Glycolysis consumes much less oxygen than oxidative phosphorylation. The consequences of the Warburg effect are that malignant cells and normal cells may behave very differently in response to PBM. In cancer cells, where ATP supply is quite limited, the ATP boost given by PBM may allow the cancer cells to respond to pro-apoptotic cytotoxic stimuli with more efficiently executed cell death programs which are heavily energy-dependent (require a lot of ATP). On the other hand, in normal healthy cells that have an adequate supply of ATP, the effect of PBM produces a burst of ROS that could induce protective mechanisms and reduce the damaging effects of cancer therapy on healthy tissue (Fig. 17.3). Although this favorable scenario remains a hypothesis at present, there are some published papers that suggest it could indeed be the case in some anti-cancer strategies, such as reports that PBM can potentiate the killing of cancer cells by photodynamic therapy [106] and also by radiation therapy [107]. Similarly, there are no data to suggest that PBM may protect cancer cells against the cytotoxic effects of RT. Schartinger et al. [96] observed a pro-apoptotic effect of PBM in HNSCC cells, whereas no anti-apoptotic effects occurred that might promote tumor cell resistance to cancer therapy. Increased apoptosis of human osteosarcoma cells was also induced by the administration of NIR (810 nm, continuous wave, 20 mW/cm^2, 1.5 J/cm^2) prior to NPe6-mediated photodynamic therapy as a result of increased cellular ATP and a higher uptake of the photosensitizer [108].

These researchers have reported that, in theory, PBM increases cell death in cancer cells in response to cytotoxic stimuli. Alternatively, while in normal cells, PBM will exert its protective effect as is well known in the case of neurotoxins, for example [109].

Furthermore, Schaffer et al. [110] observed that PBM increased the locoregional blood flow that contributed to better local oxygenation and hypothesized that PBM applied shortly before cancer treatment might enhance the effect of ionizing RT and local chemotherapy.

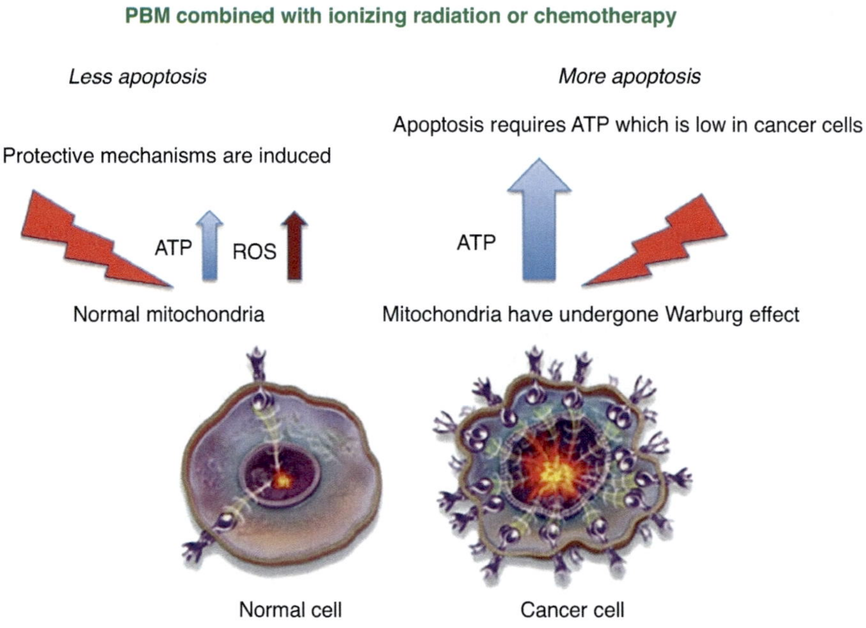

Fig. 17.3 Mechanisms of selective potentiation of cytotoxicity against cancer cells while preserving normal cells

The third mechanism, by which PBM could be beneficial to cancer patients, is its possible role in stimulation of the immune system to fight against the cancer. Ottaviani et al. [111] showed in a mouse model of melanoma that PBM using three different protocols (660 nm, 50 mW/cm^2, 3 J/cm^2; 800 nm or 970 nm, 200 mW/cm^2, 6 J/cm^2, once a day for 4 days) could all reduce tumor growth, increase the recruitment of immune cells (in particular T lymphocytes and dendritic cells secreting type I interferons). PBM also reduced the number of highly angiogenic macrophages within the tumor mass and promoted vessel normalization, which is another strategy to control tumor progression.

17.3.4 Is There Evidence of Clinical Efficacy Using PBM for Cancer in Humans?

A very interesting recent paper [112] reported that PBM could actually increase treatment outcome and progression-free survival in cancer patients. Ninety-four patients diagnosed with oropharynx, nasopharynx, and hypopharynx cancer were subjected to conventional radiotherapy plus cisplatin every 3 weeks. Preventive PBM was applied to nine points on the oral mucosa daily, from Monday to Friday, and lasted on average of 45.7 days. The PBM parameters were 660 nm, 100 mW, 4 J/cm^2, and spot size of 0.24 cm^2. Over a follow-up period of 41 months, patients receiving PBM had a statistically significant better complete response to treatment than those in the placebo group ($p = 0.013$). Patients subjected to PBM had better progression-free survival than those in the placebo group ($p = 0.030$) and had a tendency for better overall survival. The mechanism(s) for this effect require more investigation. It could be that the avoidance of oral mucositis led to better nutrition and more complete chemoradiotherapy, while it is also possible that the PBM exerted a direct anti-cancer effect.

Santana-blank et al. [113] carried out a Phase 1 trial of PBM on 17 patients suffering from a variety of "advanced malignancies." They used a 3 MHz pulsed laser (904 nm delivering 45 J/cm^2 at an average power of 35 mW) applied to a 1 cm^2 spot on the chest described as "biologically closed electric circuit and the vascular interstitial closed circuit" [114]. Patients were given a laser device to use at home each day and were allowed to remain in the trial as long as possible. Patients were asked to keep a journal over the length of their time in the trial and to record the time and duration of each PBM application as well as any sign, symptom, or problem/side effect experienced. No dose-limiting toxicity was observed. Five patients reported occasional headaches (grade 2), and four referred local pain (grade 2). Statistically significant increases in Karnovsky performance status (KPS) and quality-of-life (QLI) were observed in all of the follow-up intervals compared with pretreatment values. In the six surviving patients, one patient had a complete response, one partial response, four stable disease >12 months, and one progressive disease. In the patients that died during the trial, significant increases in QLI were observed during the first two intervals. Eight patients had stable disease >6 months and two had progressive disease. The mechanisms operating in this clinical study require more investigation, but if it can be repeated, it could be very promising.

Finally, Russian investigators have reported use of PBM in cancer patients, but it is difficult to retrieve details of the studies [115, 116].

17.4 Clinical Applications of PBM for Cancer Therapy Side Effects

A wide variety of cancer therapy side effects have been proposed to be amenable to treatment or amelioration with various kinds of photobiomodulation therapy as shown in Fig. 17.4.

17.4.1 Oral Mucositis

Oral mucositis affects virtually all patients undergoing CRT for HNC. Clinically, the manifestations of OM form a continuum, with erythematous mucosal changes when mild and ulcerative lesions that expose the submucosa when severe. The detrimental effects of OM upon QoL and functional status are significant [7].

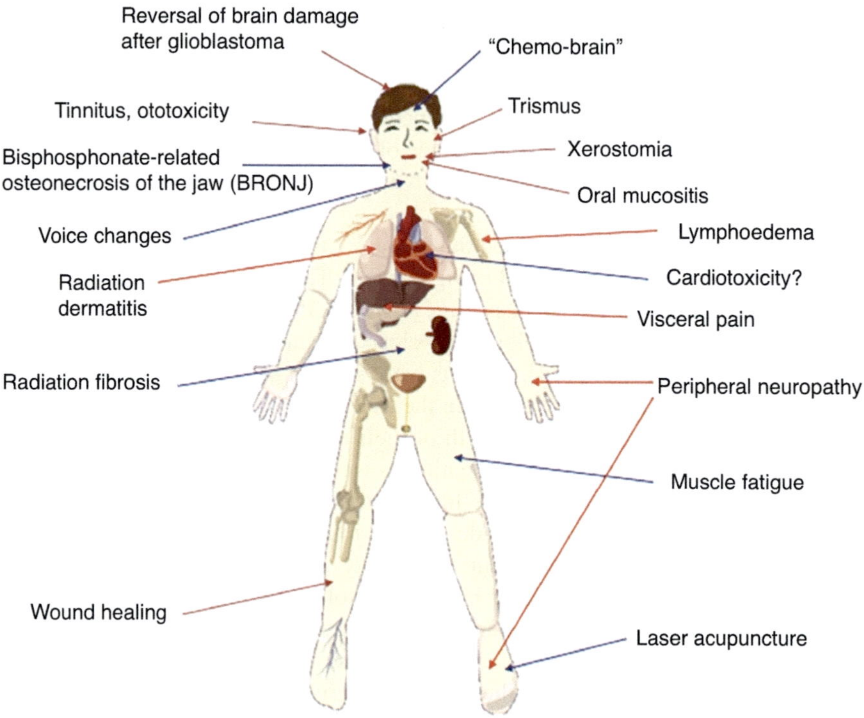

Fig. 17.4 A variety of cancer therapy side effects that may be treated with photobiomodulation therapy

The current understanding of the pathogenesis of OM is largely based on animal models, which have shown the multifactorial nature of the condition and have implicated a cascade of interrelated events in multiple tissue compartments. These observations lead to the five-phase model of OM, based on the sequence of events following cytotoxic treatment [117]. The formation of excessive ROS and activation of NF-κB are the key factors in its pathobiology. Subsequent studies implicated microvascular injury, formation of proinflammatory cytokines, host–microbiome interactions, and extracellular matrix alterations in mucositis pathogenesis [118]. In addition, EGFR inhibitors and tyrosine kinase receptor inhibitors (TKI) administered as single drugs or combined with CRT may enhance OM or cause additional symptoms [5, 6]. Effective management options for OM are limited [119], and pain control is typically inadequate [7].

A Cochrane meta-analysis concluded that PBM may prevent severe OM [11]. A systematic review and meta-analysis of 11 RCTs in HNC patients treated with CT and/or RT concluded that there was consistent evidence that PBM applied with doses of 1–6 J per point reduced OM prevalence, severity and duration, and its associated pain [13]. Another meta-analysis including RCTs in various cancer treatment settings showed that PBM reduced OM risk and decreased its severity and duration [14]. The efficacy appeared to be similar for red (630–670 nm) and

NIR (780–830 nm) light, although the optimal doses seemed to vary between these wavelengths. Similarly, a systematic review and meta-analysis including 18 RCTs reported that prophylactic PBM reduced severe OM and associated pain in patients treated for HNC or undergoing HSCT [16]. The Clinical Practice Guidelines of the Multinational Association of Supportive Care in Cancer and International Society for Oral Oncology (MASCC/ISOO) Mucositis Study Group found evidence for PBM prevention of OM in patients undergoing HSCT and patients treated with RT for HNC [15, 120]. Evidence was derived from high-quality studies using specific PBM parameters and the authors noted that there remains a need to identify optimal PBM parameters per cancer type and cancer treatment modality (see Chap. 5 for PBM recommendations for oral mucositis).

17.4.2 Dermatitis

Radiation dermatitis occurs in the majority of patients with locoregionally advanced HNC treated with RT. The pathobiology of acute radiation dermatitis is complex and partially overlaps that of OM. Irradiation of the skin leads to direct tissue injury and inflammatory cell recruitment, involving damage to epidermal basal cells, endothelial cells, and vascular components [121]. Radiation-induced generation of free radicals induces DNA injury and release of inflammatory cytokines (mainly IL-1 and IL-6) [122, 123]. This process leads to development of erythema, edema, and possible ulceration. Late RT-induced changes involving skin are characterized by the disappearance of follicular structures, an increase in collagen and damage to elastic fibers in the dermis, and a fragile epidermal covering [124]. TGF-β is considered to play a central role in mediating RT-induced tissue fibrosis [51, 125, 126].

The severity of skin reactions is dependent on the total radiation dose, the dose per fraction, the overall treatment time, beam type and energy, the surface area of the skin exposed to radiation, the use of combined chemoradiotherapy with or without targeted therapies, and individual risk factors [122]. The severity of acute reactions has been shown to predict late effects. Radiation dermatitis impacts adversely on cosmesis and function, especially in patients who develop secondarily infected dermatitis, and reduces QoL [121].

Patients with SCC of the head and neck treated with an EGFR inhibitor may develop an acneiform skin rash in addition to radiation dermatitis [6, 124]. Based on the effects of PBM on the epidermis and dermis (reduced inflammation and improved wound healing), and on the shared similarities in pathobiology with OM, it is reasonable to assume that PBM may reduce the severity and/or prevalence of radiation dermatitis [127, 128]. A study in pigs suggested that multi-wavelength PBM ameliorated the development of late radiation damage to the skin [129]. DeLand et al. [130] reported that LED treatments immediately after IMRT reduced the incidence of radiation dermatitis in patients with breast cancer; however, Fife et al. [131] were not able to reproduce these results, although they did not specify important parameters such as irradiation time and size of area treated. A case series report described promising results for PBM treatment at an NIR wavelength (970 nm) in patients with EGFR inhibitor-induced facial rash.

17.4.3 Dysphagia

Acute and chronic dysphagia (difficulty swallowing) and odynophagia (painful swallowing) are common in HNC patients, due to primary disease (oral, oropharyngeal, laryngeal, and esophageal cancers) and those treated with RT or CRT [132, 133]. Dysphagia can be due to anatomical, mechanical, or neurological changes affecting any structure from the lips to the gastric cardia [134]. Nguyen et al. [135] found 60% of patients to have dysphagia following CRT, of which 45% had severe dysphagia a median of 17 months post-treatment, and chronic dysphagia is not likely to resolve over time [136].

Dysphagia associated with CRT has a complex pathogenesis, involving acute inflammation, edema, and fibrosis, with consequent neurological and muscular injury that may result in generalized weakness and a lack of muscle coordination while swallowing [137, 138]. Excessive fibrosis results in a loss of elasticity that may contribute to chronic dysphagia [139, 140]. In addition, hyposalivation may contribute to dysphagia following CRT [8]. Moreover, the duration of total parenteral nutrition (TPN) or nasogastric tube feeding and resulting reduced swallowing may affect the ability to return to safe, normal oral intake, since inactivity will cause atrophy of the swallowing muscles [141, 142]. Dysphagia negatively affects QoL [8, 143] and may predispose to aspiration and life-threatening pulmonary complications [136, 144].

Intensity-modulated radiation therapy (IMRT) has emerged as an effective technique to deliver the full radiation dose to the tumor and regions at risk while reducing exposure of surrounding healthy tissues. Eisbruch and coworkers [145] identified dysphagia and aspiration risk structures (DARS) as susceptible to damage during IMRT. In particular, damage to the tongue base, pharyngeal constrictors, the larynx, and the autonomic neural plexus was found to be crucial in the development of post-RT dysphagia. Studies confirmed that reducing the radiation dose to DARS decreases dysphagia risk [146–148], but dysphagia remains a significant clinical problem [149].

The potential role of PBM in the prevention and treatment of dysphagia requires further investigation. One study reported a lower incidence of severe OM and mucositis affecting the throat (contributing to acute dysphagia) when six predetermined oral sites were exposed to PBM prior to and during RT [150]. In this study, dysphagia was scored indirectly by assessing the need for TPN. Given the ability of PBM to prevent and ameliorate inflammation and pain associated with OM, and potential to control exuberant fibrosis [53], PBM delivered to the DARS structures may have a potential role in the management of acute and chronic dysphagia.

17.4.4 Hyposalivation and Xerostomia

Another significant complication of RT to the head and neck region is hyposalivation and its related complaint of xerostomia (subjective oral dryness). For all head and neck radiation regimens pooled, the weighted prevalence of xerostomia was found to be 6% before treatment, 93% during irradiation, and a slightly lower prevalence from 1 month to more than 2 years post-treatment [151]. Saliva plays an important role in maintaining mucosal integrity, promoting oral wound healing, taste perception, formation of food bolus, initiation of food ingestion, swallowing, and speech [152]. Alterations in the oral microbiome, reduced oral clearance, changes in saliva composition (e.g., decreased buffer capacity, pH, immunoglobulin concentrations, defensins), and dietary changes may increase the risk for mucosal infections and rapidly progressing dental demineralization and caries [153]. A substantial decrease in salivary function has a significant impact on QoL and results in an increased burden of long-term dental care [154, 155].

Irradiation of the salivary glands results in loss of gland function, beginning early in the course of RT [156], and has been shown to induce apoptosis in parotid glands in a dose-dependent manner. This process is p53-dependent [157]. There can be a modest improvement in xerostomia a few months after RT suggesting that an adaptation or compensatory function of non-irradiated salivary glands or recovery of some of the function occurs. However, most patients have persisting oral dryness for the rest of their life, even when 3D conformal radiotherapy is used. With IMRT preserving more of the major salivary glands, long-term oral dryness may be reduced, but a significant proportion of patients still experience xerostomia [158].

The literature on PBM for the management of hyposalivation is limited. In a study involving a variety of non-cancer patients with xerostomia, PBM was applied daily: extra-orally to the parotid and submandibular glands and intra-orally on the sublingual glands. A gradual increase in the stimulated salivary flow was found after PBM compared to controls [159]. Similar results in non-cancer patients were reported by Vidović et al. [160]. Animal studies have shown an increase in the number of duct epithelial cell mitoses and stimulation to protein synthesis in submandibular glands following PBM [161, 162]. Similarly, a study reported the use of PBM to increase salivary flow rate and amylase activity in rat parotid glands [163]. These authors also performed a study in HNC patients and reported that PBM given concurrently with RT could prevent hyposalivation and xerostomia and had an impact on the composition of saliva [164]. Less severe xerostomia was also reported following prophylactic PBM in HSCT recipients [165], and in a small RCT in HNC patients treated with RT [166], and increased salivary flow was observed in PBM-treated patients when compared to controls [167]. A recent study performed in HNC patients at least 6 months following conventional RT found no improvement of hyposalivation and xerostomia, likely due to irreversible acinar atrophy and fibrosis [168].

These results point to the potential use of PBM for prevention of hyposalivation and xerostomia; PBM may also show efficacy for the treatment of hyposalivation when there is residual gland function following current RT modalities.

17.4.5 Taste Alterations

Taste is one of the five senses and interacts with smell, touch, and other physiological cues to affect the wider perception of flavor. Disturbed taste (dysgeusia) is complex and includes difficulties with smell and touch resulting in reduced food interest and affecting appetite and QoL. Taste function is the perception derived when food molecules stimulate taste receptors of the tongue, soft palate, and the oropharyngeal region to perceive basic taste qualities (sweet, sour, salty, bitter, and umami) that can be measured via standardized methods [169].

The prevalence of dysgeusia is estimated to be 66.5% following RT alone and 76.0% after CRT; approximately 15% of patients continued to experience dysgeusia after treatment [170]. Ohrn and colleagues reported that the severity of taste alterations assessed by patients was correlated with the cumulative RT dose [171].

The mechanisms of dysgeusia during cancer therapy are not well understood: however, it is believed that CT and RT cause dysgeusia by destroying rapidly dividing taste bud cells and olfactory receptor cells [170]. Direct neurologic toxicity may also be involved, as taste recovery lags epithelial recovery and may continue indefinitely [172]. Hyposalivation may also have a significant contribution. The presence of the anterior part of the tongue in the radiation field may be predictive of taste disturbances [173].

Altered taste significantly affects overall QoL and may lead to energy and nutrient deficiencies and related complications and weight loss [8, 170]. Management options to decrease the prevalence and severity of taste problems are inadequate [172].

A pilot study reported that PBM administered to taste buds may ameliorate neurologically mediated burning mouth syndrome symptoms including taste alterations [174], but to our knowledge, there are no published studies on PBM for the management of taste problems in cancer patients. Hence, we feel that studies on the efficacy of PBM for the management of dysgeusia in patients treated for HNC should be performed.

17.4.6 Trismus

Trismus refers to reduced opening of the jaws caused by spasm of the muscles of mastication, or may generally refer to all causes of limited mouth opening of less than 40 or less than 20 mm, whereas less restrictive classifications also have been used [175].

Limited mouth opening may be due to tumor, local infection, tissue fibrosis, pain upon mouth opening, a tonic contraction of the muscles of mastication, or intrinsic changes in the temporomandibular joint.

The weighted prevalence of trismus is estimated to be 25% following conventional RT, 5% following IMRT, and 31% for CRT [176]. Patients may have limitations in jaw opening associated with tumor invasion of the masticatory muscles or the temporomandibular joint or may develop trismus following RT to these structures [175, 177]. Cumulative radiation doses above 60 Gy are more likely to cause trismus [178], while the inclusion of the lateral pterygoid muscles in the high-dose fields appears to be the most decisive factor [179]. Trismus typically develops 3–6 months post RT and frequently becomes a lifelong problem [177, 180].

Studies have demonstrated that fibrosis is an important initial event in RT-induced trismus. Additionally, there may be scar tissue from surgery, nerve damage, or a combination of these factors [177]. Mandibular hypomobility ultimately results in muscle contraction and potentially temporomandibular joint dysfunction [176].

Trismus and orofacial pain interfering with function may have significant health implications including reduced nutritional intake, difficulty speaking, compromised oral health, and poor QoL [181]. Aside from avoiding RT to the masticatory structures, early interventions are indicated to prevent or minimize trismus [3, 148, 182].

Concerning muscle spasms following oral surgery, a reduction was found in several studies using PBM [183, 184]. To our knowledge, PBM to prevent or reduce the severity of RT-induced trismus in HNC patients has not been reported. The potential of PBM to reduce fibrosis and to promote muscle regeneration forms the main rationale for a potential clinical benefit.

17.4.7 Soft Tissue Necrosis and Osteoradionecrosis

Soft tissue and/or osteoradionecrosis (ORN) may occur as a consequence of RT. ORN is a process of radiation-induced vascular occlusion leading to loss of osteocytes and bone necrosis following RT [185]. The incidence of ORN has declined with proper pre-treatment dental care and advances in RT; in conventional RT, mandibular ORN prevalence ranges from 5% to 15%, but in the era of IMRT, less than 5% of patients are affected [177, 186].

The pathogenesis of ORN is not completely understood. It has been proposed that ORN occurs following a radiation-induced fibroatrophic process, including free radical formation, endothelial dysfunction, inflammation, microvascular thrombosis, fibrosis and remodeling, and finally bone and tissue necrosis [187]. Common triggers of necrosis are inflammatory dental disease, trauma to soft tissue, and dental surgical procedures in sites of high-dose radiation exposure to bone. Removing diseased teeth after RT is considered a critical risk factor for ORN, but the lesion can also emerge due to periodontal disease or trauma or spontaneously [188–190].

Prevention of ORN is mainly based on extractions of compromised teeth before RT and adequate dental care during and following cancer therapy [1, 185].

Over the last years, angiogenesis inhibitors have been introduced in the treatment of advanced HNC [191]. Bevacizumab, an antibody that blocks VEGF, may induce jaw osteonecrosis possibly as a result of tissue ischemia [192–194]. Bevacizumab may impair wound healing and can cause oral mucosal breakdown and exposure of necrotic jawbone [195]. Sunitinib, a tyrosine kinase inhibitor that blocks several pathways central to angiogenesis and tumor cell proliferation, has also been associated with osteonecrosis of the jaw [196, 197].

PBM has a biostimulation effect on irradiated rat bone when applied before and during RT [198], and similar results were reported by El-Maghraby et al. [199]. However, an in vivo study found that PBM was not able to reverse RT-induced bone damage [200]. To our knowledge, there are no clinical studies on the effects of PBM for RT-induced jaw osteonecrosis. However, multiple studies suggest there was a benefit from PBM in the management of bisphosphonate-related osteonecrosis of the jaw (BRONJ) [201–203]. Vescovi et al. proposed a prophylactic protocol including PBM for reducing BRONJ incidence following tooth extractions [204]. A study in a rodent wound healing model found evidence that both laser and LED were capable of stimulating angiogenesis in vivo [205]. These findings point to a possible role of PBM in the management of jaw osteonecrosis induced by RT or angiogenesis inhibitors.

17.4.8 Head and Neck Lymphedema

A commonly neglected late effect in patients treated for HNC is secondary lymphedema [206], although these complications may be reduced with IMRT. Patients may develop lymphedema externally, on the face and neck, and/or internally involving the larynx and pharynx. External lymphedema may have a profound effect on appearance and body image [207], whereas internal lymphedema may impact breathing, contribute to dysphagia and trismus, and may affect speech [208].

In a single center study on 81 HNC patients, 75% had lymphedema. Of those, 10% had external, 39% had internal, and 51% had both types of lymphedema [208]. Individuals with pharyngeal carcinoma were at highest risk [209]. Lymphedema typically develops 2–6 months after the completion of RT and may resolve spontaneously in some patients, but not in all. Assessment and measurement of head and neck lymphedema remain challenging [210].

Lymphedema is initiated by disruption of lymphatic structures by surgery or RT, resulting in the accumulation of lymph fluid in the interstitial tissues. This leads to infiltration of inflammatory cells, and, because of the lymphatic dysfunction, cytokines and chemokines remain in the tissue and recruit additional inflammatory cells from the circulation. This ongoing inflammatory response results in additional soft tissue damage and fibrosis, which further adversely affects lymphatic function [211].

Low level laser therapy has been identified as a potential treatment for post-mastectomy lymphedema, as it stimulates lymphangiogenesis, enhances lymphatic motility, and reduces lymphostatic fibrosis [212]. Patients received additional benefits from PBM when used in conjunction with standard lymphedema treatment [213]. Systematic reviews found evidence suggesting that PBM reduced limb volume in patients with lymphedema following treatment for breast cancer [214–216].

It was concluded that future research should be performed comparing PBM with standard practices and to establish the duration of laser application, number of treatment sessions, energy settings, power density, and dose. In addition, longer follow-up was considered necessary [215].

It has been proposed by Lee and coworkers that PBM may also have a role in the management of lymphedema associated with HNC [217].

17.4.9 Voice and Speech Alterations

Voice and speech are important communication tools and form part of a person's identity and personality. Voice quality mainly depends on the movement and characteristics of the vocal cords and speech on the resonance characteristics of the vocal tract. Speech is based on the volitional coordinated movements of the articulator structures and can be affected by any alteration in muscle or tissue properties of these structures. Although voice and speech dysfunctions significantly affect QoL, these complications have received little attention and are likely under-reported in efforts to preserve organ function after cancer therapy [218–220].

Currently, there is limited information on the prevalence of speech and voice dysfunction in advanced HNC patients treated with (C)RT, and prospective studies are needed, including baseline measurements and standardized multidimensional assessment of functional aspects of voice and speech [219].

The etiology of voice and speech problems resembles that of dysphagia and may include neuromuscular weakness as a result of tumor invasion. CRT-induced voice and/or speech dysfunction can result from mucositis of the soft palate and laryngeal soft tissues, fibrosis or vocal fold atrophy, edema and atrophy of laryngeal and pharyngeal tissues, and altered saliva or hyposalivation [221, 222].

New RT delivery techniques, including IMRT, designed to spare anatomical structures that are involved with voice and/or speech functions may prevent long-term functional impairment and early speech rehabilitation [223].

We are not aware of any studies on the effect of PBM on the quality of speech and voicing in HNC patients. They PBM may preserve function of the anatomical structures involved directly and could have indirect benefits by decreasing hyposalivation.

17.5 Conclusion

Acute and chronic complications induced by RT and CRT in patients with HNC represent a significant clinical challenge [1]. There are similarities with respect to pathophysiology across different complications, and patients may suffer from multiple concurrent and interrelated problems. There is anecdotal evidence suggesting that the inflammation associated with acute complications is a harbinger for chronic complications. This observation suggests that preventive approaches starting before, and in the early phases of treatment with RT and CRT, may reduce not only the risk for developing acute problems but may also have an impact on the risk for late complications.

PBM has shown effectiveness in the management of OM and elicits several potentially beneficial effects, including reduction of inflammation and pain, promotion of tissue repair, reduction of fibrosis, and protection and regeneration of nerves. Therefore, there is a clear motivation for the application of PBM to treat a broad range of acute and chronic complications associated with RT or CRT in HNC patients. RCTs should be conducted to assess the feasibility and efficacy of PBM for prophylactic and therapeutic management of the head and neck complications of cancer therapy.

We hope that this chapter will serve as the basis for establishing a platform for facilitating future collaborations among clinicians and researchers, which will then create firm scientific evidence for the use of PBM in patients with HNC. PBM and/or LED protocols should be administered using parameters that are likely to affect the anatomic structures at risk. The parameters (including the wavelengths) we have proposed are largely based on evidence derived from studies using PBM for the management of OM (typically 633–685 nm or 780–830 nm). However, trials directed to other (non-head and neck) indications for the use of PBM suggest that a broader range of wavelengths (590–1064 nm) has efficacy for healing, and for reducing inflammation and pain. Future investigations should be conducted to better define optimal photobiomodulation parameters for each of the complications of HNC treatment. In addition, the ideal timing and frequency of PBM/LED administration should be determined as well as how long PBM should be continued following the completion of cancer treatment. PBM parameters should be reported in detail. Validated outcome measures must be identified and employed to assess the effect of prophylaxis and therapy, from the time of diagnosis through active treatment and survival.

Despite the potential benefits and plausible safety of PBM for supportive care in HNC patients, vigilance remains warranted. While the reported results of in vitro studies of PBM on malignant cells vary, and clinical reports have shown little or no adverse reactions, there is a paucity of robust data regarding potential protection and promotion of tumor. Even less data are available on potential beneficial effects of BPM by enhancing the efficacy of (C)RT or immunologic antitumor reactivity. It is thus imperative that further investigations be directed to elucidating the effects of PBM on oncology treatment outcomes and to obtaining more insight into the mechanisms for the host tumor responses to PBM.

Acknowledgments Michael R. Hamblin was supported by US NIH grant R01AI050875.

Bibliography

1. Epstein JB, et al. Oral complications of cancer and cancer therapy: from cancer treatment to survivorship. CA Cancer J Clin. 2012;62(6):400–22.
2. Rosenthal DI, Lewin JS, Eisbruch A. Prevention and treatment of dysphagia and aspiration after chemoradiation for head and neck cancer. J Clin Oncol. 2006;24(17):2636–43.
3. van der Molen L, et al. Functional outcomes and rehabilitation strategies in patients treated with chemoradiotherapy for advanced head and neck cancer: a systematic review. Eur Arch Otorhinolaryngol. 2009;266(6):889–900.
4. Rapidis AD, Vermorken JB, Bourhis J. Targeted therapies in head and neck cancer: past, present and future. Rev Recent Clin Trials. 2008;3(3):156–66.
5. Watters AL, Epstein JB, Agulnik M. Oral complications of targeted cancer therapies: a narrative literature review. Oral Oncol. 2011;47(6):441–8.
6. Lacouture ME, et al. Clinical practice guidelines for the prevention and treatment of EGFR inhibitor-associated dermatologic toxicities. Support Care Cancer. 2011;19(8):1079–95.
7. Elting LS, et al. Patient-reported measurements of oral mucositis in head and neck cancer patients treated with radiotherapy with or without chemotherapy: demonstration of increased frequency, severity, resistance to palliation, and impact on quality of life. Cancer. 2008;113(10):2704–13.
8. Cooperstein E, et al. Vanderbilt Head and Neck Symptom Survey version 2.0: report of the development and initial testing of a subscale for assessment of oral health. Head Neck. 2012;34(6):797–804.
9. Hunter KU, et al. Toxicities affecting quality of life after chemo-IMRT of oropharyngeal cancer: prospective study of patient-reported, observer-rated, and objective outcomes. Int J Radiat Oncol Biol Phys. 2013;85(4):935–40.
10. Raber-Durlacher JE, Scully C. Oral cancer: comprehending the condition, causes, controversies, control and consequences. 14. Mucositis. Dent Update. 2012;39(2):145–7.
11. Clarkson JE, et al. Interventions for treating oral mucositis for patients with cancer receiving treatment. Cochrane Database Syst Rev. 2010;(8):CD001973.
12. Worthington HV, et al. Interventions for preventing oral mucositis for patients with cancer receiving treatment. Cochrane Database Syst Rev. 2011;4:CD000978.
13. Bjordal JM, et al. A systematic review with meta-analysis of the effect of low-level laser therapy (LLLT) in cancer therapy-induced oral mucositis. Support Care Cancer. 2011;19(8):1069–77.
14. Bensadoun RJ, Nair RG. Low-level laser therapy in the prevention and treatment of cancer therapy-induced mucositis: 2012 state of the art based on literature review and meta-analysis. Curr Opin Oncol. 2012;24(4):363–70.
15. Migliorati C, et al. Systematic review of laser and other light therapy for the management of oral mucositis in cancer patients. Support Care Cancer. 2013;21(1):333–41.
16. Oberoi S, et al. Effect of prophylactic low level laser therapy on oral mucositis: a systematic review and meta-analysis. PLoS One. 2014;9(9):e107418.
17. Hodgson BD, et al. Amelioration of oral mucositis pain by NASA near-infrared light-emitting diodes in bone marrow transplant patients. Support Care Cancer. 2012;20(7):1405–15.
18. Hudson DE, et al. Penetration of laser light at 808 and 980 nm in bovine tissue samples. Photomed Laser Surg. 2013;31(4):163–8.
19. Bjordal JM, et al. Low-level laser therapy in acute pain: a systematic review of possible mechanisms of action and clinical effects in randomized placebo-controlled trials. Photomed Laser Surg. 2006;24(2):158–68.
20. Hashmi JT, et al. Effect of pulsing in low-level light therapy. Lasers Surg Med. 2010;42(6):450–66.
21. Mester E, et al. Effect of laser rays on wound healing. Am J Surg. 1971;122(4):532–5.

22. Woodruff LD, et al. The efficacy of laser therapy in wound repair: a meta-analysis of the literature. Photomed Laser Surg. 2004;22(3):241–7.
23. Hawkins D, Abrahamse H. Biological effects of helium-neon laser irradiation on normal and wounded human skin fibroblasts. Photomed Laser Surg. 2005;23(3):251–9.
24. Oron U, et al. Low-energy laser irradiation reduces formation of scar tissue after myocardial infarction in rats and dogs. Circulation. 2001;103(2):296–301.
25. Rizzi CF, et al. Effects of low-level laser therapy (LLLT) on the nuclear factor (NF)-kappaB signaling pathway in traumatized muscle. Lasers Surg Med. 2006;38(7):704–13.
26. Barolet D, Boucher A. Prophylactic low-level light therapy for the treatment of hypertrophic scars and keloids: a case series. Lasers Surg Med. 2010;42(6):597–601.
27. Oliveira FA, et al. Low-level laser therapy decreases renal interstitial fibrosis. Photomed Laser Surg. 2012;30(12):705–13.
28. Meneguzzo DT, et al. Prevention and treatment of mice paw edema by near-infrared low-level laser therapy on lymph nodes. Lasers Med Sci. 2013;28(3):973–80.
29. Luo L, et al. Effects of low-level laser therapy on ROS homeostasis and expression of IGF-1 and TGF-beta1 in skeletal muscle during the repair process. Lasers Med Sci. 2013;28(3):725–34.
30. Bjordal JM, et al. A systematic review of low level laser therapy with location-specific doses for pain from chronic joint disorders. Aust J Physiother. 2003;49(2):107–16.
31. Chow RT, et al. Efficacy of low-level laser therapy in the management of neck pain: a systematic review and meta-analysis of randomised placebo or active-treatment controlled trials. Lancet. 2009;374(9705):1897–908.
32. Chow R, et al. Inhibitory effects of laser irradiation on peripheral mammalian nerves and relevance to analgesic effects: a systematic review. Photomed Laser Surg. 2011;29(6):365–81.
33. Song S, Zhou F, Chen WR. Low-level laser therapy regulates microglial function through Src-mediated signaling pathways: implications for neurodegenerative diseases. J Neuroinflammation. 2012;9:219.
34. Huang YY, et al. Transcranial low level laser (light) therapy for traumatic brain injury. J Biophotonics. 2012;5(11–12):827–37.
35. Karu TI. Multiple roles of cytochrome c oxidase in mammalian cells under action of red and IR-A radiation. IUBMB Life. 2010;62(8):607–10.
36. Khakh BS, Burnstock G. The double life of ATP. Sci Am. 2009;301(6):84–90, 92.
37. Murrell GA, Francis MJ, Bromley L. Modulation of fibroblast proliferation by oxygen free radicals. Biochem J. 1990;265(3):659–65.
38. Antunes F, Boveris A, Cadenas E. On the mechanism and biology of cytochrome oxidase inhibition by nitric oxide. Proc Natl Acad Sci U S A. 2004;101(48):16774–9.
39. Chung H, et al. The nuts and bolts of low-level laser (light) therapy. Ann Biomed Eng. 2012;40(2):516–33.
40. Karu TI, Kolyakov SF. Exact action spectra for cellular responses relevant to phototherapy. Photomed Laser Surg. 2005;23(4):355–61.
41. Karu T. Photobiology of low-power laser effects. Health Phys. 1989;56(5):691–704.
42. Assis L, et al. Low-level laser therapy (808 nm) reduces inflammatory response and oxidative stress in rat tibialis anterior muscle after cryolesion. Lasers Surg Med. 2012;44(9):726–35.
43. Karu TI, Pyatibrat LV, Kalendo GS. Photobiological modulation of cell attachment via cytochrome c oxidase. Photochem Photobiol Sci. 2004;3(2):211–6.
44. Fujimaki Y, et al. Low-level laser irradiation attenuates production of reactive oxygen species by human neutrophils. J Clin Laser Med Surg. 2003;21(3):165–70.
45. Silveira PC, et al. Effects of low-level laser therapy (GaAs) in an animal model of muscular damage induced by trauma. Lasers Med Sci. 2013;28(2):431–6.
46. de Lima FM, et al. Dual effect of low-level laser therapy (LLLT) on the acute lung inflammation induced by intestinal ischemia and reperfusion: action on anti- and pro-inflammatory cytokines. Lasers Surg Med. 2011;43(5):410–20.

47. Lohr NL, et al. Enhancement of nitric oxide release from nitrosyl hemoglobin and nitrosyl myoglobin by red/near infrared radiation: potential role in cardioprotection. J Mol Cell Cardiol. 2009;47(2):256–63.
48. Lopes NN, et al. Cyclooxygenase-2 and vascular endothelial growth factor expression in 5-fluorouracil-induced oral mucositis in hamsters: evaluation of two low-intensity laser protocols. Support Care Cancer. 2009;17(11):1409–15.
49. Lopes NN, et al. Effects of low-level laser therapy on collagen expression and neutrophil infiltrate in 5-fluorouracil-induced oral mucositis in hamsters. Lasers Surg Med. 2010;42(6):546–52.
50. Mendenhall WM, et al. Advances in radiotherapy for head and neck cancer. Semin Surg Oncol. 1995;11(3):256–64.
51. Mancini ML, Sonis ST. Mechanisms of cellular fibrosis associated with cancer regimen-related toxicities. Front Pharmacol. 2014;5:51.
52. Fillipin LI, et al. Low-level laser therapy (LLLT) prevents oxidative stress and reduces fibrosis in rat traumatized Achilles tendon. Lasers Surg Med. 2005;37(4):293–300.
53. Lev-Tov H, et al. Inhibition of fibroblast proliferation in vitro using low-level infrared light-emitting diodes. Dermatol Surg. 2013;39(3 Pt 1):422–5.
54. Huang YY, et al. Biphasic dose response in low level light therapy. Dose Response. 2009;7(4):358–83.
55. Sommer AP, et al. Biostimulatory windows in low-intensity laser activation: lasers, scanners, and NASA's light-emitting diode array system. J Clin Laser Med Surg. 2001;19(1):29–33.
56. (WALT), W.A.f.L.T. Available from: http://www.waltza.co.za/.
57. Gouvea de Lima A, et al. Oral mucositis prevention by low-level laser therapy in head-and-neck cancer patients undergoing concurrent chemoradiotherapy: a phase III randomized study. Int J Radiat Oncol Biol Phys. 2012;82(1):270–5.
58. Bjordal JM. Low level laser therapy (LLLT) and World Association for Laser Therapy (WALT) dosage recommendations. Photomed Laser Surg. 2012;30(2):61–2.
59. Jenkins PA, Carroll JD. How to report low-level laser therapy (LLLT)/photomedicine dose and beam parameters in clinical and laboratory studies. Photomed Laser Surg. 2011;29(12):785–7.
60. Guirro RR, Weis LC. Radiant power determination of low-level laser therapy equipment and characterization of its clinical use procedures. Photomed Laser Surg. 2009;27(4):633–9.
61. Simpson DR, Mell LK, Cohen EE. Targeting the PI3K/AKT/mTOR pathway in squamous cell carcinoma of the head and neck. Oral Oncol. 2015;51(4):291–8.
62. Chang L, et al. Acquisition of epithelial-mesenchymal transition and cancer stem cell phenotypes is associated with activation of the PI3K/Akt/mTOR pathway in prostate cancer radioresistance. Cell Death Dis. 2013;4:e875.
63. Nagata Y, et al. Effect of rapamycin, an mTOR inhibitor, on radiation sensitivity of lung cancer cells having different p53 gene status. Int J Oncol. 2010;37(4):1001–10.
64. Pellicioli AC, et al. Laser phototherapy accelerates oral keratinocyte migration through the modulation of the mammalian target of rapamycin signaling pathway. J Biomed Opt. 2014;19(2):028002.
65. Sperandio FF, et al. Low-level laser therapy can produce increased aggressiveness of dysplastic and oral cancer cell lines by modulation of Akt/mTOR signaling pathway. J Biophotonics. 2013;6(10):839–47.
66. Pardali K, Moustakas A. Actions of TGF-beta as tumor suppressor and pro-metastatic factor in human cancer. Biochim Biophys Acta. 2007;1775(1):21–62.
67. Siegel PM, Massague J. Cytostatic and apoptotic actions of TGF-beta in homeostasis and cancer. Nat Rev Cancer. 2003;3(11):807–21.
68. Prime SS, et al. The role of TGF-beta in epithelial malignancy and its relevance to the pathogenesis of oral cancer (part II). Crit Rev Oral Biol Med. 2004;15(6):337–47.
69. Hwang YS, Park KK, Chung WY. Stromal transforming growth factor-beta 1 is crucial for reinforcing the invasive potential of low invasive cancer. Arch Oral Biol. 2014;59(7):687–94.
70. Dang Y, et al. The 800-nm diode laser irradiation induces skin collagen synthesis by stimulating TGF-beta/Smad signaling pathway. Lasers Med Sci. 2011;26(6):837–43.

71. Chen YK, et al. Overexpression of Smad proteins, especially Smad7, in oral epithelial dysplasias. Clin Oral Investig. 2013;17(3):921–32.
72. Dhillon AS, et al. MAP kinase signalling pathways in cancer. Oncogene. 2007;26(22): 3279–90.
73. Cui X, et al. Significance of elevated ERK expression and its positive correlation with EGFR in Kazakh patients with esophageal squamous cell carcinoma. Int J Clin Exp Pathol. 2014;7(5):2382–91.
74. Feng J, Zhang Y, Xing D. Low-power laser irradiation (LPLI) promotes VEGF expression and vascular endothelial cell proliferation through the activation of ERK/Sp1 pathway. Cell Signal. 2012;24(6):1116–25.
75. Kawano Y, et al. The production of VEGF involving MAP kinase activation by low level laser therapy in human granulosa cells. Laser Ther. 2012;21(4):269–74.
76. Gupta A, et al. Superpulsed (Ga-As, 904 nm) low-level laser therapy (LLLT) attenuates inflammatory response and enhances healing of burn wounds. J Biophotonics. 2015;8(6):489–501.
77. Kushibiki T, et al. Regulation of miRNA expression by low-level laser therapy (LLLT) and photodynamic therapy (PDT). Int J Mol Sci. 2013;14(7):13542–58.
78. Png KJ, et al. A microRNA regulon that mediates endothelial recruitment and metastasis by cancer cells. Nature. 2012;481(7380):190–4.
79. Shabbir M, et al. Purinergic receptor-mediated effects of ATP in high-grade bladder cancer. BJU Int. 2008;101(1):106–12.
80. Marchesini R, et al. Effect of low-energy laser irradiation on colony formation capability in different human tumor cells in vitro. Lasers Surg Med. 1989;9(1):59–62.
81. Kreisler M, et al. Low-level 809 nm GaAlAs laser irradiation increases the proliferation rate of human laryngeal carcinoma cells in vitro. Lasers Med Sci. 2003;18(2):100–3.
82. de Castro JL, et al. The effect of laser therapy on the proliferation of oral KB carcinoma cells: an in vitro study. Photomed Laser Surg. 2005;23(6):586–9.
83. Schaffer M, et al. Biomodulative effects induced by 805 nm laser light irradiation of normal and tumor cells. J Photochem Photobiol B. 1997;40(3):253–7.
84. Pinheiro AL, et al. Effects of low-level laser therapy on malignant cells: in vitro study. J Clin Laser Med Surg. 2002;20(1):23–6.
85. Werneck CE, et al. Laser light is capable of inducing proliferation of carcinoma cells in culture: a spectroscopic in vitro study. Photomed Laser Surg. 2005;23(3):300–3.
86. Renno AC, et al. The effects of laser irradiation on osteoblast and osteosarcoma cell proliferation and differentiation in vitro. Photomed Laser Surg. 2007;25(4):275–80.
87. Powell K, et al. The effect of laser irradiation on proliferation of human breast carcinoma, melanoma, and immortalized mammary epithelial cells. Photomed Laser Surg. 2010;28(1):115–23.
88. Gomes Henriques AC, et al. Low-level laser therapy promotes proliferation and invasion of oral squamous cell carcinoma cells. Lasers Med Sci. 2014;29(4):1385–95.
89. Coombe AR, et al. The effects of low level laser irradiation on osteoblastic cells. Clin Orthod Res. 2001;4(1):3–14.
90. Liu YH, et al. Effects of diode 808 nm GaAlAs low-power laser irradiation on inhibition of the proliferation of human hepatoma cells in vitro and their possible mechanism. Res Commun Mol Pathol Pharmacol. 2004;115–116:185–201.
91. Sroka R, et al. Effects on the mitosis of normal and tumor cells induced by light treatment of different wavelengths. Lasers Surg Med. 1999;25(3):263–71.
92. Murayama H, et al. Low-power 808-nm laser irradiation inhibits cell proliferation of a human-derived glioblastoma cell line in vitro. Lasers Med Sci. 2012;27(1):87–93.
93. Al-Watban FA, Andres BL. Laser biomodulation of normal and neoplastic cells. Lasers Med Sci. 2012;27(5):1039–43.
94. Crous AM, Abrahamse H. Lung cancer stem cells and low-intensity laser irradiation: a potential future therapy? Stem Cell Res Ther. 2013;4(5):129.
95. Mester E, Szende B, Gartner P. [The effect of laser beams on the growth of hair in mice]. Radiobiol Radiother (Berl). 1968;9(5):621–6.

96. Schartinger VH, et al. Differential responses of fibroblasts, non-neoplastic epithelial cells, and oral carcinoma cells to low-level laser therapy. Support Care Cancer. 2012;20(3):523–9.
97. Liu TC, Zhang J, Li XE. The balance between normal and tumor tissues in phototherapy of tissues harboring cancer. Photomed Laser Surg. 2013;31(3):93–4.
98. Monteiro JSC, et al. Influence of laser phototherapy (lambda660 nm) on the outcome of oral chemical carcinogenesis on the hamster cheek pouch model: histological study. Photomed Laser Surg. 2011;29(11):741–5.
99. Frigo L, et al. The effect of low-level laser irradiation (In-Ga-Al-AsP - 660 nm) on melanoma in vitro and in vivo. BMC Cancer. 2009;9:404.
100. Myakishev-Rempel M, et al. A preliminary study of the safety of red light phototherapy of tissues harboring cancer. Photomed Laser Surg. 2012;30(9):551–8.
101. Kiro NE, Hamblin MR, Abrahamse H. Photobiomodulation of breast and cervical cancer stem cells using low-intensity laser irradiation. Tumour Biol. 2017;39(6):1010428317706913.
102. Wu S, et al. Cancer phototherapy via selective photoinactivation of respiratory chain oxidase to trigger a fatal superoxide anion burst. Antioxid Redox Signal. 2014;20(5):733–46.
103. Wu S, et al. High fluence low-power laser irradiation induces mitochondrial permeability transition mediated by reactive oxygen species. J Cell Physiol. 2009;218(3):603–11.
104. Lu C, et al. Phototherapy-induced antitumor immunity: long-term tumor suppression effects via photoinactivation of respiratory chain oxidase-triggered superoxide anion burst. Antioxid Redox Signal. 2016;24(5):249–62.
105. Kalyanaraman B. Teaching the basics of cancer metabolism: developing antitumor strategies by exploiting the differences between normal and cancer cell metabolism. Redox Biol. 2017;12:833–42.
106. Tsai SR, et al. Low-level light therapy potentiates NPe6-mediated photodynamic therapy in a human osteosarcoma cell line via increased ATP. Photodiagnosis Photodyn Ther. 2015;12(1):123–30.
107. Djavid GE, et al. Photobiomodulation leads to enhanced radiosensitivity through induction of apoptosis and autophagy in human cervical cancer cells. J Biophotonics. 2017;10(12):1732–42.
108. Tsai SR, et al. Low-level light therapy potentiates NPe6-mediated photodynamic therapy in a human osteosarcoma cell line via increased ATP. Photodiagn Photodyn Ther. 2015;12(1):123–30.
109. Wong-Riley MT, et al. Photobiomodulation directly benefits primary neurons functionally inactivated by toxins: role of cytochrome c oxidase. J Biol Chem. 2005;280(6):4761–71.
110. Schaffer M, et al. Effects of 780 nm diode laser irradiation on blood microcirculation: preliminary findings on time-dependent T1-weighted contrast-enhanced magnetic resonance imaging (MRI). J Photochem Photobiol B. 2000;54(1):55–60.
111. Ottaviani G, et al. Laser therapy inhibits tumor growth in mice by promoting immune surveillance and vessel normalization. EBioMedicine. 2016;11:165–72.
112. Antunes HS, et al. Long-term survival of a randomized phase III trial of head and neck cancer patients receiving concurrent chemoradiation therapy with or without low-level laser therapy (LLLT) to prevent oral mucositis. Oral Oncol. 2017;71:11–5.
113. Santana-Blank LA, et al. Phase I trial of an infrared pulsed laser device in patients with advanced neoplasias. Clin Cancer Res. 2002;8(10):3082–91.
114. Nordenstrom BE. Fleischner lecture. Biokinetic impacts on structure and imaging of the lung: the concept of biologically closed electric circuits. AJR Am J Roentgenol. 1985;145(3):447–67.
115. Zimin AA, et al. [Application of low-power visible and near infrared radiation in clinical oncology]. Vopr Kurortol Fizioter Lech Fiz Kult. 2009;(6):49–52.
116. Zhevago NA, et al. [The efficacy of polychromatic visible and infrared radiation used for the postoperative immunological rehabilitation of patients with breast cancer]. Vopr Kurortol Fizioter Lech Fiz Kult. 2012;(4):23–32.
117. Sonis ST. A biological approach to mucositis. J Support Oncol. 2004;2(1):21–32; discussion 35–6.
118. Al-Dasooqi N, et al. Emerging evidence on the pathobiology of mucositis. Support Care Cancer. 2013;21(11):3233–41.

119. Lalla RV, et al. MASCC/ISOO clinical practice guidelines for the management of mucositis secondary to cancer therapy. Cancer. 2014;120(10):1453–61.
120. Zadik Y, Arany PR, Fregnani ER, Bossi P, Antunes HS, Bensadoun RJ, et al. Systematic review of photobiomodulation for the management of oral mucositis in cancer patients and clinical practice guidelines. Support Care Cancer. 2019;27(10):3969–83.
121. Dorr W, Hendry JH. Consequential late effects in normal tissues. Radiother Oncol. 2001;61(3):223–31.
122. Hymes SR, Strom EA, Fife C. Radiation dermatitis: clinical presentation, pathophysiology, and treatment 2006. J Am Acad Dermatol. 2006;54(1):28–46.
123. Kim JH, et al. Mechanisms of radiation-induced skin injury and implications for future clinical trials. Int J Radiat Biol. 2013;89(5):311–8.
124. Bernier J, et al. Consensus guidelines for the management of radiation dermatitis and coexisting acne-like rash in patients receiving radiotherapy plus EGFR inhibitors for the treatment of squamous cell carcinoma of the head and neck. Ann Oncol. 2008;19(1):142–9.
125. Martin M, Lefaix J, Delanian S. TGF-beta1 and radiation fibrosis: a master switch and a specific therapeutic target? Int J Radiat Oncol Biol Phys. 2000;47(2):277–90.
126. Westbury CB, Yarnold JR. Radiation fibrosis—current clinical and therapeutic perspectives. Clin Oncol. 2012;24(10):657–72.
127. Avci P, et al. Low-level laser (light) therapy (LLLT) in skin: stimulating, healing, restoring. Semin Cutan Med Surg. 2013;32(1):41–52.
128. Costa MM, et al. Phototherapy 660 nm for the prevention of radiodermatitis in breast cancer patients receiving radiation therapy: study protocol for a randomized controlled trial. Trials. 2014;15:330.
129. Rezvani M, et al. Modification of late dermal necrosis in the pig by treatment with multi-wavelength light. Br J Radiol. 1993;66(782):145–9.
130. DeLand MM, et al. Treatment of radiation-induced dermatitis with light-emitting diode (LED) photomodulation. Lasers Surg Med. 2007;39(2):164–8.
131. Fife D, et al. A randomized, controlled, double-blind study of light emitting diode photomodulation for the prevention of radiation dermatitis in patients with breast cancer. Dermatol Surg. 2010;36(12):1921–7.
132. Raber-Durlacher JE, et al. Swallowing dysfunction in cancer patients. Support Care Cancer. 2012;20(3):433–43.
133. Russi EG, et al. Swallowing dysfunction in head and neck cancer patients treated by radiotherapy: review and recommendations of the supportive task group of the Italian Association of Radiation Oncology. Cancer Treat Rev. 2012;38(8):1033–49.
134. Leslie P, Carding PN, Wilson JA. Investigation and management of chronic dysphagia. BMJ. 2003;326(7386):433–6.
135. Nguyen NP, et al. Dysphagia following chemoradiation for locally advanced head and neck cancer. Ann Oncol. 2004;15(3):383–8.
136. Nguyen NP, et al. Aspiration rate following chemoradiation for head and neck cancer: an underreported occurrence. Radiother Oncol. 2006;80(3):302–6.
137. Mittal BB, et al. Swallowing dysfunction—preventative and rehabilitation strategies in patients with head-and-neck cancers treated with surgery, radiotherapy, and chemotherapy: a critical review. Int J Radiat Oncol Biol Phys. 2003;57(5):1219–30.
138. Langmore SE. Evaluation of oropharyngeal dysphagia: which diagnostic tool is superior? Curr Opin Otolaryngol Head Neck Surg. 2003;11(6):485–9.
139. Murphy BA, Gilbert J. Dysphagia in head and neck cancer patients treated with radiation: assessment, sequelae, and rehabilitation. Semin Radiat Oncol. 2009;19(1):35–42.
140. Murphy BA, et al. Reliability and validity of the Vanderbilt Head and Neck Symptom Survey: a tool to assess symptom burden in patients treated with chemoradiation. Head Neck. 2010;32(1):26–37.
141. van der Molen L, et al. A randomized preventive rehabilitation trial in advanced head and neck cancer patients treated with chemoradiotherapy: feasibility, compliance, and short-term effects. Dysphagia. 2011;26(2):155–70.

142. Ganzer H, et al. Symptom burden in head and neck cancer: impact upon oral energy and protein intake. Support Care Cancer. 2013;21(2):495–503.
143. Langendijk JA, et al. Impact of late treatment-related toxicity on quality of life among patients with head and neck cancer treated with radiotherapy. J Clin Oncol. 2008;26(22):3770–6.
144. Nguyen NP, et al. Effectiveness of the cough reflex in patients with aspiration following radiation for head and neck cancer. Lung. 2007;185(5):243–8.
145. Eisbruch A, et al. Objective assessment of swallowing dysfunction and aspiration after radiation concurrent with chemotherapy for head-and-neck cancer. Int J Radiat Oncol Biol Phys. 2002;53(1):23–8.
146. Langendijk JA, et al. A predictive model for swallowing dysfunction after curative radiotherapy in head and neck cancer. Radiother Oncol. 2009;90(2):189–95.
147. Roe JW, et al. Swallowing outcomes following Intensity Modulated Radiation Therapy (IMRT) for head & neck cancer - a systematic review. Oral Oncol. 2010;46(10):727–33.
148. van der Molen L, et al. Dysphagia and trismus after concomitant chemo-Intensity-Modulated Radiation Therapy (chemo-IMRT) in advanced head and neck cancer; dose-effect relationships for swallowing and mastication structures. Radiother Oncol. 2013;106(3):364–9.
149. Kraaijenga SA, et al. Effects of strengthening exercises on swallowing musculature and function in senior healthy subjects: a prospective effectiveness and feasibility study. Dysphagia. 2015;30(4):392–403.
150. Gautam AP, et al. Low level laser therapy for concurrent chemoradiotherapy induced oral mucositis in head and neck cancer patients - a triple blinded randomized controlled trial. Radiother Oncol. 2012;104(3):349–54.
151. Jensen SB, et al. A systematic review of salivary gland hypofunction and xerostomia induced by cancer therapies: prevalence, severity and impact on quality of life. Support Care Cancer. 2010;18(8):1039–60.
152. Pedersen AM, et al. Saliva and gastrointestinal functions of taste, mastication, swallowing and digestion. Oral Dis. 2002;8(3):117–29.
153. Vissink A, et al. Clinical management of salivary gland hypofunction and xerostomia in head-and-neck cancer patients: successes and barriers. Int J Radiat Oncol Biol Phys. 2010;78(4):983–91.
154. Epstein JB, et al. Quality of life and oral function in patients treated with radiation therapy for head and neck cancer. Head Neck. 2001;23(5):389–98.
155. Shiboski CH, et al. Management of salivary hypofunction during and after radiotherapy. Oral Surg Oral Med Oral Pathol Oral Radiol Endod. 2007;103(Suppl):S66–19.
156. Burlage FR, et al. Parotid and submandibular/sublingual salivary flow during high dose radiotherapy. Radiother Oncol. 2001;61(3):271–4.
157. Avila JL, et al. Radiation-induced salivary gland dysfunction results from p53-dependent apoptosis. Int J Radiat Oncol Biol Phys. 2009;73(2):523–9.
158. Vissink A, et al. Current ideas to reduce or salvage radiation damage to salivary glands. Oral Dis. 2015;21(1):e1–10.
159. Loncar B, et al. The effect of low-level laser therapy on salivary glands in patients with xerostomia. Photomed Laser Surg. 2011;29(3):171–5.
160. Vidovic JD, et al. Effects of low-level laser treatment on mouth dryness. Coll Antropol. 2010;34(3):1039–43.
161. Plavnik LM, De Crosa ME, Malberti AI. Effect of low-power radiation (helium/neon) upon submandibulary glands. J Clin Laser Med Surg. 2003;21(4):219–25.
162. Takeda Y. Irradiation effect of low-energy laser on rat submandibular salivary gland. J Oral Pathol. 1988;17(2):91–4.
163. Simoes A, et al. Effect of defocused infrared diode laser on salivary flow rate and some salivary parameters of rats. Clin Oral Investig. 2008;12(1):25–30.
164. Simoes A, et al. Laser phototherapy as topical prophylaxis against radiation-induced xerostomia. Photomed Laser Surg. 2010;28(3):357–63.

165. Cowen D, et al. Low energy Helium-Neon laser in the prevention of oral mucositis in patients undergoing bone marrow transplant: results of a double blind randomized trial. Int J Radiat Oncol Biol Phys. 1997;38(4):697–703.
166. Arbabi-Kalati F, Arbabi-Kalati F, Moridi T. Evaluation of the effect of low level laser on prevention of chemotherapy-induced mucositis. Acta Med Iran. 2013;51(3):157–62.
167. Oton-Leite AF, et al. Effect of low level laser therapy in the reduction of oral complications in patients with cancer of the head and neck submitted to radiotherapy. Spec Care Dentist. 2013;33(6):294–300.
168. Saleh J, et al. Effect of low-level laser therapy on radiotherapy-induced hyposalivation and xerostomia: a pilot study. Photomed Laser Surg. 2014;32(10):546–52.
169. Boltong A, et al. A prospective cohort study of the effects of adjuvant breast cancer chemotherapy on taste function, food liking, appetite and associated nutritional outcomes. PLoS One. 2014;9(7):e103512.
170. Hovan AJ, et al. A systematic review of dysgeusia induced by cancer therapies. Support Care Cancer. 2010;18(8):1081–7.
171. Ohrn KE, Wahlin YB, Sjoden PO. Oral status during radiotherapy and chemotherapy: a descriptive study of patient experiences and the occurrence of oral complications. Support Care Cancer. 2001;9(4):247–57.
172. Epstein JB, Barasch A. Taste disorders in cancer patients: pathogenesis, and approach to assessment and management. Oral Oncol. 2010;46(2):77–81.
173. Yamashita H, et al. Relation between acute and late irradiation impairment of four basic tastes and irradiated tongue volume in patients with head-and-neck cancer. Int J Radiat Oncol Biol Phys. 2006;66(5):1422–9.
174. Romeo U, et al. The low level laser therapy in the management of neurological burning mouth syndrome. A pilot study. Ann Stomatol. 2010;1(1):14–8.
175. Dijkstra PU, Huisman PM, Roodenburg JL. Criteria for trismus in head and neck oncology. Int J Oral Maxillofac Surg. 2006;35(4):337–42.
176. Bensadoun RJ, et al. A systematic review of trismus induced by cancer therapies in head and neck cancer patients. Support Care Cancer. 2010;18(8):1033–8.
177. Vissink A, et al. Oral sequelae of head and neck radiotherapy. Crit Rev Oral Biol Med. 2003;14(3):199–212.
178. Teguh DN, et al. Trismus in patients with oropharyngeal cancer: relationship with dose in structures of mastication apparatus. Head Neck. 2008;30(5):622–30.
179. Goldstein M, et al. The effects of antitumor irradiation on mandibular opening and mobility: a prospective study of 58 patients. Oral Surg Oral Med Oral Pathol Oral Radiol Endod. 1999;88(3):365–73.
180. Wang CJ, et al. The degree and time-course assessment of radiation-induced trismus occurring after radiotherapy for nasopharyngeal cancer. Laryngoscope. 2005;115(8):1458–60.
181. Dijkstra PU, Kalk WW, Roodenburg JL. Trismus in head and neck oncology: a systematic review. Oral Oncol. 2004;40(9):879–89.
182. Carnaby-Mann G, et al. "Pharyngocise": randomized controlled trial of preventative exercises to maintain muscle structure and swallowing function during head-and-neck chemoradiotherapy. Int J Radiat Oncol Biol Phys. 2012;83(1):210–9.
183. Carrillo JS, et al. A randomized double-blind clinical trial on the effectiveness of helium-neon laser in the prevention of pain, swelling and trismus after removal of impacted third molars. Int Dent J. 1990;40(1):31–6.
184. Aras MH, Gungormus M. Placebo-controlled randomized clinical trial of the effect two different low-level laser therapies (LLLT)—intraoral and extraoral—on trismus and facial swelling following surgical extraction of the lower third molar. Lasers Med Sci. 2010;25(5):641–5.
185. Chrcanovic BR, et al. Osteoradionecrosis of the jaws—a current overview—Part 1: Physiopathology and risk and predisposing factors. Oral Maxillofac Surg. 2010;14(1):3–16.
186. Epstein J, et al. Postradiation osteonecrosis of the mandible: a long-term follow-up study. Oral Surg Oral Med Oral Pathol Oral Radiol Endod. 1997;83(6):657–62.

187. Delanian S, Lefaix JL. The radiation-induced fibroatrophic process: therapeutic perspective via the antioxidant pathway. Radiother Oncol. 2004;73(2):119–31.
188. Bagan JV, et al. Osteonecrosis of the jaws by intravenous bisphosphonates and osteoradionecrosis: a comparative study. Med Oral Patol Oral Cir Bucal. 2009;14(12):e616–9.
189. Madrid C, Abarca M, Bouferrache K. Osteoradionecrosis: an update. Oral Oncol. 2010;46(6):471–4.
190. Schuurhuis JM, et al. Evidence supporting pre-radiation elimination of oral foci of infection in head and neck cancer patients to prevent oral sequelae. A systematic review. Oral Oncol. 2015;51(3):212–20.
191. Kurzweg T, et al. Current treatment options for recurrent/metastatic head and neck cancer: a post-ASCO 2011 update and review of last year's literature. Eur Arch Otorhinolaryngol. 2012;269(10):2157–67.
192. Estilo CL, et al. Osteonecrosis of the jaw related to bevacizumab. J Clin Oncol. 2008;26(24):4037–8.
193. Brunamonti BP, et al. Osteonecrosis of the jaws and bevacizumab therapy: a case report. Int J Immunopathol Pharmacol. 2012;25(3):789–91.
194. Sivolella S, et al. Denosumab and anti-angiogenetic drug-related osteonecrosis of the jaw: an uncommon but potentially severe disease. Anticancer Res. 2013;33(5):1793–7.
195. Santos-Silva AR, et al. Osteonecrosis of the mandible associated with bevacizumab therapy. Oral Surg Oral Med Oral Pathol Oral Radiol. 2013;115(6):e32–6.
196. Koch FP, et al. Osteonecrosis of the jaw related to sunitinib. Oral Maxillofac Surg. 2011;15(1):63–6.
197. Nicolatou-Galitis O, et al. Gingival bleeding and jaw bone necrosis in patients with metastatic renal cell carcinoma receiving sunitinib: report of 2 cases with clinical implications. Oral Surg Oral Med Oral Pathol Oral Radiol. 2012;113(2):234–8.
198. Da Cunha SS, et al. Effect of laser therapy on bone tissue submitted to radiotherapy: experimental study in rats. Photomed Laser Surg. 2007;25(3):197–204.
199. El-Maghraby EM, El-Rouby DH, Saafan AM. Assessment of the effect of low-energy diode laser irradiation on gamma irradiated rats' mandibles. Arch Oral Biol. 2013;58(7):796–805.
200. Batista JD, et al. Effect of low-level laser therapy on repair of the bone compromised by radiotherapy. Lasers Med Sci. 2014;29(6):1913–8.
201. Scoletta M, et al. Effect of low-level laser irradiation on bisphosphonate-induced osteonecrosis of the jaws: preliminary results of a prospective study. Photomed Laser Surg. 2010;28(2):179–84.
202. Romeo U, et al. Observation of pain control in patients with bisphosphonate-induced osteonecrosis using low level laser therapy: preliminary results. Photomed Laser Surg. 2011;29(7):447–52.
203. Vescovi P, et al. Surgical approach and laser applications in BRONJ osteoporotic and cancer patients. J Osteoporos. 2012;2012:585434.
204. Vescovi P, et al. Tooth extractions in high-risk patients under bisphosphonate therapy and previously affected with osteonecrosis of the jaws: surgical protocol supported by low-level laser therapy. J Craniofac Surg. 2015;26(3):696–9.
205. de Sousa AP, et al. Laser and LED phototherapies on angiogenesis. Lasers Med Sci. 2013;28(3):981–7.
206. Smith BG, Lewin JS. Lymphedema management in head and neck cancer. Curr Opin Otolaryngol Head Neck Surg. 2010;18(3):153–8.
207. McGarvey AC, et al. Lymphoedema following treatment for head and neck cancer: impact on patients, and beliefs of health professionals. Eur J Cancer Care (Engl). 2014;23(3):317–27.
208. Deng J, et al. Prevalence of secondary lymphedema in patients with head and neck cancer. J Pain Symptom Manag. 2012;43(2):244–52.
209. Deng J, et al. Factors associated with external and internal lymphedema in patients with head-and-neck cancer. Int J Radiat Oncol Biol Phys. 2012;84(3):e319–28.
210. Deng J, et al. Assessment and measurement of head and neck lymphedema: state-of-the-science and future directions. Oral Oncol. 2015;51(5):431–7.

211. Deng J, Ridner SH, Murphy BA. Lymphedema in patients with head and neck cancer. Oncol Nurs Forum. 2011;38(1):E1–E10.
212. Lau RW, Cheing GL. Managing postmastectomy lymphedema with low-level laser therapy. Photomed Laser Surg. 2009;27(5):763–9.
213. Dirican A, et al. The short-term effects of low-level laser therapy in the management of breast-cancer-related lymphedema. Support Care Cancer. 2011;19(5):685–90.
214. Omar MT, Shaheen AA, Zafar H. A systematic review of the effect of low-level laser therapy in the management of breast cancer-related lymphedema. Support Care Cancer. 2012;20(11):2977–84.
215. E Lima EL, et al. Low-level laser therapy in secondary lymphedema after breast cancer: systematic review. Lasers Med Sci. 2014;29(3):1289–95.
216. Smoot B, et al. Effect of low-level laser therapy on pain and swelling in women with breast cancer-related lymphedema: a systematic review and meta-analysis. J Cancer Surviv. 2015;9(2):287–304.
217. Wigg J, Lee N. Redefining essential care in lymphoedema. Br J Community Nurs. 2014;(Suppl):S20, s22, s24–7.
218. Dwivedi RC, et al. Evaluation of speech outcomes following treatment of oral and oropharyngeal cancers. Cancer Treat Rev. 2009;35(5):417–24.
219. Jacobi I, et al. Voice and speech outcomes of chemoradiation for advanced head and neck cancer: a systematic review. Eur Arch Otorhinolaryngol. 2010;267(10):1495–505.
220. van der Molen L, et al. Pre- and posttreatment voice and speech outcomes in patients with advanced head and neck cancer treated with chemoradiotherapy: expert listeners' and patient's perception. J Voice. 2012;26(5):664–33.
221. Meleca RJ, et al. Functional outcomes following nonsurgical treatment for advanced-stage laryngeal carcinoma. Laryngoscope. 2003;113(4):720–8.
222. Johns MM, et al. Radiation fibrosis of the vocal fold: from man to mouse. Laryngoscope. 2012;122(Suppl 5):S107–25.
223. de Bruijn MJ, et al. Objective acoustic-phonetic speech analysis in patients treated for oral or oropharyngeal cancer. Folia Phoniatr Logop. 2009;61(3):180–7.

GPSR Compliance

The European Union's (EU) General Product Safety Regulation (GPSR) is a set of rules that requires consumer products to be safe and our obligations to ensure this.

If you have any concerns about our products, you can contact us on ProductSafety@springernature.com

In case Publisher is established outside the EU, the EU authorized representative is:

Springer Nature Customer Service Center GmbH
Europaplatz 3
69115 Heidelberg, Germany

Batch number: 10732044

Printed by Printforce, the Netherlands